Malaria and the red cell

The Ciba Foundation is an international scientific and educational charity. It was established in 1947 by the Swiss chemical and pharmaceutical company of CIBA Limited—now CIBA-GEIGY Limited. The Foundation operates independently in London under English trust law.

The Ciba Foundation exists to promote international cooperation in medical and chemical research. It organizes international multidisciplinary meetings on topics that seem ready for discussion by a small group of research workers. The papers and discussions are published in the Ciba Foundation series.

The Foundation organizes many other meetings, maintains a library which is open to all graduates in science or medicine who are visiting or working in London, and provides an information service for scientists. The Ciba Foundation also functions as a centre where scientists from any part of the world may stay during working visits to London.

Malaria and the red cell

Ciba Foundation symposium 94

1983

Pitman
London

© Ciba Foundation 1983

ISBN 0 272 79658 1

Published in March 1983 by Pitman Books Ltd, London. Distributed in North America by CIBA Pharmaceutical Company (Medical Education Administration), Summit, NJ 07006, USA.

Suggested series entry for library catalogues:
Ciba Foundation symposia.

Ciba Foundation symposium 94
x + 257 pages, 42 figures, 20 tables

Malaria and the red cell.—(Ciba Foundation
  symposium; 94)
  1. Malaria—Congresses
  I. Evered, David   II. Whelam, Julie
  III. Series
  616.9'362   RC156

Text set in 10/12 pt Linotron 202 Times, printed and bound in Great Britain at The Pitman Press, Bath

Contents

Participants

M. AIKAWA Institute of Pathology, Case Western Reserve University, Cleveland, Ohio 44106, USA

R. F. ANDERS Immunoparasitology Laboratory, The Walter and Eliza Hall Institute of Medical Research, Royal Melbourne Hospital, Melbourne, Victoria 3050, Australia

L. H. BANNISTER Department of Anatomy, Guy's Hospital Medical School, London Bridge, London SE1 9RT, UK

J. W. BARNWELL Laboratory of Parasitic Diseases, National Institute of Allergy and Infectious Diseases, National Institutes of Health, Bethesda, Maryland 20205, USA

K. N. BROWN Division of Parasitology, National Institute for Medical Research, The Ridgeway, Mill Hill, London NW7 1AA, UK

Z. I. CABANTCHIK Department of Biological Chemistry, Institute of Life Sciences, Hebrew University, Jerusalem—91904, Israel

S. COHEN Department of Chemical Pathology, Guy's Hospital Medical School, London Bridge, London SE1 9RT, UK

C. A. FACER Department of Haematology, London Hospital Medical College, Turner Street, London E1 2AD, UK

C. D. FITCH Department of Internal Medicine, Division of Endocrinology, St Louis University School of Medicine, 1402 S Grand Boulevard, St Louis, Missouri 63104, USA

M. J. FRIEDMAN Department of Medicine, HSE-1504, School of Medicine, University of California, San Francisco, California 94143, USA

B. M. GREENWOOD MRC Laboratories, Fajara, P.O. Box 273, Banjul, The Gambia

A. HOLDER Wellcome Research Laboratories, Langley Court, Beckenham, Kent BR3 3BS, UK

R. J. HOWARD Laboratory of Parasitic Diseases, National Institute of Allergy and Infectious Diseases, National Institutes of Health, Bethesda, Maryland 20205, USA

W. JARRA Division of Parasitology, National Institute for Medical Research, The Ridgeway, Mill Hill, London NW7 1AA, UK

M. JUNGERY Nuffield Department of Clinical Medicine, John Radcliffe Hospital, Headington, Oxford OX3 9DU, UK

L. LUZZATTO Department of Haematology, Royal Postgraduate Medical School, University of London, Hammersmith Hospital, Du Cane Road, London W12 0HS, UK

Sir Ian McGREGOR Department of Tropical Medicine, Liverpool School of Tropical Medicine, Pembroke Place, Liverpool L3 5QA, UK

G. PASVOL Tropical Medicine Unit, Nuffield Department of Clinical Medicine, John Radcliffe Hospital, Headington, Oxford OX3 9DU, UK

R. S. PHILLIPS Department of Zoology, University of Glasgow, Glasgow G12 8QQ, UK

I. W. SHERMAN Department of Biology, University of California, Riverside, California 92521, USA

M. J. A. TANNER Department of Biochemistry, University of Bristol Medical School, University Walk, Bristol, Avon BS8 1TD, UK

D. F. H. WALLACH Radiobiology Division, Department of Therapeutic Radiology, Tufts University School of Medicine, New England Medical Center Hospital, 171 Harrison Avenue, Boston, Massachusetts 02111, USA

D. J. WEATHERALL Nuffield Department of Clinical Medicine, John Radcliffe Hospital, Headington, Oxford OX3 9DU, UK

R. J. M. WILSON   Division of Parasitology, National Institute for Medical Research, The Ridgeway, Mill Hill, London NW7 1AA, UK

D. J. WYLER   Department of Medicine, Division of Geographic Medicine, Tufts University School of Medicine, 136 Harrison Avenue, Boston, Massachusetts 02111, USA

Introduction

D.J. WEATHERALL

Nuffield Department of Clinical Medicine, John Radcliffe Hospital, Headington, Oxford, OX3 9DU, UK

This meeting was first suggested to the Ciba Foundation by Neil Brown. I think that there are excellent reasons for holding it at this particular time. In the last few years there has been a remarkable increase in knowledge about the physiology and pathology of the red cell, and in particular we are starting to gain some insight into the structure and function of the red cell membrane. At the same time a great deal of new and fascinating information has appeared about the immunological aspects of malarial parasites and how various antigens appear during different specific phases of development. Even more important for the subject of this meeting are the recent observations which suggest that these changes may be associated with specific alterations in the red cell itself.

On the broader biological front, there is no question that the high frequency of many of the common single-gene disorders in the world population, sickle cell anaemia and thalassaemia for example, is due to the protection which is afforded to heterozygous carriers against malaria. I was thinking about this recently when some of my colleagues in Papua New Guinea asked us to look at the globin genes in a population that is still highly malarious. We found that approximately 80% of the population are missing one or two β globin genes. If, as seems likely, this extraordinarily high gene frequency reflects protection against malarial infection, the malarial parasite is a remarkably sophisticated organism. Certainly no haematologist can identify a red cell which is missing one β globin gene! During the meeting we shall hear about attempts to identify some of the factors both in the red cell and on its surface which may make these genetically variant cells less attractive to the parasite. The feedback from that information may help us to understand a little bit more about parasite interactions with red cells.

Although this is not a clinical meeting on malaria we should keep in mind that a lot of what we shall be talking about has important clinical relevance. We shall have vaccines in the back of our minds, of course, but beyond that, my feeling is that much of what we will discuss will underline the need to rethink a lot of the pathophysiology of malaria over the next year or two. Thinking about some of

1983 Malaria and the red cell. Pitman, London (Ciba Foundation symposium 94) p 1-2

1

the recent studies on cerebral blood flow in cerebral malaria, and about our old ideas about the cerebral microcirculation being crammed with parasitized red cells, my guess is that one of the most exciting areas for study over the next few years will be the way in which changes on the surface of parasitized red cells cause them to interact with vascular endothelium. I hope that we shall be able to keep all these different aspects of this fascinating subject in mind over the next couple of days.

Erythrocyte membrane structure and function

M. J. A. TANNER

Department of Biochemistry, University of Bristol, Bristol, BS8 1TD, UK

Abstract The structure and function of the proteins of the human erythrocyte membrane are discussed. The major integral proteins comprise the anion transport protein (band 3), the glucose transporter and four sialic acid-rich polypeptides. The anion transport protein equilibrates Cl^- and HCO_3^- between the plasma and red cell and also provides an anchorage site for peripheral proteins including those in the red cell cytoskeleton. The sialic acid-rich proteins are predominantly exposed at the surface of the cell. The bulk of the peripheral proteins are organized in a complex fashion to form a skeletal meshwork at the cytoplasmic surface of the membrane which maintains the shape and deformability of the red cell. The changes in membrane components during differentiation of the red cell are discussed.

The erythrocyte is highly specialized for the transport of oxyhaemoglobin complexes and carbon dioxide between the lungs and tissues. Many of the special properties of the cell are attributable to proteins associated with the flexible membrane surrounding the cell. This paper briefly reviews the biochemistry of the erythrocyte membrane proteins.

Figure 1 identifies the major proteins present in the human erythrocyte membrane after separation by sodium dodecyl sulphate (SDS)–gel electrophoresis and detection with a protein stain (Fig. 1a) or the periodic acid–Schiff's base (PAS) carbohydrate stain (Fig. 1b). The conventional nomenclature for the protein-staining bands of the human erythrocyte membrane is based on that of Steck (1974); however, since the functional roles of the major proteins have now been assigned, they are often referred to by more informative names. The nomenclature of the PAS-staining bands is discussed below.

The integral membrane proteins

The proteins involved in anion transport (band 3), proteins in the band 4.5 region which include the glucose transport protein, and the PAS-staining

1983 Malaria and the red cell. Pitman, London (Ciba Foundation symposium 94) p 3-23

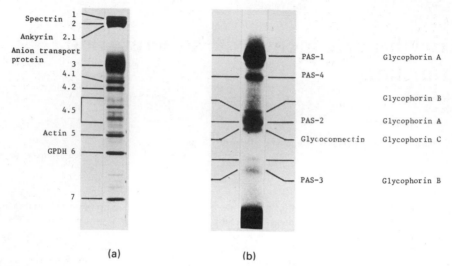

(a)　　　　　　　(b)

FIG. 1. Proteins of the human erythrocyte membrane. (a) SDS–gel electrophoresis of erythrocyte membrane proteins stained with Coomassie blue. Electrophoresis was on a gel containing a gradient of 6–20% acrylamide. (b) SDS–gel electrophoresis of erythrocyte membrane proteins stained with the PAS stain. Electrophoresis was on a gel containing 10% acrylamide. The different nomenclatures used for the bands are shown. The PAS nomenclature is from Steck (1974) and the glycophorin nomenclature from Furthmayr (1978). GPDH, glyceraldehyde-3-phosphate dehydrogenase.

glycoproteins (Fig. 1b) are the only major integral membrane proteins that are detectable on SDS–gel electrophoresis. These proteins all interact with the hydrophobic interior of the membrane since they can be solubilized only after disruption of the membrane by detergents. All these proteins are glycoproteins and contain regions which together substantially contribute to the surface structure of the erythrocyte.

The anion transport protein (band 3)

This protein increases the capacity of blood to carry CO_2 (in the form of HCO_3^-) from tissues to the lungs by allowing HCO_3^- to equilibrate between the intraerythrocytic and plasma phases of the blood. The equilibration occurs through a very rapid one-for-one exchange transport of cell HCO_3^- for plasma Cl^- and vice versa. The transport process has been shown to involve the band 3 protein and has been extensively studied (see Knauf 1979 for a detailed review). This protein is the predominant integral polypeptide of the membrane and makes up about 25% of the membrane protein, which is equivalent to 1.2×10^6 copies per red blood cell (Steck 1974).

The band 3 protein is made up of two domains of clearly different character. The N-terminus of the protein consists of a $40\,000\,M_r$ portion located entirely within the cytoplasm which can be readily rendered water-soluble by mild proteolysis, while the C-terminal domain is intercalated into the membrane (Fig. 2). The cytoplasmic domain can associate with many of

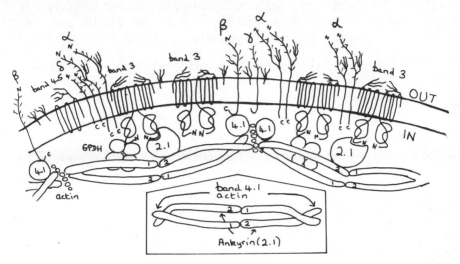

FIG. 2. Organization of the human erythrocyte membrane. Highly schematic diagram of the interactions between the components of the human erythrocyte membrane. There is evidence that the anion transport protein (band 3) is present as dimeric and possibly more highly aggregated oligomers, and that the sialoglycoproteins α (and possibly δ) are associated with these oligomers; α and δ may themselves be dimers. The anion transport protein/sialoglycoprotein aggregates probably form the intramembranous particles visualized by freeze-fracture electron microscopy. The glycoprotein oligosaccharides are shown as tree-like structures extending from the polypeptide chains. The small tree-like structures directly attached to the outer surface of the membrane represent glycolipids. The inset shows the sites of interaction of other components with the spectrin tetramer.

the peripheral proteins found in red cell membranes (see review by Gillies 1982). The glycolytic enzymes aldolase and glyceraldehyde-3-phosphate dehydrogenase bind electrostatically to a highly acidic segment of polypeptide close to the N-terminus (Murthy et al 1981) and the extent of this association is influenced by the presence of metabolites which bind to these enzymes. This domain also binds band 4.2 and additionally forms part of the linkage between the membrane and the red cell cytoskeleton by association with ankyrin (band 2.1) (Bennett & Stenbuck 1980). Other proteins, such as phosphofructokinase and haemoglobin, can probably also bind to this region of the band 3 protein. Because of the relative abundance of the anion transport protein the individual protein ligands each bind to only a small fraction of the total number of anion transport protein molecules present. For example, only about 10% of the band 3 molecules are complexed with ankyrin (Bennett & Stenbuck 1980). It is not known whether all these components bind to the same anionic binding site at the extreme N-terminus of the anion transport protein molecule.

The C-terminal portion of the band 3 protein (M_r of approximately 55 000) carries out the anion exchange and is membrane bound. The polypeptide chain in this region traverses the membrane several times to form the

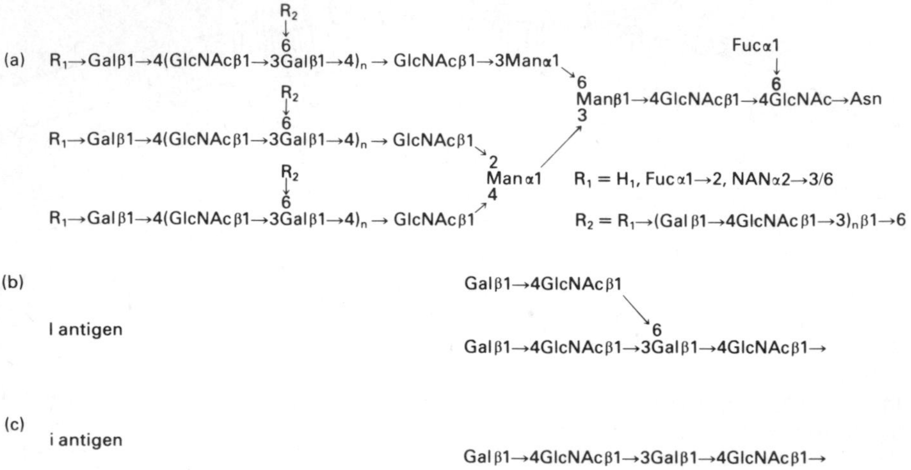

(a)
$$R_1 \rightarrow Gal\beta1 \rightarrow 4(GlcNAc\beta1 \rightarrow 3Gal\beta1 \rightarrow 4)_n \rightarrow GlcNAc\beta1 \rightarrow 3Man\alpha1$$

with R_2 substituent at position 6.

$R_1 = H_1, Fuc\alpha1 \rightarrow 2, NAN\alpha2 \rightarrow 3/6$

$R_2 = R_1 \rightarrow (Gal\beta1 \rightarrow 4GlcNAc\beta1 \rightarrow 3)_n\beta1 \rightarrow 6$

(b) I antigen

$$Gal\beta1 \rightarrow 4GlcNAc\beta1 \searrow 6$$
$$Gal\beta1 \rightarrow 4GlcNAc\beta1 \rightarrow 3Gal\beta1 \rightarrow 4GlcNAc\beta1 \rightarrow$$

(c) i antigen

$$Gal\beta1 \rightarrow 4GlcNAc\beta1 \rightarrow 3Gal\beta1 \rightarrow 4GlcNAc\beta1 \rightarrow$$

FIG. 3. Structure of band 3 and band 4.5 oligosaccharide. Suggested structures for the N-linked oligosaccharide containing repeating N-acetyllactosamine disaccharide units (Fukuda & Fukuda 1981). (a) General structure of lactosaminoglycan oligosaccharide. (b) Structure of I antigen found on adult erythrocytes. The antigenic determinant is the terminus of branched chains ending in galactose residues. (c) Structure of i antigen found on fetal erythrocytes. The antigenic determinant is the terminus of linear chains ending in galactose residues.

anion-transporting structure (see, for example, Tanner et al 1980). The band 3 protein carries a single N-linked oligosaccharide which is heterogeneous in size and gives rise to the diffuse character of the band on SDS gel electrophoresis (Fig. 1a). This oligosaccharide contains a variable number of repeating N-acetyllactosamine disaccharide units (Gal $\beta1 \rightarrow 4$ GlcNAc)$_n\beta1 \rightarrow 3$ which are branched in adult erythrocytes and are substituted into the N-linked oligosaccharide core. The structure suggested for these lactosaminoglycan chains by Fukuda & Fukuda (1981) is shown in Fig. 3a. The branched chains found in adult erythrocytes terminate in galactose residues and give rise to the blood group I antigenic determinant (Fig. 3b). These chains can also carry blood group ABH antigens (Finne 1980). In fetal erythrocytes the oligosaccharide is not branched (it lacks the R_2 substituents in Fig. 3a) and the linear chains which terminate in galactose residues give rise to the i blood group antigenic determinant (Fig. 3c). There is a further level of heterogeneity in this oligosaccharide in that a proportion of the protein molecules appear to have no repeating N-acetyllactosamine units, but only the core structure mannose residues substituted to different extents with GlcNAc and Gal-GlcNAc structures (Tsuji et al 1981). In erythrocytes which lack the major sialoglycoprotein α (En(a−) erythrocytes) (see below), the anion transport protein has a significantly increased relative molecular mass (M_r) which appears to result from an increase in the average number of (Gal $\beta1 \rightarrow 4$ GlcNAc)$\beta1 \rightarrow 3$ repeating units present in the oligosaccharide (Tanner et al 1976).

The band 4.5 region and glucose transport

The band 4.5 region contains a diffuse band of protein which has a similar heterogeneous lactosaminoglycan oligosaccharide to that found on the anion transport protein. Studies using reconstitution and the binding of cytochalasin B, the glucose transport inhibitor, have shown that one of the components in this band is involved in transporting glucose into the erythrocyte (see Baldwin & Lienhard 1981 for a recent review). Immunological studies suggest that this component is distinct from the anion transport protein and its fragments. However, this protein is likely to be of a similar structural type to the anion transport protein, although it is not clear whether this protein associates as extensively with peripheral membrane proteins as the anion transport protein.

The PAS-staining glycoproteins

Four sialic acid-rich glycoproteins are present in the human erythrocyte membrane (denoted α, β, γ, δ; Fig. 1b, see Anstee et al 1979 for nomenclature). These sialoglycoproteins give a complex pattern of bands on SDS–gel electrophoresis because two of them, α (glycophorin A) and δ (glycophorin B), form complexes with themselves and each other (Fig. 1b). The major sialoglycoprotein, α, is a well-characterized amphiphilic membrane protein orientated in the membrane with the N-terminus extracellular and C-terminus on the cytoplasmic side of the membrane (Fig. 2). The complete amino acid

sequence (Fig. 4) of the protein is known (Tomita et al 1978). It contains a
23-residue hydrophobic segment which forms an apolar α-helix that traverses
the membrane (Schulte & Marchesi 1979). The extracellular N-terminal
domain is densely glycosylated and contains 15 O-linked sialotetrasaccharides
(with the structure shown in Fig. 5a; Thomas & Winzler 1969), most of which
are located close to the N-terminus of the protein. A single larger N-linked

δ (Glycophorin B) Leu-Ser-Thr-Thr-Glu-Val-Ala-Met-His-Thr-Ser-Thr-Ser-Ser-Ser-Val-Thr-Lys-Ser-Tyr-Ile-Ser-Ser-Gln-Thr-
                                                        (Thr)   (Ser)

          S Met 30
          Asn-Gly-Glu-   -Gly-Gln-Leu-Val-His-Arg-
                s Thr   (Glu)

          M Ser   Gly   10   20
α (Glycophorin A) -Ser-Thr-Thr-   -Val-Ala-Met-His-Thr-Thr-Thr-Ser-Ser-Ser-Val-Ser-Lys-Ser-Tyr-Ile-Ser-Ser-Gln-Thr-
          N Leu   Glu
          ‡   30   40   50
          Asn-Asp-Thr-His-Lys-Arg-Asp-Thr-Tyr-Ala-Ala-Thr-Pro-Arg-Ala-His-Glu-Val-Ser-Glu-Ile-Ser-Val-Arg-Thr-

                                60   70
          Val-Tyr-Pro-Pro-Glu-Glu-Glu-Thr-Gly-Glu-Arg-Val-Gln-Leu-Ala-His-His-Phe-Ser-Glu-Pro-Glu-Ile-Thr-Leu-

                        80   90   100
          Ile-Ile-Phe-Gly-Val-Met-Ala-Gly-Val-Ile-Gly-Thr-Ile-Leu-Leu-Ile-Ser-Tyr-Gly-Ile-Arg-Arg-Leu-Ile-Lys-

                                110   120
          Lys-Ser-Pro-Ser-Asp-Val-Lys-Pro-Leu-Pro-Ser-Pro-Asp-Thr-Asp-Val-Pro-Leu-Ser-Ser-Val-Glu-Ile-Glu-Asn-

                        130
          Pro-Glu-Thr-Ser-Asp-Gln

FIG. 4. Amino acid sequences of sialoglycoproteins α and δ. The partial amino acid sequence of
δ (Furthmayr 1978, Dahr et al 1980a,b) and the complete sequence of α (Tomita et al 1978) are
shown. The hydrophobic membrane-penetrating portion of α is between residues 73 and 92. The
regions of homology between α and δ (apart from the N-terminal identity between residues 1 and
26) are shown underlined (Dahr et al 1980b). The amino acids in the sequence of δ that are shown
in parentheses are those found by Furthmayr (1978), who also suggests a slightly different
sequence for residues 28–31 of δ. *indicates the presence of an O-linked oligosaccharide; ≠
indicates the location of the N-linked oligosaccharide in the sequence of α.

oligosaccharide is present at asparagine-26. The structure shown in Fig. 5b
predominates but related structures are also present (Yoshima et al 1980).
    The blood group M, N antigens are located on α. Although the antigenic
determinants involve both the polypeptide chain and part of the carbohydrate
on the protein, the blood group M and blood group N antigenic forms of the
protein differ only in the amino acids present at residues 1 and 5 of the
polypeptide chain (Fig. 4; and see review by Anstee 1981). The α and δ
sialoglycoproteins have unusually closely related amino acid sequences (Fig.
4). The sequence of the N-terminal 26 residues of δ is identical to the same
portion of blood group N type α, and so, as might be expected, δ carries
blood group N antigen activity. The glycosylation sites of both α and δ in this
N-terminal region are also similar except that δ lacks the complex mannose-
containing oligosaccharide at asparagine-26. The remaining nine residues of

the sequence of δ which have so far been determined (residues 27–35) show homology with two sequences at residues 56–64 and 59–67 of α (Dahr et al 1980a,b). The δ sialoglycoprotein carries blood group S and blood group s antigen activity, which is associated with the presence of methionine and threonine respectively at residue 29 (Fig. 4; Dahr et al 1980b).

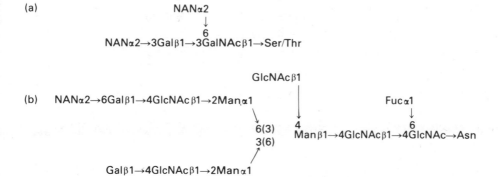

FIG. 5. Structure of the oligosaccharides present in α. (a) Structure of the O-linked sialotetra-saccharide (Thomas & Winzler 1969). (b) Structure of the N-linked oligosaccharide (Yoshima et al 1980). The major structure is shown but a related structure in which both peripheral chains terminate in sialic acid was also found.

The N-terminal sequence of the sialoglycoprotein β (glycophorin C) differs completely from that of α (Furthmayr 1978, Dahr et al 1980b). This protein has been called 'glycoconnectin', since there is evidence that it may be associated with the erythrocyte cytoskeleton network by attachment to band 4.1 (Mueller & Morrison 1980). The sialoglycoprotein γ is poorly characterized at the present time.

Sialoglycoprotein variants

Several different types of sialoglycoprotein variants occur which involve alterations in the α and δ sialoglycoproteins (see Anstee et al 1982a for a review). Table 1 shows some of the variants that have been studied. As might be expected, most of these are associated with altered blood group MN and Ss antigens. The Mg and Mc variants contain rare simple alleles of α and involve changes in the N-terminal five residues of the protein which appear to be immunologically dominant. The Mc form of α appears to be intermediate between the M and N forms, since it contains the serine-1 characteristic of blood group M-type α as well as the glutamic acid-5 characteristic of N-type

TABLE 1 Sialoglycoprotein variants of human erythrocytes

	Cell type[a]	Alteration[b]
Variants involving α		
Altered α	M^g	Thr*-4 → Asn-4[c]
	M^c	Res. 1 → Ser, Res. 5 → Glu
Loss of α	En(a−)	? Deletion
Variants involving δ		
Altered δ(s)	MiIII	Allelic forms of δ with approx. 15 K
Altered δ(S)	MiIV	increase in M_r
Loss of δ	S−s−	? New component also present
Variants involving both α and δ		
Loss of α and δ	M^k	? Deletion
(δ–α) hybrid with α and δ still present	Ph	Anti-Lepore type hybrid resulting from
	St^a	cross-over event[d]
(α–δ) hybrid with loss of α and δ	MiV	Lepore-type hybrid with deletion of α and δ genes resulting from cross-over event

[a] MiIII, MiIV, MiV: Miltenberger classes III, IV and V.
[b] See review by Anstee et al (1982a) for a more comprehensive bibliography and discussion of the variants described in this table.
[c] Thr* denotes the replacement of an *O*-glycosylated threonine residue in the M^g variant (Furthmayr et al 1981).
[d] The St^a variant is discussed by Anstee et al (1982b).

α. The Lepore-like and anti-Lepore-like variants (Ph, St^a and MiV) probably result from mispairing between δ and α genes and cross-over within the sequences coding for residues 27–35 of δ and the internal homologies at residues 56–64 or 59–67 of α (see Anstee et al 1982a for a more detailed discussion). There are no known deleterious effects on the health of the individuals carrying any of the variant erythrocytes shown in Table 1, and the functional roles of α and δ are not at all clear. In contrast, erythrocytes lacking β (and also band 4.1) appear to have defective cytoskeleton networks (see review by Cohen & Branton 1981).

The discussion so far concerns the most predominant of the integral proteins of the erythrocyte membrane. Many less abundant integral proteins are also present. These include transporters such as the Na$^+$, K$^+$-ATPase, enzymes like acetylcholinesterase, and several blood group antigenic proteins such as Rh. At present there is little structural information available on most of these components.

The peripheral membrane proteins and the red cell cytoskeleton

Many of the 'peripheral' proteins of the red cell membrane appear to be involved in the formation of an extensive submembrane reticulum which is usually called the red cell cytoskeleton (see Lux 1979, Gratzer 1981, Cohen & Branton 1981 for recent reviews). The major components of this cytoskeletal network are bands 1 and 2 (spectrin), band 2.1 (ankyrin), band 4.1, and band 5 (actin). This cytoskeleton is believed to control the shape, integrity and flexibility of the erythrocyte membrane. Removal of this complex from erythrocyte membranes causes the membranes to fragment into small vesicles. Treatment of erythrocyte membranes with non-ionic detergent (which solubilizes the lipid bilayer and the integral membrane proteins) leaves a structure containing the cytoskeletal proteins which also retains the discoid shape of the red cell.

The spectrin bands 1 and 2 are both fibrous molecules about 100 nm long which associate with each other at one end to form a heterodimer. The open ends of two dimers associate tail-to-tail to give the spectrin tetramer (see inset to Fig. 2), which appears to be the building block of the cytoskeleton. Electron microscopy has shown that band 4.1 associates with the ends of the tetramer, while band 2.1 binds to the band 2 chain nearer to the centre of the spectrin tetramer. The association between spectrin tetramers to form a two-dimensional network appears to involve both band 4.1 and short actin 'protofilaments' in the formation of a polyvalent linkage between spectrin tetramers. This meshwork is connected to the lipid bilayer by the association of band 2.1 with the N-terminal region of the anion transport protein, and perhaps also by the association of band 4.1 with the C-terminal cytoplasmic portion of the sialoglycoprotein β (glycoconnectin). A schematic view of the overall structure of the cytoskeleton is shown in Fig. 2 (p 5).

The importance of the cytoskeleton in erythrocyte viability is emphasized by increasing evidence that several types of haemolytic anaemia (which usually involve misshapen erythrocytes) are associated with different molecular defects in the cytoskeleton system (see Cohen & Branton 1981). Whether the cytoskeleton system simply provides a mechanical restraint to stabilize the membrane against excessive deformation and vesicularization, or whether more subtle mechanisms operate, is not at all clear.

Changes in membrane components during erythrocyte differentiation

The earliest recognizable cell of the erythroid line, the pronormoblast, matures by division through three successive nucleated cell stages. These stages, the basophilic, polychromatic and orthochromatic normoblast, all normally remain in the bone marrow. The orthochromatic normoblast then expels its nucleus and the anucleate reticulocyte is subsequently released from the bone marrow into the circulation, where it matures into the erythrocyte.

The erythrocyte membrane proteins are made at different times during erythropoiesis. Spectrin and the other high M_r proteins are synthesized during the nucleated cell stages in the bone marrow (Chang et al 1976). The synthesis of these is essentially complete by the reticulocyte stage, with only peripheral membrane proteins being synthesized in reticulocytes (Light & Tanner 1978). The surface of the developing erythrocyte undergoes its most marked changes during the nucleated cell stages between the pronormoblast and orthochromatic normoblast. Both the major sialoglycoprotein α (Gahmberg et al 1978) and the anion transport protein (Foxwell & Tanner 1981) appear at the cell surface in increasing amounts during these stages, and their incorporation is complete by the time the cells mature to the reticulocyte. Interestingly, the membrane loss which occurs during the decrease in size of the reticulocyte as it becomes an erythrocyte appears to occur by endocytosis of spectrin-free areas of the plasma membrane (Zweig et al 1981). During enucleation of the orthochromatic normoblast, spectrin is also excluded from the membrane surrounding the expelled nucleus. Zweig et al (1981) suggest that loss of spectrin-free membrane occurs until the density of spectrin in the cytoskeleton reaches a sufficiently high concentration for the membrane to reach the stable state in the erythrocyte. Perhaps the predilection of certain malaria parasites for young cells results from the natural instability and tendency towards endocytosis of the membrane of the immature cells.

The invasion of the erythrocyte by the malarial parasite involves both interaction with an erythrocyte surface receptor and the disruption, or dissociation from the membrane, of the erythrocyte cytoskeleton. The detailed biochemical information available on these components and on the structure of the red cell membrane should make it possible to test specific hypotheses about the way in which the parasite gains entry into the red cell. For example, is it possible that the histidine-rich protein, which is released by the parasite during invasion, enters the cell and because of its strongly cationic nature binds to the strongly anionic N-terminus of the anion transport protein? This might cause the displacement of ankyrin from the anion transport protein with the dissociation of the cytoskeleton from the membrane, so destabilizing the local area of membrane and rendering it more susceptible to endocytosis. Clearly, there are many other ways in which the parasite could achieve the same end, but specific hypotheses like these are directly amenable to experimental test and should help to increase our understanding of the invasion process.

Acknowledgements

The work from my laboratory was supported at different stages by grants from The Wellcome Trust and the Medical Research Council.

REFERENCES

Anstee DJ 1981 The blood group MN Ss-active sialoglycoproteins. Semin Hematol 18:13-31

Anstee DJ, Mawby WJ, Tanner MJA 1979 Abnormal blood group Ss-active sialoglycoproteins in the membranes of Miltenberger Class III, IV and V human erythrocytes. Biochem J 183:193-203

Anstee DJ, Mawby WJ, Tanner MJA 1982a Structural variation in human erythrocyte sialoglycoproteins. In: Martonosi A (ed) Membranes and transport. Plenum Press, New York, vol 2:427-432

Anstee DJ, Mawby WJ, Parsons SF, Tanner MJA, Giles CM 1982b A novel hybrid sialoglycoprotein in St[a] positive human erythrocytes. J Immunogenet (Oxf) 9:51-55

Baldwin SA, Lienhard GE 1981 Glucose transport across plasma membranes: facilitated diffusion systems. Trends Biochem Sci 6:208-211

Bennett V, Stenbuck PJ 1980 Association between ankyrin and the cytoplasmic domain of band 3 isolated from the human erythrocyte membrane. J Biol Chem 255:6424-6432

Chang H, Langer PJ, Lodish HF 1976 Asynchronous synthesis of erythrocyte membrane proteins. Proc Natl Acad Sci USA 72:3206-3210

Cohen CM, Branton D 1981 The normal and abnormal red cell cytoskeleton: a renewed search for molecular defects. Trends Biochem Sci 6:260-268

Dahr W, Gielen W, Beyreuther K, Krüger J 1980a Structure of the Ss blood group antigens. I. Isolation of Ss-active glycopeptides and differentiation of the antigens by modification of methionine. Hoppe-Seyler's Z Physiol Chem 361:145-152

Dahr W, Beyreuther K, Steinbach H, Gielan W, Krüger J 1980b Structure of the Ss blood group antigens. II: A methionine/threonine polymorphism within the N-terminal sequence of the Ss glycoprotein. Hoppe-Seyler's Z Physiol Chem 361:895-906

Finne J 1980 Identification of the blood group ABH active glycoprotein components of human erythrocyte membrane. Eur J Biochem 104:181-189

Foxwell BMJ, Tanner MJA 1981 Synthesis of the erythrocyte anion transport protein. Biochem J 195:129-137

Fukuda M, Fukuda MN 1981 Changes in cell surface glycoproteins and carbohydrate structures during the development and differentiation of human erythroid cells. J Supramol Struct 17:313-324

Furthmayr H 1978 Glycophorins A, B and C. A family of sialoglycoproteins. J Supramol Struct 9:79-95

Furthmayr H, Metaxas MN, Metaxas-Buhler M 1981 M^g and M^c: mutations within the amino terminal region of glycophorin A. Proc Natl Acad Sci USA 78:631-635

Gahmberg CG, Jokinen M, Andersson LC 1978 Expression of the major sialoglycoprotein (glycophorin) in erythroid cells in human bone marrow. Blood 52:379-387

Gillies RJ 1982 The binding site for aldolase and G3PDH in erythrocyte membranes. Trends Biochem Sci 37:45-46

Gratzer W 1981 The red cell cytoskeleton. Biochem J 198:1-8

Knauf PA 1979 Erythrocyte anion exchange and the band 3 protein. Curr Top Membr Transp 12:251-363

Light ND, Tanner MJA 1978 Erythrocyte membrane proteins. Sequential accumulation in the membrane during reticulocyte maturation. Biochem Biophys Acta 508:571-576

Lux SE 1979 Dissecting the red cell membrane cytoskeleton. Nature (Lond) 281:426-429

Mueller TJ, Morrison M 1980 Glycoconnectin (PAS 2), a component of the cytoskeleton of the human erythrocyte membrane. J Cell Biol 87:202a (abstr)

Murthy SNP, Lie T, Kaul RJ, Kohler H, Steck TL 1981 The aldolase binding site of the human erythrocyte membrane is at the NH_2-terminus of band 3. J Biol Chem 256:11203-11208

Schulte TH, Marchesi VT 1979 Conformation of human erythrocyte glycophorin A and its constituent peptides. Biochemistry 18:275-280

Steck TL 1974 The organization of the proteins in the human red blood cell membrane. J Cell Biol 62:1-19

Tanner MJA, Jenkins RE, Anstee DJ, Clamp JR 1976 Abnormal carbohydrate composition of the major penetrating membrane protein of En(a−) human erythrocytes. Biochem J 155:701-703

Tanner MJA, Williams DG, Jenkins RE 1980 Structure of the erythrocyte anion transport protein. Ann NY Acad Sci 341:455-464

Thomas DB, Winzler RJ 1969 Structural studies on human erythrocyte glycoproteins: alkalilabile oligosaccharides. J Biol Chem 244:5943-5946

Tomita M, Furthmayr H, Marchesi VT 1978 Primary structure of human erythrocyte glycophorin A. Biochemistry 17:4756-4770

Tsuji T, Irimura T, Osawa T 1981 The carbohydrate moiety of band 3 glycoprotein of human erythrocyte membranes. J Biol Chem 256:10497-10502

Yoshima H, Furthmayr H, Kobata A 1980 Structures of the asparagine-linked sugar chains of glycophorin A. J Biol Chem 255:9713-9718

Zweig SE, Tokuyasa KT, Singer SJ 1981 Membrane associated changes during erythropoiesis. On the mechanism of maturation of reticulocytes to erythrocytes. J Supramol Struct 17:163-181

DISCUSSION

Wallach: It has recently been shown that hereditary elliptocytosis is due to a defect in the ability of spectrin to form tetramers (Liu et al 1982). This has always been considered a possibility, but now this has been shown not only for spherocytosis but for elliptocytosis. I am interested in the loss of red cell membrane during maturation. Is the membrane exocytosed, or endocytosed?

Tanner: It seems that the lost membrane goes into the cell in reticulocytes. Zweig et al (1981) have observed vesicles in reticulocytes which are spectrin-free and derived from the plasma membrane. The reticulocyte is rapidly degrading its intracellular structures, so presumably there is a membrane-degrading system for dealing with the endocytosed membrane.

Pasvol: Is the endocytosed membrane glycophorin-free as well?

Tanner: Zweig et al (1981) did not determine whether there was any exclusion of integral membrane proteins from the endocytosed membrane. However, if the cytoskeleton limits membrane protein mobility in the reticulocyte as it does in the intact red cell, even if only by simple entrapment of the proteins, the absence of spectrin from the endocytosed membrane makes it likely that the major integral membrane proteins are also absent.

Pasvol: In your hypothesis about the histidine-rich protein and its ability to dissociate cytoskeleton from membrane, would there be a requirement on the part of the red cell for either the uncoupling process or re-instating the *status quo* ? Can the fact that young red cells are more likely to be invaded than older cells depend on the red cell's metabolic activity, rather than the parasite's predilection for young cells or other structural aspects of the cell, such as the availability of 'receptors'?

Tanner: Several different factors may determine the overall likelihood of invasion of a cell. The endocytosis that occurs in immature cells may tip the balance in favour of a younger cell being invaded because its membrane is intrinsically less stable, so that parasite endocytosis is helped by the natural endocytic mechanism present in the immature cell.

Weatherall: What do you really mean by saying that the young cell is more susceptible to endocytosis?

Tanner: The interpretation at the molecular level is that there is insufficient spectrin present to form a cytoskeleton which will cover the surface of the additional membrane that is present in immature cells. As a result there will be spectrin-free areas of the immature cell membrane which may then spontaneously be endocytosed (Zweig et al 1981).

Weatherall: So the final cell size is related to the density of spectrin?

Tanner: Yes, cell size is related to the amount of cytoskeleton present. When the ratio of cytoskeleton to membrane surface area reaches a critical value, the membrane becomes stable. Presumably this is when all the membrane is covered by cytoskeleton.

Wallach: You didn't discuss the linkages that have been suggested between band 3 and membrane-associated haemoglobin (Eisinger et al 1982).

Tanner: Band 3 has a very anionic N-terminus and in appropriate conditions I suspect that anything can be made to stick to it. I am not certain how to interpret those experiments.

Wallach: The evidence is quite strong. Shaklai et al (1981) have shown the linkage in viable intact cells. The point is important, because it relates to the issue of why certain haemoglobins protect against malaria. This linkage would be one way in which the message could be transmitted to the invading parasite.

Tanner: The mechanism by which this might give protection against malaria is not at all clear to me.

Cabantchik: As a general comment on such interactions, many of the studies done on isolated proteins and membranes, or membrane vesicles containing primarily band 3, have been done at low ionic strength. Most of the reported interactions were observed in these artificial conditions but at normal ionic strength, they were not. I therefore think that the physiological relevance of these interactions has still to be demonstrated. For the specific case of haemoglobin, there is indirect evidence about molecular interactions with band 3 in the intact cell membrane.

Wallach: There is so much haemoglobin in the red cell that transient interactions are almost inevitable. A very high affinity association is not required. The haemoglobin–membrane interaction occurs in undamaged cells at physiological intracellular potassium concentrations, at normal shear levels, and is much greater with sickle cell haemoglobin than with non-sickling haemoglobin in deoxygenated conditions. Whether there is high affinity binding or not is not the main issue with so much haemoglobin present.

Cabantchik: So there may not be specific sites on band 3 for the binding of these soluble proteins, but even with low affinity binding sites, there could be substantial binding of a major component such as haemoglobin? Is that the point?

Wallach: It is a point to keep in mind. We have to consider the effect of abnormal haemoglobins on malarial invasion. This still appears a mystery, but we may be coming close to solving the mystery. High affinity binding may not be involved. It may be sufficient to have haemoglobin present in the red cell for it to exert a transmembrane effect that can be sensed by the invading parasite.

Pasvol: Band 3 was once said to be concerned with glucose transport as well as anion transport. How similar are these two proteins, band 3 and band 4.5?

Tanner: There are some similarities between band 3 and band 4.5; however, the evidence suggests that glucose transport is mediated by band 4.5 and that this molecule is not a degradation product of band 3 but a separate component.

Wilson: What are the current ideas on the relationship between intramembranous particles and the integral membrane proteins? In terms of molecular dimensions, how many molecules of, say, band 3 would be required to form an intramembranous particle commensurate with those seen in freeze-fracture studies?

Tanner: The anion transport protein dimer is thought to be part of the intramembranous particle. It is likely that the particles represent only the portions of the proteins which are within the lipid bilayer. This would be substantial in the case of the anion transport protein. There is also evidence that higher oligomers of band 3 than the dimer are also present in the membrane (Weinstein et al 1980). There is indirect evidence that the α sialoglycoprotein is associated with band 3 (Nigg et al 1980) and therefore this protein may also be a component of the particles. The intramembranous particles of En(a−) red cells (which lack sialoglycoprotein α) do not differ in size or shape from those of normal erythrocytes (Bachi et al 1977). Since the sialoglycoprotein contains only a single transmembrane helix, it probably contributes little to the mass of the particles.

Sherman: I was interested in your hypothesis that the histidine-rich protein plays a specific role in parasite invasion, ultimately destabilizing the red cell membrane and making it more prone to endocytosis. There has been an assumption that this protein, which is found in granules in *P. lophurae* growing in duckling erythrocytes, is present in the rhoptries and/or the micronemes. The only direct evidence for that comes from autoradiographs made after labelling the parasitized red cells with tritiated histidine. Silver grains were seen over some of those organelles, but they were also present over other parts of the cell. Thus, the identification of the material in the rhoptries and microncmes as the histidine-rich protein is not firmly established. When Hewitt (1942) first described the granules, which he called 'orange granules', he noted that they were put into the residual body and then dumped into the bloodstream when the merozoitcs were released. If the material of the granules *is* in fact incorporated into the rhoptries, then only a small part of it would be incorporated. The histidine-rich protein has an M_r of about 43 000 and for it to affect band 3, as you propose, it must gain entry to the red blood cell. I think that is unlikely. However, the histidine-rich protein is interesting because of its unusual amino acid composition. The protein has haemolytic properties at low concentrations; but on treating human red cells with it we did not find the deformations (invaginations) described by Kilejian (1976) at even lower, sub-lytic concentrations. In a study by Dubremetz & Dissous (1980) on *Sarcocystis tenella* , a coccidian protozoan, a protein was identified in the micronemes with an M_r of 43 000, similar to that of the histidine-rich protein of *P. lophurae*. Unfortunately, the amino acid composition of this microneme protein wasn't studied. It might be interesting to look at other coccidians, which have these apical organelles, since these could provide larger amounts of material for analysis than does *P. lophurae* , and to determine whether in other Apicomplexans a material similar to the histidine-rich protein is involved in invagination of the host cell membrane.

Tanner: There is a simple experiment to test the hypothesis that I suggested. One can isolate the histidine-rich protein, take inside-out red cell vesicles, and see if it is possible to displace the ankyrin off band 3 with the histidine-rich protein. If this occurs, one must ask whether the protein actually enters the red cell, as you say. But I am only using this hypothesis to suggest that the biochemistry of the red cell membrane is now clear enough for one to think about doing specific experiments on invasion, given that one can isolate different components from parasites.

Brown: How would this protein get inside the red cell plasma membrane in the first place?

Tanner: Dr Sherman pointed out that it is lytic, so it might well have detergent-like properties. I imagine that it might insert itself into the red cell membrane or cause a local break in the membrane.

Brown: Is the endocytosis of the reticulocyte membrane increased in the presence of anti-red cell antibody?

Tanner: The experiments of Zweig et al (1981) were done by simply sectioning the cells and staining them with anti-spectrin antibody. As far as I am aware, nobody has studied whether there is an increase in endocytosis on treating reticulocytes with anti-red cell antibody.

Howard: In relation to the entry of proteins into the red cell, Dvorak and Miller studied the invasion of red cells by merozoites by video-microscopy (Dvorak et al 1975). The first event after reorientation of the merozoite appeared to be a transient explosive swelling and then contraction of the erythrocyte with the merozoite attached to it. The red cell then relaxed to a more normal shape and the parasite invaginated and went in. So there seems to be a time at which some water or ions go in or out, suggesting that lipids, or proteins such as histidine-rich protein, might enter at an early stage.

In relation to the hypothesis of membrane shape changes accompanying invasion being due to changes in spectrin structure, Sheetz and Singer have shown that negatively charged amphipathic drugs cause crenation of intact erythrocytes, whereas positively charged amphipathic drugs cause invaginations in the erythrocyte membrane (e.g. Sheetz et al 1976). Perhaps the malaria merozoite inserts a positively charged lipid or peptide into the inner half-layer of the bilayer membrane, thereby causing invagination. It would be interesting to know whether membrane invagination induced by lipid intercalation necessarily causes changes in spectrin structure. Has this been investigated?

Tanner: I don't know if this has been done.

Wallach: On the question of the entry of basic proteins, this area was investigated by Dr H.J. Ryser (1968), who looked at a series of synthetic basic polymers such as polylysine, polyhistidine and polyarginine (and also basic proteins). He established the relationship between polymer size and entry for various cell types. The red cell was quite intractable: it didn't let any polymer in, regardless of size. Cells capable of endocytosis, such as fibroblasts, readily took up the polymers, up to a certain size. Above that size the polymers became membrane-toxic. These results tend to exclude a known process of entry into the red cell for the histidine-rich protein.

Tanner: I wouldn't expect it to be a spontaneous process; I would imagine that the parasite has to do something positive. But we need to know whether it gets in, first, before asking *how*.

Friedman: We should recognize that histidine-rich protein is not in fact a positively charged protein. At physiological pH histidine is uncharged and is hydrophobic. The acidic groups on the histidine-rich protein (8 mol %) (Kilejian 1974) give it an overall negative charge.

Tanner: The pK of the imidazole nitrogen of histidine is 6.0, so around or above this pH every histidine residue could contribute at least $+\frac{1}{2}$ charge. Although the environment in the protein can alter amino acid pK values one would expect a protein containing 70% histidine to be strongly cationic.

Holder: What are the current ideas on the role of phosphorylation and dephosphorylation of spectrin in relation to the structure of the cytoskeleton?

Tanner: The significance of this phosphorylation and its role in the structure and function of the cytoskeleton is not clear (see Cohen & Branton 1981, Gratzer 1981 for reviews).

Holder: Is the ability of the red cell membrane to undergo deformation related to the degree of phosphorylation of cytoskeletal elements, and is this important for parasite invasion?

Tanner: This is thought to be possible, but there is no definitive evidence yet that this is the case.

Wilson: We have been doing experiments that bear on this aspect, with regard to parasite invasion. As described by Dluzewski et al (1981), we have prepared resealed red cell ghosts and looked at their susceptibility to invasion by *P. falciparum in vitro*. ATP has a significant effect on invasion. If the ghosts are made in the presence of ATP, the susceptibility to invasion can be increased from about 10% to as much as 75% of unlysed cells (Dluzewski et al 1982). This increase in susceptibility could be due to the role of ATP in phosphorylation or as a non-specific polyanion.

Facer: It is well established that *P. falciparum* maintained *in vitro* grows better in red cells collected into acid citrate dextrose (ACD, pH 5.0) if these cells are used within two weeks of collection. This correlates with the fact that ATP presentation is satisfactory for this period of time. As lactic acid accumulates, the falling pH halts glycolysis and deprives the red cell of its source of energy (Beutler 1974). The red cell requires ATP to maintain normal membrane shape and deformability and ATP-depleted cells leak potassium, accumulate sodium and calcium, and become rigid and echinocytic (Weed et al 1969) as a result of spectrin becoming more easily cross-linked. Lux (1979) presented evidence that dephosphorylation of spectrin is responsible for the maintenance of red cell shape and deformability.

Sherman: We looked at the rodent malaria *P. chabaudi* in mice with spherocytic erythrocytes to see whether the absence of spectrin influences invasion. Admittedly, we had only one mouse. I expected that the spectrin-free domains in the red cell membrane would enhance invasion, but we were unable to find parasites in this animal. Spherocytic mice are highly anaemic, and we wondered whether it was simply unsuitable as a host for *P. chabaudi*, which prefers mature erythrocytes. We found, however, that the animal was infected, because one could subinoculate from the spherocytic mouse into C57 black mice and obtain a transitory infection. We then obtained another spherocytic mouse. This time we used *P. berghei*, which prefers reticulocytes. Again we found no parasitaemia, but there was a patent infection, since we could subinoculate into non-spherocytic mice and obtain a transitory parasitaemia.

Tanner: The result with spherocytic cells is to be expected on mechanical grounds and is probably quite unrelated to the presence or absence of spectrin in the cells. Since they are spherical, the surface area:volume ratio is at a minimum in spherocytes. And since the membrane cannot stretch, the cells cannot undergo any surface deformation without increasing their volume and lysing. Spherocytes are therefore very resistant to the surface deformation required for the invagination and endocytosis of the parasite and would be expected to resist invasion.

Jarra: Is it possible, or is there any evidence that—in the presence of antibody—erythrocytes, or perhaps more likely reticulocytes, can 'cap', aggregate or reassociate components of their surface membrane?

Tanner: I know no evidence for this, in the reticulocyte or in the mature red cell. Very early reticulocytes that have just enucleated might be expected to be able to aggregate their surface components. Reticulocytes are able to take up iron from transferrin and this process may occur by receptor-mediated endocytosis. However, the erythrocyte loses this ability to take up iron.

Phillips: If reticulocytes endocytose their membranes more readily than mature red cells, does this mean that red cells stop endocytosing as they get older, or do all red cells endocytose to some extent?

Tanner: The hypothesis is that once a high enough spectrin-cytoskeleton concentration has been reached, the membrane will not endocytose any further unless there is some perturbation of the cytoskeleton.

Phillips: Can you identify when this happens as the red cell ages?

Tanner: The red cell size becomes stable once it is down to about 7 μm and one does not usually find a range of sizes in the circulation. The 'stable' level of spectrin is reached early on in red cell maturation.

Luzzatto: There are quite a number of red cell changes in acquired conditions such as microcytic anaemias. How much is known about quantitative variations in the content of spectrin? Does it tend to maintain a fixed stoichiometry, whereby, given a certain membrane size, the amount of spectrin is always adjusted to that size?

Tanner: That sort of quantitative study has not been done yet.

Wallach: In hereditary elliptocytosis the amount of spectrin per cell is normal; it is the polymerization that is defective.

Pasvol: Thinking of the cytoskeleton in a mechanical sense, you mentioned the interesting fact of sialoglycoprotein β (glycoconnectin) connecting with band 4.1. Do you think there is a strong association between α, band 3, ankyrin, and the underlying cytoskeleton? Is there any way in which one can think of these components in terms of a rod-and-pulley mechanism linking the outside of the cell with the cytoskeleton?

Tanner: There is evidence for a linkage between the α sialoglycoprotein and band 3 (Nigg et al 1980) and thus the cytoskeleton, but there is no good evidence that perturbation of one of the components on the outside of the red cell (with a ligand, for example) affects anything on the inside of the red cell.

Pasvol: What is known about the oligosaccharides of β and γ?

Tanner: β contains a lot of O-linked oligosaccharides, which are probably rather similar to the sialotetrasaccharides of the α and δ sialoglycoproteins.

Bannister: As a general point, the fact that we know so much about the red cell membrane is a great advantage, but it is also a hazard, in that we may be carried away by details. The ability of the Apicomplexan parasites to enter cells is not confined to erythrocytes; they enter a wide range of cells, from fibroblasts to neurons, and any mechanism proposed as an explanation of invasion has to take that into account. The membrane effects at entry are quite dramatic, and there is evidence that new membrane is formed or existing membrane is mobilized very rapidly (McLaren et al 1979). We should keep these points in mind when talking about the mechanism of invasion.

Weatherall: I agree with that. However, it is quite clear that the age of the red cell is a major factor in invasion, and that this effect varies widely between parasite species. We don't yet know the mechanism. Dr Tanner, what is known about glycoprotein changes during red cell ageing? Is glycoprotein lost?

Tanner: There is probably a net loss of membrane during red cell ageing. The lost membrane is probably quite similar in glycoprotein composition to the membrane as a whole. Nobody has satisfactorily shown that *in vivo* an old red cell has a significantly different membrane glycoprotein composition or significant degradation of its membrane proteins, in gross terms, compared with the younger cell. ATP depletion of erythrocytes *in vitro* (or storage under blood bank conditions) leads to the formation of microvesicles which lack spectrin but have the same content of band 3 and the sialoglycoproteins as the whole cell membrane (Lutz et al 1977).

Weatherall: So a peak concentration of glycophorin is reached at the late normoblast stage, and then it is relatively fixed through maturation.

Anders: Is there evidence for higher oligomeric states than the dimer of the α-glycoprotein *in situ* ?

Tanner: No. The existence of sialoglycoprotein α and δ dimers in the red cell membrane is inferred from the observation that the dimeric forms of the proteins are not dissociated even by SDS (Furthmayr & Marchesi 1976).

Anders: Is it possible that there are age-related changes in the aggregation properties of glycophorin?

Tanner: This could certainly be investigated.

REFERENCES

Bachi T, Whiting K, Tanner MJA, Metaxas MN, Anstee DJ 1977 Freeze-fracture electron microscopy of human erythrocytes lacking the major membrane sialoglycoprotein. Biochim Biophys Acta 464:635-639

Beutler E 1974 Experimental blood preservatives for liquid storage. In: Greenwalt TJ, Jamieson GA (eds) The human red cell *in vitro*. Grune & Stratton, New York and London

Cohen CM, Branton D 1981 The normal and abnormal red cell cytoskeleton: a renewed search for molecular defects. Trends Biochem Sci 6:260-268

Dluzewski AR, Rangachari K, Wilson RJM, Gratzer WB 1981 Entry of malaria parasites into resealed ghosts of human and simian erythrocytes. Br J Haematol 49:97-101

Dluzewski AR, Rangachari K, Wilson RJM, Gratzer WB 1982 The effect of ATP on the entry of malaria parasites into resealed ghosts of human erythrocytes. J Protozool, in press

Dubremetz JF, Dissous C 1980 Characteristic proteins of micronemes and dense granules from *Sarcocystis tenella* zoites (Protozoa, Coccidia). Mol Biochem Parasitol 1:279-289

Dvorak JA, Miller LH, Whitehouse WC, Shiroishi T 1975 Invasion of erythrocytes by malaria merozoites. Science (Wash DC) 187:748-749

Eisinger J, Flores J, Salhany JM 1982 Association of erythrocyte membranes with cytosol hemoglobin. Proc Natl Acad Sci USA 79:408-412

Furthmayr H, Marchesi VT 1976 Subunit structure of human erythrocyte glycoprotein A. Biochemistry 15:1137-1144

Gratzer W 1981 The red cell cytoskeleton. Biochem J 198:1-8

Hewitt R 1942 Studies on the host–parasite relationships of untreated infections with *Plasmodium lophurae* in ducks. Am J Hyg 36:6-38

Kilejian A 1974 A unique histidine-rich polypeptide from the malaria parasite, *Plasmodium lophurae*. J Biol Chem 249:4650-4655

Kilejian A 1976 Studies on a histidine-rich protein from *Plasmodium lophurae*. In: Van den Bossche H (ed) Parasites and host–parasite relationships. Elsevier/North-Holland Biomedical Press, Amsterdam, p 441-448

Liu S-C, Palek J, Prchal JT 1982 Defective spectrin dimer–dimer association in hereditary elliptocytosis. Proc Natl Acad Sci USA 79:2072-2076

Lutz HU, Liu S-C, Palek J 1977 Release of spectrin-free vesicles from human erythrocytes during ATP depletion. I. Characterization of spectrin-free vesicles. J Cell Biol 73:548-560

Lux SE 1979 Spectrin-actin membrane skeleton of normal and abnormal red blood cells. Semin Hematol 16:21-51

McLaren DJ, Bannister LH, Trigg PI, Butcher GA 1979 Freeze-fracture studies on the interaction between the malaria parasite and the host erythrocyte in *Plasmodium knowlesi* infections. Parasitology 79:125-139

Nigg EA, Bron C, Girardet M, Cherry RJ 1980 Band 3–glycophorin A association in erythrocyte membrane demonstrated by combining protein diffusion measurements with antibody-induced cross-linking. Biochemistry 19:1887-1893

Ryser HJ 1968 Uptake of protein by mammalian cells: an underdeveloped area. The penetration of foreign protein into mammalian cells can be measured and their functions explored. Science (Wash DC) 159:390-396

Shaklai N, Ranney HM, Sharma V 1981 Interactions of hemoglobin S with erythrocyte membranes. In: Wallach DFH (ed) The function of red blood cells: erythrocyte pathobiology. Alan R. Liss, New York, p 1-16

Sheetz MP, Painter RG, Singer SJ 1976 Biological membranes as bilayer couples. III. Compensatory shape changes induced in membranes. J Cell Biol 70:193-203

Weed RI, LaCelle PL, Merrill EW 1969 Metabolic dependence of red cell deformability. J Clin Invest 48:795-809

Weinstein RS, Khodadad JK, Steck TL 1980 The band 3 protein intramembrane particle of the human red blood cell. In: Lassen UV et al (eds) Membrane transport in erythrocytes. Munksgaard, Copenhagen (Alfred Benzon Symposium 14) p 35-50

Zweig SE, Tokuyasa KT, Singer SJ 1981 Membrane associated changes during erythropoiesis. On the mechanism of maturation of reticulocytes to erythrocytes. J Supramol Struct 17:163-181

Maturation of the intracellular parasite and antigenicity

K. N. BROWN, D. B. BOYLE and C. I. NEWBOLD

National Institute for Medical Research, Mill Hill, London NW7 1AA, UK

Abstract The protein antigens synthesized by the malarial parasite change as the parasite matures, with a number of proteins showing strict stage-specificity. A detailed correlation between the stage-specificity of protein synthesis and parasite structure has yet to be established, but a number of proteins synthesized in the cycle are lost selectively during merozoite escape and reinvasion. These antigens are presumably associated with structures utilized and ultimately lost during this process. Particular interest has focused on some >200K proteins identified as being on the surface of infected erythrocytes and internally and on the surface of merozoites. Smaller parasite proteins have also been identified in the erythrocyte membrane.

The erythrocyte itself, including its membrane, is much modified by parasite growth. Changes include the presence of new cytoplasmic structures and differences in the surface labelling and isoantigenic characteristics of the surface membrane. An appreciation of the variability and specificity of exposed parasite antigens, and their relationship to newly exposed isoantigens, is central to our understanding of protective immunity to malaria.

A merozoite entering an erythrocyte can embark on one of three alternative paths of differentiation: to asexual schizogony, to microgametogenesis and to macrogametogenesis. This paper will investigate these pathways in relation to the antigenicity of the parasite and of the parasitized erythrocyte.

Although the information available, particularly on the ring–trophozoite–schizont pathway, is increasing rapidly, this knowledge remains largely superficial with regard to many fundamental questions concerning the parasite's biology and immunology. We shall not attempt to review all the literature, but select only those papers which seem germane to the role of the parasitized erythrocyte in protective immunity. The salient characteristics of protective immunity to malaria have been discussed elsewhere (Brown 1976). Suffice it to say that under conditions of natural transmission, or after induced infections in man, and in natural and most experimental infections in other vertebrates, protective immunity is incomplete. Chronic low level infection is

1983 Malaria and red cell. Pitman, London (Ciba Foundation symposium 94) p 24–44

usual for some time after control of primary parasitaemias, even occurring in immune subjects exposed for many years to repeated infection. Recrudescences are common. We can only hope to understand the partial and unstable immunity to malaria if we understand the parasite–erythrocyte complex as an immunogen. The differentiation pathway of the parasite within the erythrocyte is reflected not only in a changing parasite structure and antigenicity, but also in modification of the erythrocyte's structure and antigenicity, both of which are important for the induction of protective immunity.

Ultrastructural aspects of differentiation

Asexual erythrocytic cycle

On entry of a merozoite into an erythrocyte, the parasite loses most of its surface coat. Soon afterwards, the inner pellicular membranes, microtubules, rhoptries, micronemes and conoid complex, all dedifferentiate (Bannister et al 1975, Aikawa 1977). Freeze-fracture studies on *Plasmodium knowlesi* have shown that in addition, the regular particle arrangement in the P face of the mature merozoite is replaced by a reticulate pattern, which persists through development up to and including the formation of merozoites. In mature merozoites, this pattern is replaced by a regular arrangement (McLaren et al 1979). Thus, the specializations concerned with merozoite release and erythrocyte invasion are lost, leaving a parasite which initially is structurally relatively simple, enclosed in a parasitophorous vacuole induced by the parasite during invasion. The erythrocyte shape is discoid, and the parasitophorous vacuole is a simple bilayer almost entirely devoid of intramembranous particles (McLaren et al 1979). During merozoite escape and reinvasion the parasite loses selectively certain proteins synthesized during the previous cell cycle (Fig. 1), although the majority are carried through to the next cycle. Apart from the presence of the young parasite the erythrocyte appears essentially normal in structure and presumably function, although preliminary changes in the erythrocyte membrane have been detected (McLaren et al 1979). In the so-called ring stage, soon after entry, protein synthesis by the parasite can be shown to include polypeptides which continue to be synthesized through the cell cycle, and others specific for the ring stage (Newbold et al 1982a). Continuous synthesis of common polypeptides, and selective synthesis of stage-specific polypeptides, continues through ring–trophozoite–schizont differentiation (Fig. 2).

As the parasite develops into a trophozoite it becomes amoeboid, haemoglobin is actively phagocytosed through a cytostome, and the dense crystalline malaria pigment is found enclosed in vesicles (Aikawa 1977). Particle density

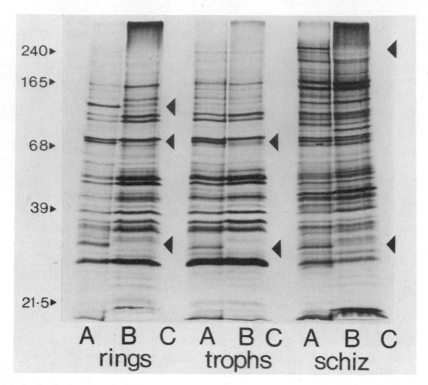

FIG. 1. Stage-specific polypeptides of *P. chabaudi* lost during schizogony and reinvasion. Sodium dodecyl sulphate–polyacrylamide gel electrophoresis and fluorographic analysis of 'one-step' ghosts (Newbold et al 1982a) of [^{35}S]methionine-labelled *P. chabaudi*. Parasitized cells at three different stages of development were labelled for 2–3 h *in vitro*, then allowed further development, schizogony and reinvasion *in vivo*. Parasitized cells were harvested after reinvasion was complete.

Track A: labelled *in vitro*, 2–3 h, [^{35}S]methionine.

Track B: recovered after schizogony and reinvasion *in vivo*.

Track C: indicates proteins lost during schizogony and reinvasion.

Equal numbers of counts were loaded. Trophs, trophozoites; schiz, schizonts.

on both the E and P faces of the parasite plasma membrane increases as the parasite develops. The erythrocyte tends to lose its discoid shape. Parasite ribosomes become clustered in polysomes, frequently attached to endoplasmic reticulum, and cisternae of the reticulum contain granular material (Ladda 1969). At this time, the parasitophorous vacuole can be shown by freeze-fracture to contain intramembranous particles (McLaren et al 1979), presumably proteins synthesized by the parasite and inserted into the membrane.

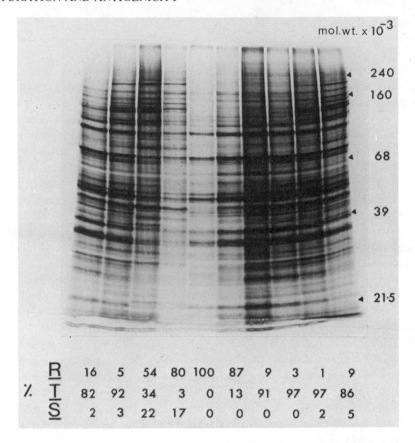

R	16	5	54	80	100	87	9	3	1	9
% T	82	92	34	3	0	13	91	97	97	86
S	2	3	22	17	0	0	0	0	2	5

FIG. 2. Stage specific polypeptide synthesis by *P. falciparum*. Sodium dodecyl sulphate–polyacrylamide gel electrophoresis and fluorographic analysis of total lysates of *P. falciparum* clone C10 cultures labelled with [^{35}S]methionine (Newbold et al 1982a). Cultures were synchronized by several rounds of sorbitol treatment. Samples taken at 6 h intervals were pulse-labelled with [^{35}S]methionine for 2 h. The percentages of rings (R), trophozoites (T) and schizonts (S) at the start of the culture period, determined from Giemsa-stained smears, are given below their corresponding track. Equal numbers of parasitized cells were used for each track. (This study was done in collaboration with Dr R. J. M. Wilson, Division of Parasitology, NIMR, London.)

One aspect of the parasitized cell that may be of particular relevance to the ultimate antigenic structure of the parasitized erythrocyte is the appearance of membrane-bound 'clefts' in the erythrocyte cytoplasm. The particle distribution in these membranes is similar to that of the parasitophorous vacuole from which they appear to arise (Aikawa et al 1975, McLaren et al 1979). Fusion of the clefts, or vesicles derived therefrom, with the erythrocyte surface has also been reported. Thus a means by which parasite antigens could be transported to the erythrocyte surface via the parasitophorous vacuole and the clefts can be imagined (Brown 1982, Howard 1982). Modifications of the erythrocyte surface become demonstrable by light and transmission electron microscopy, including the so-called excrescences on the membranes of cells parasitized by species like *P. falciparum* and *P. malariae*, and the caveola–vesicle complexes, as in *P. vivax* (Aikawa 1977). The former are found with many but not all parasites infecting predominantly mature erythrocytes, and the latter occur with parasites with a preference for reticulocytes. Thus the differences noted in surfaces of cells parasitized with different species of malaria parasite may have more to do with the type of erythrocyte parasitized than with intrinsic differences in parasite cell products modifying the host cell membrane.

The surface membrane of parasitized cells also becomes selectively changed with regard to its antigenic and isoantigenic (Brown et al 1982) and surface-labelling characteristics (Howard 1982), and the distribution of particles in the membrane changes (McLaren et al 1979). Parasite-specific antigens are detected in the membrane (Brown 1976), sometimes apparently in close juxtaposition to exposed isoantigens (Brown et al 1982). These modifications increase as the parasite goes into schizogony.

As happens earlier in the cell cycle, during the late trophozoite stage and during nuclear division leading to merozoite differentiation, stage-specific proteins are synthesized (Fig. 2). Structures associated with the merozoite begin to appear—the rhoptries, micronemes, subpellicular membranes and microtubules, the conoid complex and ultimately the merozoite surface coat. Fine granular material is present in the void between the dividing parasite and the parasitophorous vacuole (Ladda 1969).

The function of these organelles is not clear. The conoid, rhoptries and micronemes are apparently concerned with erythrocyte penetration but the details are not understood. The subpellicular membranes may be concerned with cell shape (Aikawa 1977), but connections between this structure and rhoptry-like bodies have been reported in gametocytes (Aikawa et al 1969). The fact that there are two types of organelles, rhoptries and micronemes, with apparent secretory function present in merozoites, suggests that at least two types of molecule concerned with merozoite release and erythrocyte penetration may be produced.

Final disruption of the erythrocyte membranes and parasitophorous vacuole leads to the release into the circulation of the merozoites, the residual body containing pigment, the contents of the parasitophorous vacuole and the erythrocyte, the parasitophorous membrane, the 'clefts' and the much-modified erythrocyte membrane. All of these are complex potential immunogens.

Gametocytogenesis

Ultrastructural observations on gametocytogenesis are few, mostly by Sinden and his associates. The most detailed study is that of Sinden (1982) on *P. falciparum*. When considering this excellent and valuable study, it should however be remembered that *P. falciparum* is unusual among mammalian malarias in that gametogenesis is much prolonged, taking six or more days. In most species it apparently takes only a few hours longer than the asexual cell cycle (Hawking et al 1968).

Gametocytes are generally distinguishable from trophozoites by their more regular shape. Initially, like the asexual parasite, they have a single plasmalemma, but the subpellicular sac of unit membranes subtended by microtubules, also typical of merozoite differentiation late in the asexual cycle, begins to differentiate quite early in gametocytes. Phagotrophic vacuoles are common; protein synthesis is active, as judged by the presence of numerous polysomes, some attached to endoplasmic reticulum. Membrane-bound 'clefts' appear in the host cell cytoplasm and, with *P. falciparum* gametocytes, the erythrocyte shape becomes deformed. Excrescences do not appear on the membranes of erythrocytes infected with *P. falciparum* gametocytes, but with *P. malariae* they are present (Aikawa 1977). As development proceeds, the subpellicular membrane complex and microtubules differentiate further. Sexual dimorphism soon becomes apparent, for in the macrogametocyte there is marked proliferation of the mitochondria, Golgi vesicles and dense spherules, by comparison with presumptive microgametocytes. Vesicles containing membrane whorls appear in the cytoplasm of the erythrocyte and the amount of haemoglobin is much reduced.

Gametocyte differentiation to maturity results in increased sexual dimorphism, characterized by nuclear differences, and the presence of an extensive network of rough endoplasmic reticulum in the macrogametocyte, contrasting with the predominantly smooth-membraned reticulum of the microgametocyte. Osmiophilic bodies, more numerous in the macrogametocyte, appear to arise from the Golgi vesicles. At gamete release these appear to be concerned with dissociation of the erythrocyte membrane (Sinden et al 1976).

Antigenicity

It is evident from this very brief description of the differentiation of erythrocytic parasites that, apart from differences among species, within one species the structure of the parasite (and therefore presumably its antigenicity) differs substantially in a number of respects between asexual forms and gametocytes, and between micro- and macrogametocytes. These differences may be reflected not only in the macromolecules synthesized, but also in the sequence in which similar molecules are synthesized and expressed either within the parasite, or at the parasite or parasitized cell surface. In attempting to relate our knowledge of antigenicity of the parasite and the parasitized erythrocyte to parasite maturation, two main types of problem arise: (i) differences among parasite species and host–parasite combinations used and their biological behaviour, and (ii) limitation of discrimination and sensitivity of the techniques so far used. Practically all the available information relates to the asexual forms.

The stage-specificity of protein antigen synthesis through the asexual cycle has been examined by a number of workers (Deans et al 1978, Kilejian 1980a, Freeman et al 1980, Perrin & Dayal 1982). The most detailed studies are those of Newbold et al (1982a) on *P. chabaudi*, and by D. B. Boyle, C. I. Newbold and R. J. M. Wilson, illustrated in this paper (Fig. 2), on *P. falciparum*. Assigning a biological function to these numerous polypeptides is a formidable task, and not surprisingly most interest has concentrated on those proteins likely to be exposed to immune attack at the surface of infected erythrocytes, schizonts and merozoites. Table 1 summarizes the antigens that have been considered, either *in vitro* or *in vivo*, to be associated with immune inhibition of parasite growth. Since most investigations have tended to look preferentially at the schizont and merozoite stages, the results are necessarily weighted in that direction.

Particular interest has centred on some high molecular weight (M_r) antigens that are synthesized and expressed late in the cell cycle, when merozoite differentiation begins, and lost during initiation of the next cycle (Figs. 1 and 2). These are estimated at 250 K for *P. knowlesi*, *P. chabaudi* and *P. berghei* (Epstein et al 1981, Newbold et al 1982a,b), 230 and 235 K for *P. yoelii* (Holder & Freeman 1981), and 210 K for *P. falciparum* (Perrin & Dayal 1982 and Fig. 2). By surface labelling and surface immunoprecipitation they have been located at the surface of erythrocytes infected with schizonts of *P. falciparum* (Perrin & Dayal 1982), *P. chabaudi* and *P. berghei* (Newbold et al 1982b), and by immunofluorescence and agglutination on the surface of merozoites of *P. yoelii* (Holder & Freeman 1982), *P. knowlesi* (Epstein et al 1981) and *P. chabaudi* (D. B. Boyle, personal communication). The 235 K protein of *P. yoelii* has been tentatively localized in the internal organs of the merozoite. From the ultrastructural evidence and the timing of their differentiation, two distinct secretory organelles, the rhoptries and micronemes, appear to be particularly concerned with the escape of merozoites from the erythrocyte and their entry into fresh cells. This evidence would suggest that more than one protein may be directly involved in these processes, conclusions perhaps relevant to the description of two >200 K proteins in *P. yoelii* (Holder & Freeman 1981).

TABLE 1 Plasmodium antigens with possible protective significance

Species	M_r $(10^{-3} K)$	Location	Technique	Authors
P. berghei	250	Surface of PE[a]/merozoites	Surface immunoprecipitation	Newbold et al 1982b
P. chabaudi	250	Surface of PE/merozoites	Monoclonal, immunofluorescent, surface immunoprecipitation, in vivo protection	Newbold et al 1982b; D. B. Boyle (personal communication)
P. falciparum	80	Excrescences on PE	Immuno EM and metabolic labelling	Kilejian 1980a,b
	>200, 140, 82, 41	Surface of PE	Monoclonal antibody Surface labelling Metabolic labelling In vitro multiplication inhibition	Perrin & Dayal 1982
P. knowlesi	66	Merozoite surface	Monoclonal antibody In vitro multiplication inhibition	J. A. Deans et al (personal communication)
	65	Surface PE	Surface/metabolic labelling, in vivo immunization	Schmidt-Ullrich et al 1981
	250	Surface of merozoite	Monoclonal antibody agglutination In vitro multiplication inhibition	Epstein et al 1981
P. yoelii	230 235	Surface merozoite Internal merozoite	Immunofluorescence In vivo protection	Holder & Freeman 1981

[a] Parasitized erythrocytes.

Kilejian et al (1975) described a 40 K protein containing 73% histidine in the avian parasite *P. lophurae*, with the property of agglutinating erythrocytes and modifying their shape (Kilejian 1976). She also described a somewhat similar histidine-enriched 80 K protein in *P. falciparum* which can be demonstrated in the excrescences on the surface of infected erythrocytes (Kilejian 1980b). The question arises as to how far the histidine-enriched protein of 80 K of Kilejian, and the 82 K and 41 K proteins identified by Perrin & Dayal (1982) as being exposed on the surface of *P. falciparum*-infected erythrocytes, are related one to another; and, indeed, whether they are processed or degraded fragments of the >200 K proteins. Processing of the large polypeptides in *P. yoelii* has been considered possible by Holder & Freeman (1981). Some of the *P. falciparum* results, unlike those obtained with the other species, were obtained with parasites maintained continuously *in vitro* in aged erythrocytes. At this stage we have no idea whether the age and condition of the erythrocyte affects the degree of exposure of parasite-derived proteins in the erythrocyte membrane, and how far these *in vitro* results necessarily correspond to the situation *in vivo*.

There is now a substantial body of evidence demonstrating that the major exposed antigens on malaria parasites show phenotypic antigenic variation (Brown 1976, McLean et al 1982). It is quite extraordinary how the question of phenotypic variation is often totally neglected (Perrin & Dayal 1982), or relegated to a minor role (Howard 1982), in spite of the extensive and detailed evidence on the subject. Yet to ignore this question seems to make interpretation of protection experiments almost meaningless. The reality of protective immunity to malaria readily allows a role for phenotypic variation (Brown 1976, Brown et al 1976). Only under special and rare experimental conditions is a sterilizing immune response generated that transcends phenotypic and strain, but not species, differences. Even then, it is frequently accompanied by extensive anaemia, suggesting an autoimmune component related to the parasite modification of host erythrocytes, either during entry or during parasite maturation (Brown 1977). Thus it is important that exposed antigens be examined critically for their specificity and potential for variability.

Although much of the evidence for phenotypic variation comes from serum transfer and cross-protection tests, apparently only with *P. knowlesi* in the rhesus monkey can this variation be detected by the schizont-infected cell agglutination (SICA) test. It is difficult at the moment to explain this discrepancy, which may be related in some way to the curiously limited immunogenic properties of rhesus erythrocyte alloantigens for rhesus monkeys (Stone et al 1980). In *P. berghei*, binding of parasite-specific antibodies is apparently blocked by cold-reacting haemagglutinins to isoantigens (Brown et al 1982).

As stated above, the antigens present in the erythrocyte membrane of *P. falciparum* include the histidine-enriched protein described by Kilejian. Synthesis of this protein correlates with the presence of excrescences on the erythrocyte membrane, and there is ultrastructural evidence that this protein is antigenic and exposed at these sites. Some lines of *P. falciparum* maintained *in vitro* fail to synthesize this protein and to produce excrescences on the erythrocyte membrane. Erythrocytes infected with *P. falciparum* gametocytes also lack excrescences and thus presumably gametocytes of this species do not synthesize the histidine-rich protein. The apparent absence of this protein in the membrane of erythrocytes infected with *P. falciparum* gametocytes may be a reflection of the protracted gametocytogenesis by this species (Sinden 1982), where the presence of exposed antigen could result in their removal from the circulation before maturation. Erythrocytes infected with *P. malariae* gametocytes do have excrescences and therefore presumably synthesize the protein.

As indicated previously, the specificity of the exposed portion of the histidine-rich protein is also a matter of extreme interest. Although rabbit anti-*P. lophurae* histidine-rich protein serum cross-reacts at low titre (Kilejian 1980b), it is difficult to escape the conclusion that in normal circumstances the histidine-rich protein is poorly immunogenic or is phenotypically variable. If not, parasitized erythrocytes would be readily removed from the circulation and infection rapidly terminated.

There may however be non-variable parasite-derived molecules, antibodies to which may inhibit but not completely prevent parasite development and multiplication. Taliaferro & Taliaferro (1944) have described a reduction in the number of merozoites per schizont in chronic infections of *P. brasilianum*, and Perrin & Dayal (1982) have isolated monoclonal antibodies which partially inhibit the *in vitro* growth of several geographical isolates of *P. falciparum*. There is indirect evidence that a parasite-derived transport protein(s) may be inserted into the erythrocyte membrane, for the transport characteristics of infected erythrocytes change markedly and selectively during parasite maturation; in *P. falciparum* this metabolic change occurs about 15 hours into the cell cycle (B. C. Elford, personal communication). Such proteins are possible sites for inhibitory antibody action. If this is the case, however, the tendency towards repeated attacks of malaria, the chronic recrudescent nature of the infection, and the *in vitro* results, all indicate that the inhibitory response to any putative exposed transport protein, or any non-variable antigens exposed to immune attack, is only partial and unstable. The presence of non-variable antigens exposed to avid antibody binding does not appear consistent with the strain-specific, chronic, recrudescent and persistent nature of malaria infections in subjects exposed under all types of conditions and frequency.

The structural changes which occur in the membrane of infected erythrocytes can include exposure of isoantigens as well as parasite-derived antigens.
The possible significance of these isoantigens for the immunology of malaria,
and particularly for protective immunity, is only beginning to be explored
(see W. Jarra, this volume). In addition, changes in erythrocyte membrane
configuration may occur more readily, or be more extensive, in cells with
haemoglobinopathies or enzyme deficiencies which become parasitized, since
these conditions can in themselves affect erythrocyte membrane structure
(see Brown 1982). Such changes may render the cells more immunogenic and
therefore enhance protective responses to malaria, conferring significant
survival value on these polymorphisms.

Conclusions

Parasite maturation involves changes not only in structure but also in
antigenicity. Although many protein antigens are synthesized throughout the
cell cycle, others are specific for particular stages of development. Practically
all studies of antigens have been confined to the asexual parasites, while
ultrastructural observations indicate that gametocytes will differ antigenically
in many respects from asexual forms, both in the presence of type-specific
antigens, and in the sequence in which similar antigens are synthesized.

Parasite maturation also results in the appearance of new structures in the
erythrocyte cytoplasm and in changes in the erythrocyte membrane. Parasite-
derived antigens appear in the membrane, and the erythrocyte membrane
may itself become isoantigenic. Both these types of antigen, parasite-derived
and isoantigens, and their specificity, variability and relationship to one
another, are probably important in the induction of protective immunity.

Acknowledgements

The experiments referred to in this paper were supported in part by the UNDP/World
Bank/WHO Special Programme for Research and Training in Tropical Diseases under the
Scientific Working Group on the immunology of malaria.

REFERENCES

Aikawa M 1977 Variations in structure and function during the life cycle of malarial parasites.
   Bull WHO 55:139-156
Aikawa M, Huff CG, Sprinz H 1969 Comparative fine structure study of gametocytes of avian,
   reptilian and mammalian malarial parasites. J Ultrastruct Res 26:316-331

Aikawa M, Miller LH, Rabbege J 1975 Caveola–vesicle complexes in the plasmalemma of erythrocytes infected by *Plasmodium vivax* and *P. cynomolgi*. Am J Pathol 79:285-300

Bannister LH, Butcher GA, Dennis ED, Mitchell GH 1975 Structure and invasive behaviour of *Plasmodium knowlesi* merozoites *in vitro*. Parasitology 71:483-491

Brown KN 1976 Resistance to malaria. In: Cohen S, Sadun E (eds) Immunology of parasitic infections. Blackwell Scientific Publications, Oxford, p 268-295

Brown KN 1977 Antigenic variation in malaria. In: Miller LH et al (eds) Immunity to blood parasites of animals and man. Plenum Press, New York, p 5-25

Brown KN 1982 Host resistance to malaria. Crit Rev Trop Med 1: in press

Brown KN, Jarra W, Hills LA 1976 T cells and protective immunity to *Plasmodium berghei* in rats. Infect Immun 14:858-871

Brown KN, McLaren DJ, Hills LA, Jarra W 1982 The binding of antibodies from *Plasmodium berghei*-infected rats to isoantigens and parasite-specific antigenic sites on the surfaces of infected erythrocytes. Parasite Immunol 4:21-31

Deans JA, Dennis ED, Cohen S 1978 Antigenic analysis of sequential erythrocyte stages of *Plasmodium knowlesi*. Parasitology 77:333-344

Epstein N, Miller LH, Kaushel DC, Udeinya IJ, Rener J, Howard RJ, Asofsky R, Aikawa M, Hess RL 1981 Monoclonal antibodies against a specific surface determinant on malarial (*Plasmodium knowlesi*) merozoites block erythrocyte invasion. *J. Immunol* 127:212-217

Freeman RR, Holder AA, Avril JT, Cross GAM 1980 Monoclonal antibodies against the rodent malarial parasite *Plasmodium yoelii*. In: Van den Bossche H (ed) The host–invader interplay. Elsevier/North-Holland Biomedical Press, Amsterdam, p 121-124

Hawking F, Worms MJ, Gammage K 1968 24- and 48-hour cycles of malaria parasites in the blood; their purpose, production and control. Trans R Soc Trop Med Hyg 62:731-765

Holder AA, Freeman RR 1981 Immunization against blood stage rodent malarias using purified parasite antigens. Nature (Lond) 294:361-364

Howard RJ 1982 Alterations in the surface membrane of red blood cells during malaria. Immunol Rev 61:67-107

Jarra W 1983 Protective immunity to malaria and anti-erythrocyte autoimmunity. This volume p 137-153

Kilejian A 1976 Does a histidine-rich protein from *Plasmodium lophurae* have a function in merozoite penetration? J Protozool 23:272-277

Kilejian A 1980a Stage-specific proteins and glycoproteins of *Plasmodium falciparum*: identification of antigens unique to schizonts and merozoites. Proc Natl Acad Sci USA 77:3695-3699

Kilejian A 1980b Homology between a histidine-rich protein from *Plasmodium lophurae* and a protein associated with the knob-like protrusions on membranes of erythrocytes infected with *Plasmodium falciparum*. J Exp Med 151:1534-1538

Kilejian A, Liao TH, Trager W 1975 On the primary structure and biosynthesis of histidine-rich polypeptide from malaria parasite *Plasmodium lophurae*. Proc Natl Acad Sci USA 72:3057-3059

Ladda RL 1969 New insights into the fine structure of rodent malaria parasites. Milit Med 134:825-865

McLaren DJ, Bannister LH, Trigg PI, Butcher GA 1979 Freeze fracture studies on the interaction between the malaria parasite and the host erythrocyte in *Plasmodium knowlesi* infections. Parasitology 79:125-139

McLean SA, Pearson CD, Phillips RS 1982 *Plasmodium chabaudi*: evidence of antigenic variation by the parasite during recrudescent parasitaemias in mice. Exp Parasitol, in press

Newbold CI, Boyle DB, Smith CC, Brown KN 1982a Stage-specific protein and nucleic acid synthesis during the asexual cycle of the rodent malaria *Plasmodium chabaudi*. Mol Biochem Parasitol 5:33-44

Newbold CI, Boyle DB, Smith CC, Brown KN 1982b Identification of a schizont- and species-specific surface glycoprotein on erythrocytes infected with rodent malarias. Mol Biochem Parasitol 5:45-54

Perrin, LH, Dayal R 1982 Immunity to asexual erythrocytic stages of *Plasmodium falciparum*: role of defined antigens in the humoral response. Immunol Rev 61:245-269

Schmidt-Ullrich R, Miller LH, Wallach DFH, Lightholder J, Powers KG, Gwadz RW 1981 Rhesus monkeys protected against *Plasmodium knowlesi* malaria produce antibodies against a 65,000 M_r *P. knowlesi* glycoprotein at the surface of infected erythrocytes. Infect Immun 34:519-525

Sinden RE, Canning EU, Spain B 1976 Gametocytogenesis and fertilization in *Plasmodium yoelii nigeriensis*: a transmission electron microscope study. Proc R Soc Lond B Biol Sci 193:55-76

Sinden RE 1982 Gametocytogenesis of *Plasmodium falciparum in vitro*: an electron microscope study. Parasitology 84:1-11

Stone WH, Strong R, Blazkovec A, Blystad C, Houser WD 1980 Animal models of mechanisms of erythrocyte destruction: why aren't the erythrocytes of the newborn rhesus monkey (*Macaca mulatta*) destroyed by maternal antibodies? Prog Clin Biol Res 43:237-249

Taliaferro WH, Taliaferro LG 1944 The effect of immunity on the asexual reproduction of *Plasmodium brasilianum*. J Infect Dis 75:1-32

DISCUSSION

Weatherall: Apart from the transport protein, I gather that the functions of the various proteins inserted into the red cell membrane are not known?

Brown: One assumes that some of these proteins are connected with the disruption of the red cell and merozoite release, but this isn't known.

Cohen: You showed considerable changes in the number of components between ring forms and trophozoites. We had a similar impression when we studied parasites (*P. knowlesi*) synchronized *in vitro* and then biosynthetically labelled. When we loaded the wells with equal numbers of counts, however, we were surprised to find considerable identity in protein make-up between rings and trophozoites, and dramatic changes in components between trophozoites and schizonts. Were your gels loaded with comparable numbers of counts?

Brown: Yes.

Cohen: Our impression of *P. knowlesi* is that the components that can be labelled metabolically are more or less identical in young rings and trophozoites. Between the maturation of the trophozoites and the schizonts, we see several new components appearing. What is shown very nicely by your experiment is that some of those components appearing at that late stage disappear during re-invasion.

Brown: When we load equal numbers of counts or equal numbers of parasites, in several species, we get essentially the same result. There are significant changes between the rings and early trophozoites, and between trophozoites and early schizonts.

Wallach: We have been studying a surface antigen on the plasma membrane of *P. knowlesi*-infected red cells. We have been looking at messenger RNAs from various stages of erythrocyte infection and their ability to synthesize immunoprecipitable proteins. We have focused on the 74 000 M_r protein which is prominent in our system and is also prominent as translated from mRNA. This protein is synthesized *in vitro* by the parasite and is also glycosylated to a slight extent. It is transferred to the surface of the host cell, probably in vesicles. Protein, pure by electrophoretic criteria, and also by immunoprecipitation, conferred protective immunity to monkeys, so it is an immunogen *in vivo* (R. Schmidt-Ullrich, J. Lightholder & D.F.H. Wallach, unpublished results). With prolonged immunization of animals with the immunoprecipitated protein, we see immune reactions also against some of the high M_r components. We are comparing peptide maps of these high M_r components of *P. knowlesi* with that of the M_r 74 000 protein. There appears to be considerable homology. What may be happening is that a much larger protein is synthesized first, followed by cleavage to our M_r 74 000 protein. It is also possible that there are sequences in the M_r 74 000 protein which are immunogenic and also appear in the larger proteins. Alternatively, there may be polymerization of the M_r 74 000 protein.

Howard: Dr Terry Hadley and I have unpublished results which could explain the homology. We have been looking at the methods for the quantitative isolation of a *P. knowlesi* antigen of M_r 230 000, that Dr Epstein described with Dr Miller (Epstein et al 1981). They used a monoclonal antibody which reacts with the surface of merozoites—the antigen having been identified from solubilized schizont-infected cells, not from merozoites. If we extract infected cells after labelling with [^{35}S]methionine in a variety of detergents, either in the absence of protease inhibitors or with protease inhibitors such as phenyl-methylsulphonyl fluoride or EDTA, EGTA present, there is a quantitative conversion of the M_r 230 000 protein to a fragment of M_r 75 000 that is also immunoprecipitated by the monoclonal antibody characterized by Epstein and Miller. However, if we include protease inhibitors such as *p*-chloromercuribenzoate or leupeptin in the Triton X-100 solution used for solubilization, the degradation is prevented. So one possibility to explain this homology that you see is that you have degradation fragments, as you suggested, of high M_r proteins, together with your immunoprecipitated 74 000 band. Another possibility is that there is a functional significance to the proteolytic activity that results from solubilization of the cells. The protease might be required to convert high M_r proteins to biologically active cleavage products. Within intact cells its activity may be tightly controlled.

Wallach: In biology there are many examples of precursor proteins being broken down to specific proteins. We have tried unsuccessfully to link the M_r 74 000 protein to some function. We haven't found one yet.

Luzzatto: If the protein of M_r 230 000 is a precursor of the M_r 74 000 protein you should be able to show this by pulse-chase experiments.

Wallach: We have done a few of these experiments and they have not been conclusive.

Holder: We have looked at two high M_r proteins of *P. yoelii* (Holder & Freeman 1981). One of these proteins, of M_r 230 000, is processed and is recognized by a monoclonal antibody which reacts with the parasite schizont plasma membrane and the surface of merozoites. The primary protein is probably this 230 000 M_r polypeptide; this is confirmed by immunoprecipitation of this species after *in vitro* translation of *P. yoelii* mRNA (M.J. Lockyer, unpublished results). The 230 000 M_r protein is specifically processed to a series of lower molecular weight products, which can be shown by pulse chase experiments. All the lower molecular weight species react with the monoclonal antibody and can be shown by peptide mapping to be related to each other. We think that the processing is an active process involved in the maturation of the merozoite. When one attempts to surface-label merozoites in very mature schizonts most of the label goes into the lower M_r fragments with very little into the 230 000 M_r protein. This suggests that these fragments (predominantly a species of 90 000 M_r) are the functional derivatives on the surface of the merozoite.

Brown: When we do surface immunoprecipitation with *P. chabaudi* or *P. berghei*, in the undisrupted erythrocyte, we label the 250 000 protein.

Anders: This discussion suggests that there is considerable complexity in the parasite antigens that are inserted into the red cell membrane. Different methodological approaches may give a different picture. Dr Newbold and colleagues (Newbold et al 1982) have obtained in *P. chabaudi* and *P. berghei* a very simple picture of what is exposed on the infected cell surface by binding antibodies to the labelled cells before lysis with detergent and subsequent electrophoretic analysis of immunoprecipitates. We have been using 'Western' blotting, in which unlabelled antigens separated in polyacrylamide gels are electrophoretically transferred to nitrocellulose and probed with antibodies and then ^{125}I-labelled protein A (R.F. Anders & G.V. Brown, unpublished work). This also produces a simple picture of the antigens in the infected red cell membrane. A dominant protein antigen, M_r approximately 170 000, is detected, working with two different isolates of *P. falciparum*. Antibodies defined as inhibitory or not inhibitory to the growth of *P. falciparum in vitro* have been used in these studies and there does not appear to be any positive correlation of inhibitory activity with antibody titre to this membrane antigen.

Howard: There is a methodological problem with the surface-labelling techniques that we have been using with *P. knowlesi*. It relates to the altered barrier properties of the outer membrane. Various probes can be used to identify surface antigens on these red cells. A limited number of probes appear to label predominantly surface proteins of schizont-infected red cells. They are not *exclusively* surface-specific, however, especially if one uses two-dimensional electrophoresis and autoradiography for analysis. This method enables one to detect radioactivity in proteins that constitute a very small proportion of the total labelled proteins. With other probes, such as pyridoxal phosphate, it is not possible to control the degree of penetration. The outer membrane of the infected cells is extremely permeable to this and other anionic probes, resulting in very complex patterns of labelled antigens. We find simpler patterns of surface antigens by using anti-malarial antibody plus intact cells, applied *after* surface radiolabelling, rather than by first radiolabelling the cells, then solubilizing them and then doing the immunoprecipitation.

In relation to the permeability problem, there is a biological question of interest. Our results with surface radiolabelling reagents suggest that the outer membrane is relatively more permeable to some low molecular weight reagents than we would expect. We have no evidence for haemoglobin leaking out of the cell, however, and we wonder whether the apparently altered permeability properties of the outer membrane have real functional significance. Perhaps those doing transport studies with parasitized cells are in fact measuring the barrier properties of the parasitophorous vacuole, or the parasite plasmalemma? The outer membrane of the infected red cell may not be the real barrier membrane to some low molecular weight compounds.

Wallach: I shall talk about that in my paper. The point becomes important during intracellular maturation of the parasite. Amazingly enough, the membrane potential, which is as close as you can get to measuring permeability, remains stable until late in maturation. There are, as you suggest, two membrane potentials. I am talking about the red cell plasma membrane potential. An additional potential can be separated out which sums the contributions of the parasitophorous vacuole membrane and the parasite plasma membrane.

Cabantchik: There clearly must be definite changes in the permeability properties of host cell membrane, or you would not be able to lyse trophozoites or schizonts selectively by the sorbitol method. (Sorbitol penetrates non-infected cells very poorly.) In my opinion, the permeability barrier of the schizont to salt relative to water is retained (but not the barrier to other molecules), or there would be no osmotic lysis of these cells by hexitols, amino acids, etc. (Ginsburg et al 1982). So the statements of Dr Howard and Dr Wallach are not mutually exclusive. I believe that what Dr Howard implies is that the red cell membrane, which is highly permeable to small anions (Cabantchik et al 1982), becomes permeable to larger anionic substances (Kutner et al 1982). Yet, the membrane may retain its selectivity towards cationic substances, affecting the membrane potential only minimally.

Wallach: We don't find a change in the thiocyanate potential until shortly before lysis.

Cabantchik: Thiocyanate is a lipophilic anion, which is bad for measuring the plasma membrane potential because it distributes rapidly across membranes.

The fact that one doesn't observe changes in the Nernst potential, which is determined from anion distributions across infected cells, does not exclude the possibility that the permeability towards anions and neutral molecules might be considerably increased relative to that towards cations. Parenthetically, how do you know you are measuring the potential across the plasma membrane of the red blood cell?

Wallach: The results with thiocyanate fit those obtained with lipophilic cations. SCN is in fact a very good marker for the plasma membrane potential of erythrocytes. In numerous studies with different cell types, including erythrocytes, SCN distribution has been shown to reflect the membrane potential across the plasma membrane. Because it is excluded from intracellular compartments of high negative membrane potential, such as mitochondria, its transmembrane distribution almost entirely reflects the membrane potential of the plasma membrane.

Cabantchik: To go back to Dr Brown's paper, a dramatic change in anion permeability with parasite maturation was mentioned. What were you alluding to, specifically?

Brown: I was referring to experiments on glutamine transport by Dr Elford. He has found a stage-specific increase in [^{3}H]L-glutamine uptake by cells parasitized with *P. falciparum*.

Cabantchik: One doesn't want to confuse the normal pathway of anion penetration that Michael Tanner attributed to the band 3 anion transport protein, with a possibly completely different permeation pathway which appears in the cell membrane at the trophozoite stage.

Dr Brown, what is the chemical nature of the knobs that appear on the parasitized red cell, and are they of parasite origin, or produced by the red blood cell?

Brown: Little is known about the make-up of the knobs that appear on red cells parasitized by e.g. *P. falciparum*, except that a histidine-rich protein is localized there (Kilejian 1980).

McGregor: You mentioned that antigens and other substances are shed into the host's circulation at schizogony. Clark (1978) has suggested that parasites may release substances like bacterial endotoxin which can activate non-antibody mediators that are capable of killing intracellular parasites. He and his colleagues (1981) have further shown that there develop in the sera of malarious mice which have also received a small dose of endotoxin a number of macrophage-derived mediators, such as tumour necrosis factor, lymphocyte activating factor (interleukin 1) and interferon. These could be involved in the killing of parasites and also in the pathogenesis of some features of malaria, such as fever, bone marrow depression and glucocorticoid antagonism. Clark has also drawn attention to the similarity between the clinical effects of enhanced tolerance to endotoxin in animals and the 'antitoxic' immunity to

malaria that children in hyperendemic areas exhibit, prior to the development
of effective anti-parasitic immunity (Clark 1982).

Wallach: We have looked at the biosynthesis of lipids, protein and carbohy-
drates by *P. knowlesi*, and have analysed them. We have not detected endotoxin.

Greenwood: One can find an endotoxin-like substance in the plasma of some
patients with *P. falciparum* malaria (Tubbs 1980), but one has no means of
knowing that it comes from the parasite. There is evidence that in malaria the
denaturation of endotoxin by the liver is impaired (Loose et al 1971). Thus
endotoxin in plasma may have come from the gut or from bacteria elsewhere in
the body. So far as I am aware, nobody has conclusively demonstrated that
endotoxin is produced by malaria parasites.

Wyler: To my knowledge, the only evidence for endotoxin in serum of
malarious patients is the presence of activity which can induce gelation of
Limulus amoebocyte lysates *in vitro*. However, a variety of other compounds,
including thrombin, thromboplastin, polynucleotides and ribonuclease, can
also induce gelation (Elin & Wolff 1973). Such compounds could theoretically
be parasite-derived. In studies which I did with Dr Charles Oster, the potential
role of endotoxin in host defence and pathogenesis was investigated in rodent
malarias (D.J. Wyler & C.N. Oster, unpublished results). We assessed the
course of infection (parasitaemia) and mortality of *P. chabaudi adami* (408
XZ), *P. c. adami* (556 KA), *P. vinckei petteri* and *P. berghei* (chloroquine-
resistant strain) in endotoxin-responsive (C3H/HeN) and endotoxin-non-
responsive (C3H/HeJ) mice. The parasitacmia patterns were the same in both
mouse strains. Mortality due to *P. c. adami* (556 KA) and *P. v. petteri* was also
the same in the two mouse strains. Mortality was substantially greater in
endotoxin-responsive mice than unresponsive mice infected with *P. c. adami*
(408 XZ), whereas the converse was the case for infections with *P. berghei*. We
concluded that endotoxin is unlikely *consistently* to play an important role in
host defence or mortality in rodent malaria. Certainly, the importance of
endotoxin in malaria remains an unsettled issue.

You alluded to the possibility that antibody might be getting into the vesicles
on the surface of parasitized erythrocytes. Is there any evidence that these
vesicles are transported back into the parasitophorous vacuole?

Brown: There is evidence that the vesicles of the caveola–vesicle complexes
derive from the surface of the erythrocyte and move inwards, but nobody
knows whether they reach the parasite.

Bannister: Our attempts to label this sort of transport mechanism with
ferritin and other particles have failed so far (L.H. Bannister, G.H. Mitchell &
G.A. Butcher, unpublished work). It is of course impossible to distinguish in a
simple section between a vesicle that is being transported and one that is merely
an invagination of the erythrocyte plasmalemma.

Aikawa: I agree with you, but our experiment (Aikawa et al 1975) demonstrated that *P. vivax-* and *P. cynomolgi*-infected erythrocytes suspended in a medium containing cationized ferritin particles showed ferritin depositions in the vesicles. This suggests that these vesicles are pinocytic in origin.

Tanner: The indentations (which you term 'caveolae') look almost like the clathrin-coated pits found in many other cells. It would be interesting to know if clathrin is present in these structures.

Howard: Is there any *biochemical* evidence for isoantigens in the outer membrane of malaria-infected erythrocytes? Is there an antibody in serum from immunized or infected animals that immunoprecipitates an altered host protein only from infected red cells and not from normal red cells?

Brown: No. We can simply show a selective cold agglutination of infected reticulocytes. The whole question of the isoantigenicity of infected erythrocytes has to be looked at with markers, because it would be strange if, with all the changes found in the red cell membrane, there wasn't a change in antigenicity. And if there is such a change, what is it saying to the immune system?

Howard: I would agree, especially as there is evidence suggesting considerable proteolytic activity in plasma during malaria infection, particularly when the red cells rupture. One would imagine that at that time, especially in a synchronous infection, there is much proteolysis of host proteins. Some determinants on degraded proteins would presumably be recognized as new antigens.

Brown: The redistribution of membrane proteins and loss of some of those proteins would surely expose normally cryptic antigens.

Cohen: One antigen that seems to be exposed on the outside of *P. knowlesi*-infected cells, at least, is the variant-specific antigen. Has that antigen been isolated and characterized yet?

Howard: We are well advanced! Dr Barnwell will be describing our efforts at the biological level on the preparation of cloned parasites of defined variant phenotype. We now have the appropriate variant-specific antibodies to these clones and are attempting to identify radiolabelled antigens from each clone that are immunoprecipitated only by sera which agglutinate the infected erythrocytes.

Sherman: We have been interested in plasmodial proteases from the point of view of identifying protease inhibitors to add to our red cell membrane fractions. A dominant protease in *P. lophurae* seems to be a cathepsin D, with a pH optimum against haemoglobin of 3.5. It is inhibited by pepstatin (Sherman & Tanigoshi 1981). This inhibition did not occur at physiological pH. We tested this enzyme against red cell membranes, preparing sealed and unsealed red cell ghosts, and found that this protease worked at physiological pH and affected the cytoskeleton of the red cell. That is, only in the unsealed ghosts did we find proteolysis, and the bands degraded were those conventionally called cytoskeleton. It may be that late in the infection, when the residual body is formed, some proteases, including this one, get out of the parasite food vacuoles, cross the parasitophorous vacuolar membrane and affect the red cell membrane so as to assist merozoite liberation from the red cell. This may be an enzyme that does two jobs: it digests haemoglobin and then assists in the liberation of merozoites.

Secondly, there is an interesting correlation between the levels of SICA antigen and many of the antigens that appear on the surface of the infected red blood cell. This correlation is found in schizogony, when the cells are already leaky to some extent. Is it possible that what is identified as being *in* the red cell membrane is an exudate from the parasite that leaks out on the surface of red blood cells, late in development of the parasite, and is not really intercalated into the membrane?

Wilson: We have made membrane preparations from infected red cells and found that these can absorb out variant-specific antibody to *P. knowlesi* (Vincent & Wilson 1980). This suggests that SICA antigen associated with the membrane must be reasonably tightly bound to it.

Wallach: The proteins that we are looking at are transmembrane proteins, with the tail in the cytoplasm.

Barnwell: You can detect the variant antigen on the surface of *P. knowlesi*-infected cells as the parasite reaches the late trophozoite stage, when the infected cells are not as permeable as at the schizont stage. Because the infected erythrocytes agglutinate at this late trophozoite stage, if you have a high-titred immune serum, it is not likely that parasite molecules are simply leaking out onto the red cell surface.

Anders: One change that has implications for the immunogenicity of the infected cell membrane is the increased expression of histocompatibility antigens on the surface of infected reticulocytes in murine systems (A.N. Jayawardena, unpublished work).

Brown: Our preliminary experiments on the immunogenicity of *P. chabaudi* in reticulocytes and in mature red cells do suggest that *P. chabaudi* in reticulocytes may be more immunogenic than parasites in mature erythrocytes. We wanted to know whether the fact that reticulocytes have a higher density of histocompatibility antigens on their surface than mature cells might be related to the induction of protection. We feel that perhaps parasitized reticulocytes do differ significantly from parasitized mature cells.

REFERENCES

Aikawa M, Miller LH, Rabbege J 1975 Caveola–vesicle complexes in the plasmalemma of erythrocytes infected by *Plasmodium vivax* and *Plasmodium cynomolgi*: unique structures related to Schuffner's dots. Am J Pathol 79:285-300

Cabantchik ZI, Kutner S, Krugliak M, Ginsburg H 1982 Anion transport inhibitors as suppressors of *P. falciparum* growth in *in vitro* cultures. Mol Pharmacol, in press

Clark IA 1978 Does endotoxin cause both the disease and parasite death in acute malaria and babesiosis? Lancet 2:75- 77

Clark IA 1982 Correlation between susceptibility to malaria and babesia parasites and to endotoxicity. Trans R Soc Trop Med Hyg 76:4-7

Clark IA, Virelizier JL, Carswell EA, Wood PR 1981 Possible importance of macrophage derived mediators in acute malaria. Infect Immun 32:1058-1066

Elin RJ, Wolff SM 1973 Nonspecificity of the limulus amebocyte lysate test: positive reactions with polynucleotides and proteins. J Infect Dis 128:349-352

Epstein N, Miller LH, Kanshal DC, Udeinya IJ, Rener J, Howard RJ, Asofsky R, Aikawa M, Hess RL 1981 Monoclonal antibodies against a specific surface determinant on malarial (*Plasmodium knowlesi*) merozoites block erythrocyte invasion. J Immunol 127:212-217

Ginsburg H, Krugliak M, Kutner S, Cabantchik ZI 1982 Characterization of the permselectivity changes in membranes of human red blood cells infected with malaria parasites. Isr J Med Sci, in press

Holder AA, Freeman RR 1981 Immunization against blood-stage rodent malaria using purified parasite antigens. Nature (Lond) 294:361-364

Kilejian A 1980 Homology between a histidine-rich protein from *Plasmodium lophurae* and a protein associated with the knob-like protrusions on membranes of erythrocytes infected with *Plasmodium falciparum*. J Exp Med 151:1534-1538

Kutner S, Baruch D, Ginsburg H, Cabantchik ZI 1982 Alterations in membrane permeability of malaria-infected human erythrocytes are related to the growth stage of the parasite. Biochim Biophys Acta 687:113-117

Loose LD, Trejo R, Di Luzio NR 1971 Impaired endotoxin detoxification as a factor in the enhanced endotoxin sensitivity of malaria infected mice. Proc Soc Exp Biol Med 137:794-797

Newbold CI, Boyle DB, Smith CC, Brown KN 1982 Identification of a schizont- and species-specific surface glycoprotein on erythrocytes infected with rodent malarias. Mol Biochem Parasitol 5:45-54

Sherman I, Tanigoshi L 1981 The proteases of *Plasmodium*: a cathepsin D-like enzyme from *Plasmodium lophurae*. In: Slutzky GM (ed) Biochemistry of parasites. Pergamon Press, Oxford and New York, p 137-149

Tubbs H 1980 Endotoxin in human and murine malaria. Trans R Soc Trop Med Hyg 74:121-123

Vincent HM, Wilson RJM 1980 Malarial antigens on infected erythrocytes. Trans R Soc Trop Med Hyg 74:452-455

Structural alteration of the erythrocyte membrane during malarial parasite invasion and intraerythrocytic development

MASAMICHI AIKAWA and LOUIS H. MILLER*

*Institute of Pathology, Case Western Reserve University, Cleveland, OH 44106 and *Laboratory of Parasitic Diseases, National Institute of Allergy and Infectious Diseases, Bethesda, MD 20205, USA*

Abstract Erythrocyte entry by malarial merozoites causes structural alteration of the erythrocyte membrane. First, entry into erythrocytes by merozoites requires the formation of a junction between the erythrocyte membrane and the apical end of the merozoite. Secondly, migration of the junction parallel to the long axis of the merozoite brings the merozoite into an invagination of the erythrocyte membrane. Freeze-fracture studies show that the junction consists of a narrow band of rhomboidally arrayed intramembrane particles (IMP) on the P face of the erythrocyte membrane and matching rhomboidally arrayed pits on the E face. IMP on the P face of the erythrocyte membrane disappear beyond this junction, resulting in the absence of IMP from the P face of the parasitophorous vacuole membrane which originated from the erythrocyte membrane. The erythrocyte membrane is sealed off by fusion of the junction at the posterior end of the merozoite in the fashion of an iris diaphragm. After completing its entry into the erythrocyte the merozoite is surrounded by a parasitophorous vacuole membrane which is different in its molecular organization from the original erythrocyte membrane. In addition, two types of erythrocyte membrane modification are induced by intraerythrocytic parasites. They include electron-dense protrusions called knobs and caveola–vesicle complexes along the erythrocyte membrane.

Invasion of erythrocytes by malarial merozoites is the initial step in the development of the erythrocytic stages of malarial parasites. The information that has now accumulated demonstrates that the merozoites enter the erythrocytes by a definite sequence of events: (1) initial recognition of and attachment of the merozoite to the erythrocyte membrane; (2) formation of a junction between the apical end of the merozoite and the erythrocyte; (3) creation of a vacuole membrane which is continuous with the erythrocyte

1983 Malaria and the red cell. Pitman, London (Ciba Foundation symposium 94) p 45-63

membrane; (4) entry of the parasite into the vacuole by a moving junction around the merozoite; and (5) sealing of the erythrocyte and vacuole membranes after the completion of invasion (Aikawa et al 1968, Bannister et al 1975, Dvorak et al 1975).

In this chapter we shall focus on the events defined by ultrastructural studies which explain how the merozoite, which is limited in its mobility, can enter an erythrocyte, and how the structure of the erythrocyte membrane alters during these processes. In addition, we shall discuss the alterations in the erythrocyte membrane induced by the intraerythrocytic parasites.

Recognition and attachment between merozoite and erythrocyte

Since understanding the structure of the malarial merozoite is important in analysing the interaction between erythrocytes and merozoites, a brief description of the merozoite will be given here. The merozoite is surrounded by a pellicular complex of two membranes and a row of subpellicular microtubules. The apical end is a truncated conical structure demarcated by polar rings. Electron-dense rhoptries and micronemes are seen in the apical end; ductules from the rhoptries extend to the tip of the apical end.

The initial factor underlying attachment between merozoites and erythrocytes may be the difference in the surface charge of the two cells. Cytochemical studies, using positively charged colloidal ions, have indicated that the merozoite membrane is less negatively charged than the erythrocyte membrane (Seed et al 1974). Initially, merozoites can attach to erythrocytes in any orientation, but for a successful entry they reorient themselves so that the apical end of the merozoite becomes attached to the erythrocyte membrane (Dvorak et al 1975). There are several reports that indicate the presence of receptors on the erythrocyte membrane for the merozoites. These receptors include the Duffy blood group antigens for *Plasmodium knowlesi* and *P. vivax* (Miller et al 1975) and glycophorin for *P. falciparum* (Miller et al 1977, Perkins 1981).

Initially, the erythrocyte membrane becomes slightly raised at the interaction point when the apical end of the merozoite contacts the erythrocyte, but eventually a depression is created in the erythrocyte membrane (Fig. 1). The parts of the erythrocyte membrane to which the parasite is attached becomes thickened, increasing to about 15 nm (Aikawa et al 1978). This thickened membrane forms a junction with the parasite membrane in the area of close apposition between the merozoite and erythrocyte. The junctional gap between the erythrocyte membrane and merozoite membrane is about 10 nm; fine fibrils extend between the two parallel membranes.

Human erythrocytes lacking the Duffy blood group antigens are resistant to

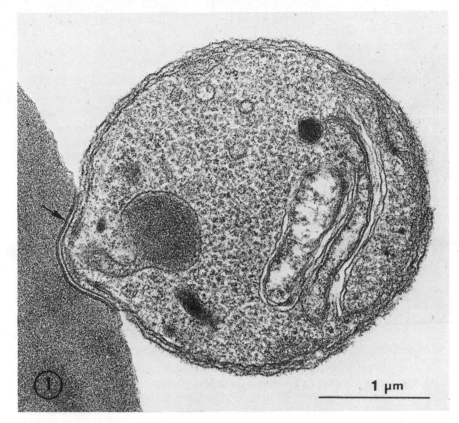

FIG. 1. Electron micrograph of a merozoite creating a depression in the erythrocyte membrane. The membrane becomes thickened at the attachment site (arrow).

invasion by the merozoites of *P. knowlesi* (Miller et al 1975). Electron microscopy showed that no junction is formed between a Duffy-negative erythrocyte and *P. knowlesi* merozoites (Miller et al 1979). The apical end of the merozoite is oriented toward the erythrocyte, but instead of a junction, the erythrocyte is about 120 nm away from the merozoite and they are connected by thin filaments (Fig. 2). Such filamentous attachments between merozoites and erythrocytes are not observed in experiments with normal rhesus monkey or human Duffy-positive erythrocytes. On the other hand, trypsin treatment of the Duffy-negative human erythrocytes permits the formation of a junction with the merozoites, and invasion (Fig. 3). The absence of junction formation with Duffy-negative human erythrocytes may indicate that the Duffy-associated antigen acts as a high affinity receptor necessary for a junction to be formed (Miller et al 1979). Recently, ovalocytic

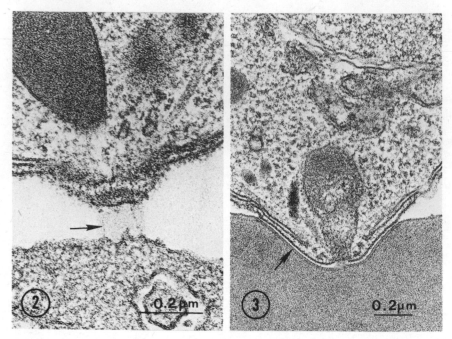

FIG. 2. *Plasmodium knowlesi* merozoite is connected with a Duffy-negative erythrocyte by fine filaments (arrow).

FIG. 3. A merozoite attaches to a trypsin-treated Duffy-negative erythrocyte by forming a junction (arrow). Note the thickened erythrocyte membrane at the site of attachment. (From Miller et al 1979 by permission of The Rockefeller University Press.)

erythrocytes have been reported to be resistant to *P. falciparum* invasion (Kidson et al 1981). This resistance may relate to an alteration in the erythrocyte cytoskeleton, preventing the redistribution of intramembrane particles (IMP) that is necessary for junction formation (Wilson 1982).

Erythrocyte entry

After the merozoite has attached to the erythrocyte membrane, products from the rhoptries and micronemes participate in the invagination of the erythrocyte membrane. Throughout the invasion, the apical end of the merozoite remains in contact with the vacuole membrane through an electron-dense band which is continuous with the common duct of the rhoptries (Aikawa et al 1978) (Fig. 4). Lower electron density in the ductule during invasion suggests that the rhoptry contents are released into the

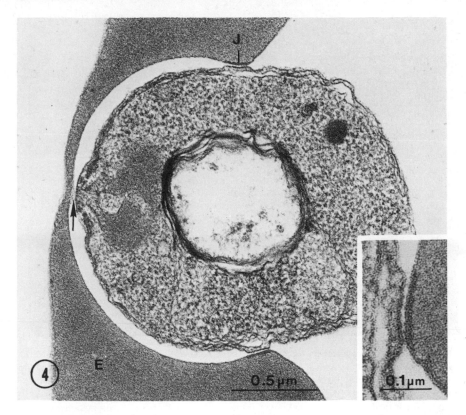

FIG. 4. An advanced stage of entry into an erythrocyte (E) by a merozoite. A junction (J) now appears at the orifice of the merozoite-induced invagination of the erythrocyte membrane. A narrow band (arrow) connects the apical end and the erythrocyte membrane. *Inset:* High magnification micrograph of the junction. (From Aikawa et al 1978 by permission of The Rockefeller University Press.)

vacuolar membrane through this band. It is likely that a histidine-rich protein is located in the rhoptries (Kilejian 1974).

As the invasion progresses, the depression of the erythrocyte membrane that was created by the apical end of the merozoite deepens and conforms to the shape of the merozoite (Aikawa et al 1978, Bannister et al 1975) (Fig. 4). The junction is no longer observed at the initial attachment point, but now appears at the orifice of the merozoite-induced invagination of the erythrocyte membrane (Fig. 4). As merozoite invasion proceeds, the junction, which is in the form of a circumferential zone of attachment between erythrocyte and merozoite, moves along the confronted membranes to maintain its position at the orifice of the parasitophorous vacuole (Aikawa et al 1978).

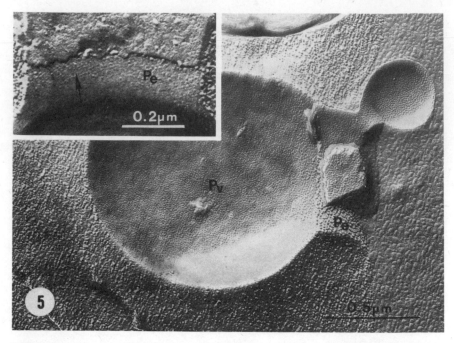

FIG. 5. Freeze-fracture electron micrograph of erythrocyte entry by a merozoite. The P face (Pe) of the erythrocyte membrane at the neck of the invagination is covered with IMP, but they disappear beyond the point where the neck of the invagination abruptly expands to form a parasitophorous vacuole (Pv). *Inset:* A narrow band of rhomboidally arrayed IMP (arrow) can be seen on the P face of the erythrocyte membrane at the orifice of the erythrocyte invagination. (From Aikawa et al 1981 by permission of The Rockefeller University Press.)

Freeze-fracture studies show a narrow circumferential band of rhomboidally arrayed IMP on the P (protoplasmic) face of the erythrocyte membrane at the orifice of the erythrocyte invagination (Fig. 5) and matching rhomboidally arrayed pits on the E face (Aikawa et al 1981) (Fig. 6). The band corresponds to the junction between the erythrocyte and merozoite membranes observed in thin sections. This finding indicates that the IMP on the erythrocyte rearrange themselves at the site of *Plasmodium* entry for local membrane specialization (Satir 1980). Studies on membrane–membrane fusions between cells have demonstrated that IMP are displaced laterally into adjacent membrane regions before the fusion process and that fusion occurs between protein-depleted lipid bilayers (Loyter & Lalazar 1980). In contrast to this lateral displacement of IMP, a reorganization of IMP occurs at the site of the erythrocyte–merozoite interaction. Apparently, this difference arises because the interaction between the erythrocyte and parasite membranes at the junction site is a transient phenomenon and is not a fusion process.

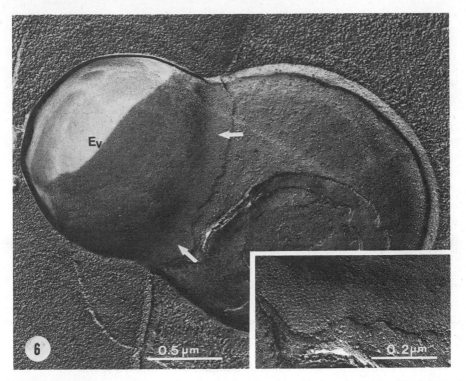

FIG. 6. Freeze-fracture electron micrograph of erythrocyte entry by a merozoite. The E face of the erythrocyte membrane at the neck of the invagination consists of a narrow circumferential band of rhomboidally arrayed pits (arrow). Ev is the E face of the vacuole membrane. *Inset:* High magnification micrograph showing a narrow band of rhomboidally arrayed pits. (From Aikawa et al 1981 by permission of The Rockefeller University Press.)

The IMP on the P face of the erythrocyte membrane disappear beyond this junction (Fig. 5). Therefore, the P face of the parasitophorous vacuole membrane, which originated from the erythrocyte membrane, is almost devoid of IMP (Aikawa et al 1981, McLaren et al 1979). By contrast, only a small difference in the number of IMP was noted between the E face of the erythrocyte membrane and the E face of the parasitophorous vacuole membrane (Aikawa et al 1981) (Table 1). A small dimple, measuring about 50 nm in diameter, is present on the P face of the parasite membrane at the tip of the apical end. This may correspond to the opening of the rhoptry duct present at the apical end of the merozoite (Aikawa et al 1981). The contents of rhoptries have been suggested to be involved in forming the relatively protein-free vacuole membrane.

From these findings one can conclude that the movement of the junction

TABLE 1 Mean densities per μm^2 of intramembrane particles (IMP) on erythrocyte and vacuole membranes

	P face	E face
Erythrocyte membrane	2109 ± 431	389 ± 100
Vacuole membrane	564 ± 148	344 ± 65

during invasion is an important component of the mechanism by which the merozoite enters the erythrocyte. This junctional movement might be the result of lateral displacement of the junction by the membrane flow on the merozoite. In fact, when erythrocytes and cytochalasin B-treated merozoites are incubated together, the merozoite attaches to the erythrocyte membrane and a junction is formed between the two, but the invasion process does not advance further and no movement of the junction occurs (Miller et al 1979). Although there is no entry of the parasite, however, the erythrocyte membrane still invaginates (Aikawa et al 1981, Miller et al 1979). A freeze-fracture study showed that the P face of the invaginated erythrocyte membrane was also almost devoid of IMP. This suggests that the attachment process in and of itself is sufficient to create a relatively IMP-free bilayer of the parasitophorous vacuole.

Sealing of erythrocyte membrane after completion of merozoite entry

When merozoite entry is completed the junction fuses at the posterior end of the merozoite, closing the orifice of the invagination in the fashion of an iris diaphragm (Aikawa et al 1978) (Fig. 7). The merozoite membrane still remains in close apposition to the thickened erythrocyte membrane at the point of final closure (Fig. 8). These observations demonstrate that the junction plays an important role in sealing the erythrocyte membrane when invasion is complete.

   When its entry into the erythrocyte is complete the merozoite is surrounded by a membrane of the parasitophorous vacuole that originated from the erythrocyte membrane, but the vacuole membrane differs in its molecular organization from the original erythrocyte membrane.

Alteration in the erythrocyte membrane during intraerythrocytic parasite development

Intraerythrocytic parasites influence not only the parasitophorous vacuole membrane but also the erythrocyte membrane itself. Two types of erythro-

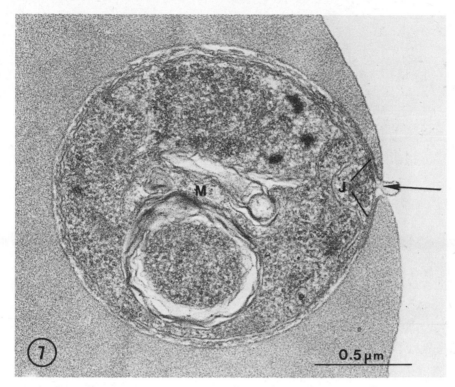

FIG. 7. Erythrocyte entry by a merozoite (M) is almost completed and a small orifice (arrow) is present at the posterior end of the merozoite. The junction (J) has now moved to the posterior end of the merozoite. (From Aikawa et al 1978 by permission of The Rockefeller University Press.)

cyte membrane modification can be seen in erythrocytes infected with certain species of malarial parasites: (1) electron-dense protrusions called knobs (Aikawa et al 1972, Luse & Miller 1971), and (2) caveola–vesicle complexes along the erythrocyte membrane (Aikawa et al 1975).

Erythrocytes infected with small trophozoites show few knobs, but they increase in number as the parasite grows within the erythrocyte (Figs. 9 and 10). The erythrocyte membrane covering the knobs is antigenically different from the rest of the erythrocyte membrane (Kilejian et al 1977, Langreth & Reese 1979). These knobs form focal junctions with the endothelial cell membranes (Fig. 11) or with the knobs of other erythrocytes, resulting in the sequestration of these infected erythrocytes along the vascular endothelium. The study of the mechanism of attachment of parasitized erythrocytes to the endothelium was made much easier when Udeinya et al (1981) demonstrated that the knobs on *P. falciparum*-infected erythrocyte membranes are the

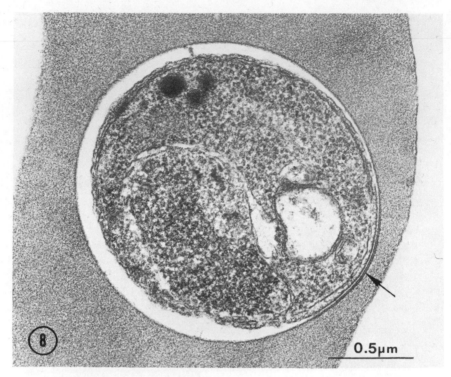

FIG. 8. Erythrocyte entry is completed and the parasite is within a parasitophorous vacuole. However, the posterior end of the merozoite is still attached (arrow) to the thickened erythrocyte membrane. (From Aikawa et al 1978 by permission of The Rockefeller University Press.)

points of attachment to *cultured* human endothelial cells. The knobs are concentrated in the area of the erythrocyte membrane in apposition to the endothelial cells and an aggregation of microfilaments in the endothelial cells is seen at the site of attachment (Fig. 11). The knobs found on the membrane of erythrocytes infected with *P. malariae* are morphologically identical to those on the membrane of *P. falciparum*-infected erythrocytes, yet cells infected with *P. malariae* do not bind to endothelial cells (Udeinya et al 1981). It is therefore conceivable that the knobs of *P. falciparum* contain components that are required for attachment to the endothelium but are not present on the knobs of *P. malariae*.

Freeze-fracture and etch techniques have been used to demonstrate that the P face of the membrane of *P. falciparum*-infected erythrocytes covering the knobs shows evenly distributed IMP without any aggregation or depletion of IMP (Fig. 10). The E face showed many indentations which correspond to the knobs. Despite the unaltered IMP distribution over the knob regions

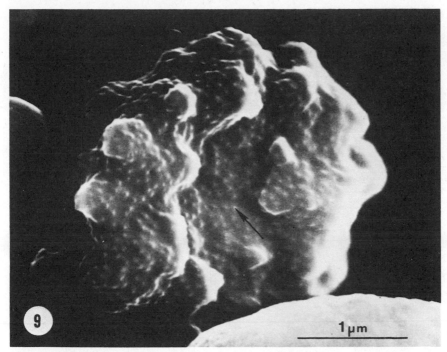

FIG. 9. Scanning electron micrograph showing numerous knobs (arrow) on the surface of the infected erythrocyte.

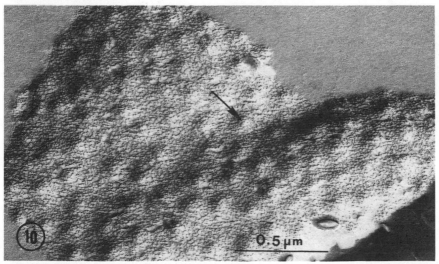

FIG. 10. Freeze-fracture electron micrograph showing knobs (arrow) on the surface of the infected erythrocyte. The distribution of IMP is not altered by the presence of these knobs.

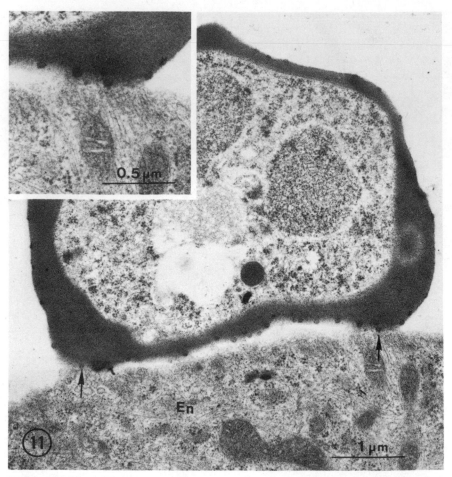

FIG. 11. Knobs on the surface of the infected erythrocyte form focal junctions (arrow) with the endothelial cell membrane (En). *Inset:* High power micrograph showing aggregation of microfilaments in the endothelial cells at the site of knob–erythrocyte attachment.

(Aikawa et al 1982), it is possible that the IMP may change their distribution pattern at the time of focal junction formation with the endothelial cells, since these particles show altered distribution at sites of junction formation (Staehelin 1974). The unaltered IMP distribution on the knob portion of the erythrocyte membrane may be correlated with the unaltered charge on the erythrocyte membrane covering the knobs induced by *P. coatneyi* infection (Miller et al 1972).

The caveola–vesicle complexes seen along the erythrocyte plasma membrane correspond to Schüffner's dots, seen in erythrocytes infected by vivax-

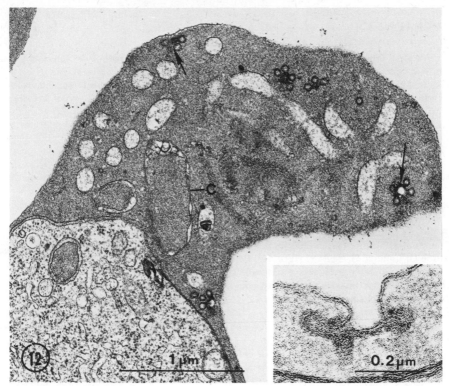

FIG. 12. Erythrocyte infected with *P. vivax* showing caveola–vesicle complexes (arrow) and clefts (C). *Inset:* High magnification micrograph showing a caveola–vesicle complex.

and ovale-type parasites by light microscopy. They consist of caveolae surrounded by small vesicles in an alveolar fashion (Aikawa et al 1975) (Fig. 12). Immunoelectron microscopy has been used to demonstrate malarial antigens within them. However, it is not clear how the malarial antigens move from the parasite to the caveola–vesicle complexes. In addition, the cytoplasm of the infected erythrocyte shows narrow clefts which correspond to the Maurer's clefts seen by light microscopy. The nature of the clefts is still unknown, but they probably originate from the parasitophorous vacuole membrane. Transmission electron microscopy showed the extension of the clefts into the parasitophorous vacuole (Aikawa et al 1975, Rudzinska & Trager 1968). The functional significance of caveola–vesicle complexes and clefts is still not clear and must await future investigation.

Acknowledgements

This work was supported in part by research grants (AI-10645 and AI-13366) from the US Public Health Service, by the US Army R & D Command (DAMD 17–79–C9029) and by the World Health Organization (T16/181/M2/52).

REFERENCES

Aikawa M, Rabbege JR, Wellde BT 1972 Junctional apparatus in erythrocytes infected with malarial parasites. Z Zellforsch Mikrosk Anat 124:72-75

Aikawa M, Miller LH, Rabbege J 1975 Caveola–vesicle complexes: the plasmalemma of erythrocytes infected by *Plasmodium vivax* and *Plasmodium cynomolgi*. Am J Pathol 79:285-300

Aikawa M, Miller LH, Johnson J, Rabbege J 1978 Erythrocyte entry by malarial parasites: a moving junction between erythrocyte and parasite. J Cell Biol 77:72-82

Aikawa M, Miller LH, Rabbege JR, Epstein N 1981 Freeze-fracture study on the erythrocyte membrane during malarial parasite invasion. J Cell Biol 92:55-62

Aikawa M, Rabbege J, Udeinya I, Miller LH 1982 Electron microscopy of knobs in *P. falciparum*-infected erythrocytes. J Parasitol, in press

Bannister LH, Butcher GA, Dennis ED, Mitchell GH 1975 Structure and invasive behaviour of *Plasmodium knowlesi* merozoites *in vitro*. Parasitology 71:483-491

Dvorak JA, Miller LH, Whitehouse WC, Shiroishi T 1975 Invasion of erythrocytes by malaria merozoites. Science (Wash DC) 187:748-750

Kidson C, Lamont G, Saul A, Nurse GT 1981 Ovalocytic erythrocytes from Melanesians are resistant to invasion by malaria parasites in culture. Proc Natl Acad Sci USA 78:5829-5832

Kilejian A 1974 A unique histidine-rich polypeptide from the malaria parasite, *Plasmodium lophurae*. J Biol Chem 249:4650-4655

Kilejian A, Abati A, Trager W 1977 *Plasmodium falciparum* and *Plasmodium coatneyi*: immunogenicity of 'knob-like protrusions' on infected erythrocyte membrane. Exp Parasitol 42:157-164

Langreth SG, Reese RT 1979 Antigenicity of the infected-erythrocyte and merozoite surfaces in *falciparum* malaria. J Exp Med 150:1241-1245

Loyter A, Lalazar A 1980 Induction of membrane fusion in human erythrocyte ghosts: involvement of spectrin in the fusion process. In: Gilula NB (ed) Membrane–membrane interactions. Raven Press, New York, p 11-26

Luse SA, Miller LH 1971 *Plasmodium falciparum* malaria: ultrastructure of parasitized erythrocytes in cardiac vessels. Am J Trop Med Hyg 20:655-660

McLaren DJ, Bannister LH, Trigg PI, Butcher GA 1979 Freeze-fracture studies on the interaction between the malaria parasite and the host erythrocyte in *Plasmodium knowlesi* infections. Parasitology 79:125-139

Miller LH, Cooper GW, Chien S, Freemount HN 1972 Surface charge on *Plasmodium knowlesi* and *P. coatneyi*-infected red cells of *Macaca mulatta*. Exp Parasitol 32:86-95

Miller LH, Mason SJ, Dvorak JA, McGinniss MH, Rothman IK 1975 Erythrocyte receptors for (*Plasmodium knowlesi*) malaria: Duffy blood group determinants. Science (Wash DC) 189:561-562

Miller LH, McAuliffe FM, Mason SJ 1977 Erythrocyte receptors for malaria merozoites. Am J Trop Med Hyg 26:204-208

Miller LH, Aikawa M, Johnson JG, Shiroishi T 1979 Interaction between cytochalasin B-treated malarial parasites and red cells. Attachment and junction formation. J Exp Med 149:172-184

Perkins M 1981 Inhibitory effect of erythrocyte membrane proteins on the *in vitro* invasion of the human malarial parasite (*Plasmodium falciparum*) into its host cell. J Cell Biol 90:563-567

Rudzinska M, Trager W 1968 The fine structure of trophozoites and gametocytes in *Plasmodium coatneyi*. J Protozool 15:73-88

Satir BH 1980 The role of local design in membrane. In: Gilula NB (ed) Membrane–membrane interactions. Raven Press, New York, p 45-58

Seed TM, Aikawa M, Sterling C, Rabbege JR 1974 Surface properties of extracellular malaria parasites: morphological and cytochemical study. Infect Immun 9:750-761
Staehelin LA 1974 Structure and function of intracellular junctions. Int Rev Cytol 39:191-283
Udeinya IJ, Schmidt JA, Aikawa M, Miller LH, Green I 1981 *Falciparum* malaria-infected erythrocytes specifically bind to cultured human endothelial cells. Science (Wash DC) 213:555-557
Wilson RJ 1982 How the malarial parasite enters the red blood cell. Nature (Lond) 295:368-369

DISCUSSION

McGregor: The knob in *P. falciparum* is obviously related to the sequestration of the parasite during the late stages of schizogony. Is there any evidence that when a knobless strain of *P. falciparum* is put into the host, there is no sequestration, and that schizogony occurs in the peripheral blood?

Barnwell: We have some evidence on this point, which we shall be presenting in our paper (p 117-132).

Anders: Is there any evidence that the number of knobs is decreased when you treat infected cells with immune serum? I was interested to see in one electron micrograph the aggregation of particles in the knob with a clear area around it.

Aikawa: The knobs do not decrease in number after treatment with immune serum. The number of knobs on the membrane of a *P. falciparum*-infected erythrocyte appears only to relate to the stage of the parasite in the erythrocyte: the more mature the parasite is, the more knobs are present on the erythrocyte membrane.

Anders: It appears then that the antiserum induces a localized redistribution of components in the area of the knob, a 'patching' phenomenon, but nothing equivalent to 'capping' which would be associated with a decrease in the number of knobs.

Howard: When the merozoite invaginates the erythrocyte membrane and enters the cell, the junctional region of electron density formed initially between the parasite apical complex and erythrocyte membrane moves as a band around the parasite. You mentioned the possibility of membrane flow, of the two membranes moving one against the other during this entry process. Have you any idea what mechanism would induce this? Have you seen any changes in microtubule orientation under the merozoite membrane that might suggest that microtubules are involved in moving the junctional complex?

Aikawa: We have no evidence for membrane flow; my statement was a suggestion only. We tried to detect microfilament changes in the merozoite, but found no such changes.

Wyler: Do normal merozoites invade cytochalasin pre-treated erythrocytes, usually?

Aikawa: Yes. When we treated erythrocytes with cytochalasin B and allowed them to interact with merozoites, the merozoites entered the cytochalasin-treated erythrocytes without any changes.

Wyler: Is anything known about the energy requirements of the merozoite for the interiorization process?

Aikawa: So far as I know, no one has demonstrated the energy requirements of the merozoite for this process.

Sherman: What is the effect of cytochalasin B on the merozoite, apart from your observation that it affects the second phase—invagination itself— but junction formation does occur? In other words, what else is known about the effect of cytochalasin on the merozoite?

Aikawa: Junction formation and the invagination of the erythrocyte membrane take place during the interaction between erythrocytes and cytochalasin B-treated merozoites. However, the movement of the junction along the membrane is blocked by cytochalasin, thereby preventing the invasion of the merozoite.

Sherman: Is there rhoptry discharge after treatment with cytochalasin? You showed somewhat less electron-dense material extruded just anterior to the rhoptries when invagination is initiated. When you look at the cytochalasin-treated merozoites, do you see such material extruded?

Aikawa: We have not noticed any changes in the appearance of the rhoptries of cytochalasin-treated merozoites.

Pasvol: The electron microscopic findings in *P. falciparum* that have been reported have been mainly to do with parasites once they are inside the red cell. Have you looked at the invasion process with *P. falciparum* and, if so, have you noted any differences from the appearances you have seen with *P. knowlesi?* Is there any technical problem with that?

Aikawa: We have not studied the interaction between erythrocytes and *P. falciparum* merozoites. However, Langreth et al (1978) reported findings almost identical to ours, during erythrocyte invasion by *P. falciparum* merozoites.

Phillips: Is any material left behind after the merozoite has gone into the red cell?

Aikawa: Our observation on erythrocyte invasion by *P. knowlesi* merozoites showed that the surface coat of the merozoite disappears at the point of the junction. However, we did not observe accumulation of the surface coat material at the site of the entry. After the junctions are fused and enclose the merozoite within the parasitophorous vacuole membrane, the thick membrane which formed a junction can no longer be seen. It therefore appears that the junction becomes part of the parasitophorous vacuole membrane.

Howard: In the scanning electron micrograph that you presented (Fig. 9), knobs were evident all over the surface of the infected red cell. There appeared to be a second-order morphological alteration of the surface as well, namely the very large protuberances, which were much larger than the knobs. I imagine that these bumps do not represent individual merozoites under the membrane, but are another type of morphological alteration of the red cell. Do you see that in other species besides *P. falciparum* ?

Aikawa: We have to be cautious about interpreting changes in erythrocyte morphology. Because erythrocytes are sensitive to hypotonic solutions, hypotonic fixatives can easily deform the shape of the erythrocyte. We have seen similar morphological changes in erythrocytes infected with other species of *Plasmodium*. Only transmission electron microscopy will answer your question. However, it is possible that this particular erythrocyte may be infected with several parasites.

Howard: Are there some knobs on ring forms?

Aikawa: There are a very few knobs in erythrocytes infected with ring forms. The number of knobs increases as the parasite matures.

Phillips: Would a red cell with two parasites have twice as many knobs? This would be a way of showing that the knobs are of parasite origin.

Aikawa: Scanning electron microscopy cannot answer this question. However, transmission electron microscopy on erythrocytes infected with two or more parasites demonstrated that the number of knobs is more closely related to the stage of the parasite than to the number of parasites within the erythrocytes. A red cell with two parasites does not have twice as many knobs.

Holder: Many micrographs of merozoites show a multilamellar, membranous body inside the parasite. Is this a structure involved in invasion, or, if not, do you know anything about its function?

Aikawa: I believe you are referring to a spherical body which is located in the posterior part of the merozoite. We do not know the function of this structure. However, since it is always closely associated with a mitochondrion, we assumed that the spherical body is an energy reservoir for the mitochondrion.

Bannister: One also sees a concentration of smooth endoplasmic reticulum in merozoites between the nucleus and the rhoptries, in well-fixed material, which corresponds to the multilamellated bodies of earlier studies. During invasion this structure is unaltered, so it probably represents a store of membrane for later development.

Jarra: Professor Aikawa, your micrograph (Fig. 11) showed interaction between parasitized erythrocytes and endothelial cells, apparently mediated by the knobs. Have you any information which suggests that the binding of antibody directed against components of the surface membrane of parasitized erythrocytes blocks this interaction, so that they don't adhere?

Aikawa: Yes, antibody against *P. falciparum* can block the binding between the endothelial cells and knobs on the membrane of *P. falciparum*-infected erythrocytes. Dr Barnwell has more information on this.

Barnwell: Dr Iroka Udeinya in our laboratory has been using endothelial and melanoma cell assays that he has developed to study the binding of infected erythrocytes. He has been able to block attachment of *P. falciparum*-infected erythrocytes, both by combining *Aotus* monkey immune sera with infected cells and then trying to attach those cells; and also by attaching the cells to the endothelium, adding antibody and eluting the attached *P. falciparum*-infected cells off. It is becoming more and more evident that the knob is a multi-component structure. We now have parasites that are knobby and will not bind to endothelial cells or melanoma cells *in vitro* (see our paper, p 117-132). There are also knobless parasites which don't attach, and there are the knobby parasites that bind. So in addition to the actual physical knob that we see, you probably also need a binding ligand molecule *on* the erythrocyte surface membrane to mediate attachment to endothelium.

Weatherall: Is this type of interaction with melanoma cells and with endothelial cells specific for these cell types, or is it a more general binding phenomenon?

Barnwell: The binding is limited to certain host cell types and is not a totally general phenomenon. Endothelial cells of human origin, some, but not all, human melanoma cell lines, and human monocyte/macrophages will bind *P. falciparum*-infected erythrocytes but many other host cell types won't. The specificity of the *parasite* in binding has been studied also. *P. falciparum*-infected erythrocytes bind (i.e. the knobby strains do), whereas *P. vivax*-infected red cells do not bind to endothelial or melanoma cells. *P. brasilianum*-infected cells have many knobs but do not become sequestered or bind to endothelium.

Anders: Do you get equivalent binding to endothelium from different host species, using *P. falciparum*-infected cells?

Barnwell: No, the *P. falciparum*-infected erythrocytes will bind to umbilical cord or aortic endothelium from humans but not bovine endothelial cells.

Luzzatto: Professor Aikawa, you mentioned the finding by Miller's group (1979) that Duffy-negative human red cells are not invaded by *P. knowlesi*; but after these red cells were treated with trypsin or other enzymes they could be infected; and you showed (Fig. 3) that normal junctions were now formed. You also suggested that the Duffy antigen may be the receptor necessary for junction formation. How do you explain that the red cell that lacks that antigen and in addition has been stripped of something else by trypsin then makes normal junctions?

Aikawa: I cannot answer your question. Evidently, we need more data to clarify this phenomenon.

Anders: Is the deformation of the red cell as seen in cinemicrophotography invariably associated with invasion? If so, at precisely what point in the sequence of events does it occur?

Aikawa: By phase microscopy, Dvorak et al (1975) demonstrated the deformation of red cells just before the invasion of the merozoite takes place. The lateral side of the merozoite bounces on the erythrocyte, resulting in its deformation. However, when the invasion process by the merozoite begins, the merozoite orients itself so that the apical end attaches to the erythrocyte membrane. At this stage, no deformation of the erythrocyte can be seen except the invagination of the erythrocyte membrane by the apical end of the merozoite.

Pasvol: How does the change occur, from the lateral attachment to the re-orientation and apical attachment?

Aikawa: We don't know how this change occurs, although Seed et al (1973) suggested that the surface charge difference between the erythrocyte and the apical end of the merozoite is responsible for this re-orientation.

REFERENCES

Dvorak JA, Miller JH, Whitehouse WC, Shiroishi T 1975 Invasion of erythrocytes by malaria merozoites. Science (Wash DC) 187:748-749

Langreth SG, Nguyen-Dinh P, Trager W 1978 *Plasmodium falciparum* in merozoite invasion *in vitro* in the presence of chloroquine. Exp Parasitol 46:235-238

Miller LH, Aikawa M, Johnson JG, Shiroishi T 1979 Interaction between cytochalasin B-treated malarial parasites and red cells. Attachment and junction formation. J Exp Med 149:172-184

Seed TM, Aikawa M, Sterling CR 1973 An electron microscope-cytochemical method for differentiating membranes of host red cells and malarial parasites. J Protozool 20:603-605

Transport of ions in erythrocytes infected by plasmodia

KAZUYUKI TANABE*, ROSS B. MIKKELSEN and DONALD F. H. WALLACH

*Tufts-New England Medical Center, Department of Therapeutic Radiology, Radiobiology Division, 171 Harrison Avenue, Boston, MA 02111, USA and *Department of Medical Zoology, Osaka City University, Medical School, Asahi-Machi, Abeno-Ku, Osaka, 545, Japan*

Abstract Throughout its erythrocytic cycle the plasmodial parasite modifies the plasma membrane of its host cell. Some changes derive from parasite metabolism. Intraerythrocytic forms use glucose at more than 10-fold normal red cell rates. The H^+ accompanying the lactate end-product is exported into the host cell cytoplasm by an electrogenic proton pump in the parasite membrane. This maintains a pH greater than 7.0 in the parasite cytoplasm, but lowers erythrocyte cytoplasmic pH from approximately 7.2 to 6.5. Ca^{2+} transport across parasite membranes is coupled to the proton pump, possibly a Ca^{2+}/H^+ antiporter.

The Ca^{2+},Mg^{2+}-ATPase and Na^+,K^+-ATPase activities of erythrocyte membranes from schizont-infected erythrocytes have been studied. Under optimal assay conditions (pH = 7.0; [ATP] = 1 mM; ±calmodulin) membranes from infected cells showed a 30% reduction in Ca^{2+},Mg^{2+}-ATPase activity but no difference from normal in Na^+,K^+-ATPase activity. The calmodulin levels of infected cells were depressed by about 30%. The [ATP] in the cytoplasm of infected erythrocytes was only 0.2 mM (as against 1.3 mM in normals) and at this ATP concentration the activities of both ATPases are only 30% of normal. Shifting the pH from 7.0 to 6.5 decreases Na^+,K^+-ATPase activity by an additional 50% but is without effect on the Ca^{2+},Mg^{2+}-ATPase. The results provide a partial explanation for the increased Ca^{2+} permeability and altered Na^+/K^+ content of plasmodia-infected erythrocytes.

The circulation of ions across the plasma membranes of prokaryotic and eukaryotic unicellular organisms is at the heart of many physiological devices that allow these cells to function as integrated units. Thus, transport of essential nutrients (e.g. amino acids) is coupled to transmembrane gradients of Na^+ and H^+, and cell regulatory processes are modulated by shifts in intracellular ion concentrations (e.g. phosphofructokinase by H^+; cyclic nucleotide metabolism enzymes by Ca^{2+}; protein synthesis by K^+ and Mg^{2+}).

1983 Malaria and the red cell. Pitman, London (Ciba Foundation symposium 94) p 64-73

Many unicellular organisms establish transmembrane ion gradients and regulate the intracellular ionic milieux by proton-extruding ATPases coupled with symport and antiport transport processes (Harold 1977).

Parasites, such as *Plasmodium*, with both intra- and extracellular cycles, represent an intriguing problem in this regard since they must adjust to the very different ionic environments of the host cell cytoplasm (high K^+; low Na^+ and Ca^{2+}) and the extracellular fluid (high Na^+ and Ca^{2+}; low K^+). Moreover, the cytoplasmic ionic composition of parasites residing within mammalian host cells depends on ion transport processes at three membrane levels—the host cell plasma membrane, the parasite vacuole membrane and the parasite plasma membrane.

Past investigations have shown altered ion contents of erythrocytes infected with plasmodial parasites. Overman (1948) and Dunn (1969) have demonstrated increased Na^+ and reduced K^+ levels in *P. falciparum*- and *P. knowlesi*-infected monkey erythrocytes. Dunn (1969) has also shown that the ouabain-sensitive efflux rate for Na^+ was reduced by 40% and the passive Na^+ influx rate increased by 30% in erythrocytes from infected animals. We (Tanabe et al 1982) have demonstrated elevated calcium levels in *P. chabaudi*-infected rat and *P. knowlesi*-infected monkey erythrocytes. Schizont-infected rat erythrocytes contain 10 times more calcium than uninfected cells.

To investigate the relative roles of the host cell membrane and parasite membranes in ion transport of *Plasmodium*-infected erythrocytes, we have examined Ca^{2+} transport processes and the membrane potential of infected cells (Tanabe et al 1982, Mikkelsen et al 1982). We have also isolated the erythrocyte plasma membrane of *P. chabaudi*-infected cells and have determined its Ca^{2+},Mg^{2+}-ATPase and Na^+,K^+-ATPase activities.

Calcium content and transport

Atomic absorption analyses of the calcium levels in *P. chabaudi*-infected rat erythrocytes fractionated, on metrizamide gradients (Tanabe et al 1982), according to the state of parasite development, revealed a two-fold increase at early (ring, early trophozoite) stages and a 10–20-fold increase at late stages (schizont, gametocyte). Most of this calcium (>90%) was localized within the parasite. Transport studies with $^{45}Ca^{2+}$ indicated that both Ca^{2+} influx and efflux processes were energy-dependent.

Influx was inhibited by about 50% and efflux enhanced by about 70% in infected but not normal erythrocytes by low concentrations of the proton ionophore, carbonylcyanide *m*-chlorophenylhydrazone (CCP; 1–10 μM) or the proton ATPase inhibitor, dicyclohexylcarbodiimide (DCCD; 5–100 μM).

In contrast, antimycin A, CN^- and N_3^- influenced Ca^{2+} influx or efflux very little, suggesting that the acristate mitochondria of schizonts contribute negligibly to Ca^{2+} transport in infected cells. Similar responses to these inhibitors were observed in measurements of the membrane potential of normal and *P. chabaudi*-infected erythrocytes, implying that Ca^{2+} transport is coupled to a membrane potential-dependent process.

The membrane potential was measured (Mikkelsen et al 1982) from the transmembrane distributions of the lipophilic cation, triphenylmethylphosphonium (TPMP) and the lipophilic anion, thiocyanate (SCN). Previous work (Hoek et al 1980, Mikkelsen & Koch 1981) has shown that the cation will concentrate in compartments of high, inside-negative membrane potential, whereas the anion accumulates in compartments that possess a less negative, depolarized, membrane potential. The simultaneous measurement of TPMP and SCN distributions provides a procedure (Mikkelsen et al 1982) for monitoring the erythrocyte membrane potential (SCN) and the parasite membrane potential (TPMP).

The SCN probe does not report a significant difference between the membrane potentials of normal (about -6.5 mV) and infected rat erythrocytes (about -6.0 mV). However, measurements with TPMP revealed a membrane potential of -35 mV for schizont-infected cells, compared to -15 mV for normal cells and -20 mV for ring-infected cells. With parasitized but not normal erythrocytes, the membrane potential reported by TPMP becomes less negative after treatment with low concentrations of CCCP and DCCD, and upon glucose deprivation. Antimycin A is effective only when the infected cells contain appreciable proportions of gametocytes.

The depolarization observed with DCCD and CCCP suggests that the membrane potential of late-stage parasites derives in part from the activity of an electrogenic proton ATPase, as has been observed for yeast and bacteria (Slayman & Slayman 1974, Schuldiner & Kaback 1975, Stroobant et al 1980). A mitochondrial contribution is unlikely since plasmodial mitochondria (except for those of gametocytes) lack cristae and the ratio of mitochondrial volume to the total parasite volume is insufficient to account for the measured TPMP accumulation.

If the E_m is a consequence of an H^+-ATPase, a ΔpH should be established across the parasite plasma membrane (plus parasitophorous vacuole). This should be sensitive to DCCD. To explore this possibility, we measured the uptake of weak acids and weak bases, and determined the pH of the erythrocytic space after saponin lysis and separation of parasites, as described by Friedman et al (1979) for *P. falciparum*. As was found by these investigators, the erythrocytic space pH of *P. chabaudi*-infected cells is appreciably lower than extracellular pH and intracellular pH of normal cells (pH 6.60 in infected cells, pH 7.22 for normal cells at extracellular pH

7.2–7.3). A low erythrocytic space pH was also detected by the weak base methylamine (pH $= 6.96 \pm 0.05$ at an external pH of 7.2 ± 0.02). However, weak acids, such as dimethyloxazolidine-2,3-dione (DMO) and acetate, give an internal pH between 7.51 and 7.62 ± 0.07. As weak bases accumulate in acidic compartments (Hinke & Menard 1978, Mikkelsen et al 1980) and weak acids concentrate in alkaline compartments, our results indicate that methylamine monitors mostly the erythrocytic space of infected cells whereas the weak acid distributions reflect an alkaline, presumably parasite compartment. Further evidence for this suggestion and support for an H^+-ATPase comes from experiments examining the effects of low concentrations of DCCD. With DCCD present, the uptake of DMO is reduced (pH internal $= 7.20 \pm 0.03$).

In additional unpublished studies a DCCD-binding protein of M_r 8000, soluble in chloroform/methanol, has been isolated from parasite membranes but not host cell membranes. The apparent molecular weight of this protein and its solubility in organic solvents corresponds to the F_0 component of H^+-ATPases isolated from bacteria and mitochondria (Kagawa et al 1980).

Overall, our experiments measuring Ca^{2+} transport and membrane potential/pH gradients suggest that Ca^{2+} transport across parasite membranes proceeds via a $Ca^{2+}:H^+$ antiporter coupled to an outwardly extruding H^+-ATPase. Evidence for the existence of such a Ca^{2+} transport mechanism has been found for yeast (Stroobant et al 1980).

Membrane ATPases

We have explored the questions of how Ca^{2+} transport through the parasite membrane relates to that through the erythrocyte membrane. Past investigations have shown that the native erythrocyte membrane is poorly permeable to Ca^{2+} and that its Ca^{2+}, Mg^{2+}-ATPase activity, which mediates Ca^{2+} efflux, is 10-fold greater than what is necessary to maintain intracellular $[Ca^{2+}]$ at or below 10^{-6} M (Sarkadi 1980).

Host membranes were isolated after $Tris/NH_4Cl$ lysis of infected cells at different stages of parasite development (Tanabe et al 1982). Using acetylcholinesterase as marker for host cell membranes and glutamate dehydrogenase as a marker for parasites and parasite lysis, we obtained a host cell membrane yield near 30%, with less than 0.1% parasite contamination and less than 5% parasite lysis (to be published). We found that, under optimal assay conditions (1 mM-ATP, 10 μM-Ca^{2+}, pH 7.0, 1 μg/ml calmodulin), the Ca^{2+}, Mg^{2+}-ATPase activity of erythrocyte membranes from schizont-infected cells was reduced by approximately 30% relative to that of membranes from uninfected cells (1396 ± 119 vs. 2088 ± 286 μmoles P_i/mg per 30 min;

$P<0.01$). In the case of late trophozoites, activity was reduced by about 20% ($1640 \pm 217\,\mu$moles P_i/mg per 30 min; $P<0.02$). At earlier stages the Ca^{2+},Mg^{2+}-ATPase activity of host cell membranes did not differ from that of normal cell membranes.

We have also investigated the responses of the Ca^{2+},Mg^{2+}-ATPase to pH, calmodulin and ATP. As noted, the pH of the erythrocyte cytoplasm lies near 6.5 in schizont-infected cells, but Ca^{2+},Mg^{2+}-ATPase activity is insensitive to pH shift between 7.0 and 6.5. We have measured the calmodulin content of normal and infected cells with a radioimmunoassay kit (CAABCO, Houston, TX) and found a 30% reduction in schizont-infected cells. The Ca^{2+},Mg^{2+}-ATPase activities of isolated membranes from normal and infected erythrocytes respond identically to calmodulin with maximal stimulation (3–4-fold) at $1\,\mu$g/ml. The significance of a 30% reduction in calmodulin levels is uncertain, since the concentration of this protein within erythrocytes is 100 times more than that necessary to activate the Ca^{2+} pump (Sarkadi 1980).

The Ca^{2+} pumps of erythrocyte membranes from normal and infected cells depend identically on ATP concentration over the range of 0.02 to 2.0 mM with maximal activities near 1.0 mM-ATP. Using a luciferin/luciferase assay for ATP (Mikkelsen & Schmidt-Ullrich 1980) we have found the ATP levels of $TrisNH_4Cl$ lysates of normal and schizont-infected erythrocytes to be 1.3 mM and 0.2 mM respectively. At 0.2 mM-ATP the Ca^{2+},Mg^{2+}-ATPase activities of both membranes are reduced by about 70%.

The reduced Ca^{2+},Mg^{2+}-ATPase activity under optimal assay conditions, and the low ATP concentrations found in the cytoplasm of infected erythrocytes, suggest that the Ca^{2+} pump of schizont-infected cells functions at only about 15–20% of normal. In view of the excess Ca^{2+},Mg^{2+}-ATPase in normal erythrocytes, this reduction in activity might appear to be insufficient to account for the elevated Ca^{2+} levels in infected cells. However, the work of Larsen et al (1981) suggests that *in vitro* studies on erythrocyte Ca^{2+} permeability may be misleading because they do not take account of the shear stresses experienced by circulating erythrocytes *in vivo*. Under physiological conditions of shear stress ($100–5000\,s^{-1}$), Ca^{2+} accumulation by ATP-depleted erythrocytes increases several fold compared with the unsheared state. With ATP-enriched cells, Ca^{2+} does not accumulate to any significant degree but Ca^{2+},Mg^{2+}-ATPase activity is greatly enhanced by shear. Na^+,K^+-ATPase activity is negligibly affected by shear stress. In light of these findings, the 80% reduction in Ca^{2+},Mg^{2+}-ATPase activity of erythrocyte membranes from schizont-infected cells may have considerable biological significance.

During our studies of Ca^{2+},Mg^{2+}-ATPase activity we also investigated the ouabain-sensitive Na^+,K^+-ATPase. Under optimal assay conditions, Na^+,K^+-ATPase activities of plasma membranes from normal and schizont-infected erythrocytes were identical (472 ± 61 vs. 469 ± 80 μmoles P_i/mg per 30 min). However, a shift of pH from 7.0 to 6.5 reduced the enzyme activity of both membranes by about 50%. At 0.2 mM-ATP (the ATP level in the cytoplasm of infected erythrocytes), the Na^+,K^+-ATPase activity of both membranes was decreased by an additional 70%. The Na^+,K^+-ATPase activity of host cell membranes is therefore about 85% less than normal. This may account for the elevated Na^+ and decreased K^+ levels in *Plasmodium*-infected erythrocytes.

Summary

Our studies indicate that the plasmodial parasite maintains ion gradients across its own plasma membrane, in part by an H^+-ATPase. They also show that ion transport across the host cell membrane is modified indirectly by parasite metabolism through its effects on H^+ and ATP levels in the erythrocyte cytoplasm.

Acknowledgement

Supported by grant AI 16087 from the National Institutes of Health (R.B.M.).

REFERENCES

Dunn MJ 1969 Alterations of red blood cell sodium transport during malarial infection. J Clin Invest 48:674-684

Friedman MJ, Roth EF, Nagel RL, Trager W 1979 *Plasmodium falciparum:* physiological interactions with the human sickle cell. Exp Parasitol 47:73-80

Harold FM 1977 Ion currents and physiological functions in microorganisms. Annu Rev Microbiol 31:181-203

Hinke JAM, Menard MR 1978 Evaluation of DMO method for measuring intracellular pH. Respiration Physiol 33:31-40

Hoek JB, Nicholls DG, Williamson JR 1980 Determination of the mitochondrial proton motive force in isolated hepatocytes. J. Biol Chem 255:1458-1464

Kagawa Y, Ohta S, Yoshida M, Sone N 1980 Functions of subunits of H^+-ATPase. Ann N Y Acad Sci 358:103-117

Larsen FL, Katz S, Roufogalis BD, Brooks DE 1981 Physiological shear stresses enhance the Ca^{2+} permeability of human erythrocytes. Nature (Lond) 294:667-668

Mikkelsen RB, Koch B 1981 Thermosensitivity of the membrane potential of normal and simian virus 40-transformed hamster lymphocytes. Cancer Res 41:209-215

Mikkelsen RB, Schmidt-Ullrich R 1980 Concanavalin A induces the release of intracellular Ca^{2+} in intact rabbit thymocytes. J Biol Chem 255:5177-5183

Mikkelsen RB, Schmidt-Ullrich R, Wallach DFH 1980 Concanavalin A induces an intraluminal alkalinization of thymocyte membrane vesicles. J Cell Physiol 102:113-117

Mikkelsen RB, Tanabe K, Wallach DFH 1982 The membrane potential of *Plasmodium*-infected erythrocytes. J Cell Biol, in press

Overman RR 1948 Reversible cellular permeability alterations in disease. *In vivo* studies on sodium, potassium and chloride concentrations in erythrocytes of the malarious monkey. Am J Physiol 152:113-121

Sarkadi B 1980 Active calcium transport in human red cells. Biochim Biophys Acta 604:159-190

Schuldiner L, Kaback HR 1975 Membrane potential and active transport in membrane vesicles from *Escherichia coli*. Biochemistry 14:5451-5461

Slayman CL, Slayman CW 1974 Depolarization of the plasma membrane of *Neurospora* during active transport of glucose: evidence for a proton-dependent co-transport system. Proc Natl Acad Sci USA 71:1935-1939

Stroobant P, Dame JB, Scarborough GA 1980 The *Neurospora* plasma membrane Ca^{2+} pump. Fed Proc 39:2437-2441

Tanabe K, Mikkelsen RB, Wallach DFH 1982 Calcium transport of *Plasmodium chabaudi*-infected erythrocytes. J Cell Biol 93:680-684

DISCUSSION

Howard: Have you looked at any effects of cation ionophores on the export of lactate from the malaria parasite? Is lactate export coupled to cation transport?

Wallach: There are several lactate export systems in the red cell. These are co-transporters, by which lactate and protons are exported together. This lactate export system is found in red cells and other cells. Our few measurements indicate a low pH and high lactate within parasitized erythrocytes.

Cabantchik: The lactate story in the red blood cell is complex. The co-transport system for protons and lactate which you mention maintains the roughly constant pH within the normal red blood cell. The additional system that moves about 5% of the total lactate produced by glycolysis is the anion transporter mentioned by Dr Tanner. The rest of the lactate, 2% or so, is exported by diffusion. These two systems are not obligatory co-transport systems and therefore may move lactate out without a proton. The hypothesis has been suggested (Ginsburg et al 1981) that if one could selectively block these lactate transport systems, there would be a decrease in pH in the red cell, primarily in the parasitized cell, which produces 200-fold more lactate than the normal red cell. Such a reduction in pH would reduce glycolysis dramatically and by a feedback type of mechanism it could block development of the parasites. Experimental support for this hypothesis has been provided in two recent studies (Ginsburg et al 1981, Cabantchik et al 1982) which demonstrated that anion transport blockers inhibited intraerythrocytic parasite growth.

Regarding infected cells, we believe that the specific lactate-H co-transporter might be working almost at saturating capacity so that a relatively higher share of the two non-specific transport systems in moving lactate out of the red cell is needed. Regarding non-infected cells, few careful studies of lactate transport have been reported (Deuticke et al 1982).

Howard: From rate measurements of lactate export from infected cells, and assuming no changes in the lactate export capacity of these three endogenous mechanisms, do we need to postulate an additional parasite-dependent change in the lactate export capacity of the erythrocyte membrane of infected cells?

Wallach: We don't have all the information needed to answer this. This is also true for glucose transport into the red cell. We have made calculations for the latter and have linked it to the export of lactate. The red cell can take up a large amount of glucose, much more than it needs—probably almost all that the parasite uses. To argue backwards, if the red cell has that kind of lactate export capacity with these three pathways, it may not need an additional component. We had thought there might be a need for an additional lactate exporter.

Cabantchik: In conditions where you block a substantial fraction of glucose transport mediated by the 'normal red cell glucose transporter', you do not affect parasite growth within the red blood cell. There is apparently a surplus of glucose transport capacity in host cell membranes.

Sherman: What about the simple diffusional entry of glucose? How much would blocking that in parasitized red cells affect their growth? All you have to do is omit glucose from the medium with infected red blood cells, and they die.

Wallach: Certainly without glucose you cannot maintain the membrane potentials of parasitized cells, nor the calcium uptake by the parasite.

Cabantchik: We are dealing here with kinetic properties. If there is a surplus of the specific glucose transporter, then partial inhibition might affect neither the import of glucose nor the intraerythrocytic growth of parasites. However, full blockade of all entry paths of glucose should definitely arrest parasite growth.

Wyler: Is there any evidence that drugs which block calcium channels, such as verapamil or nifedipine, affect calcium transport in parasitized erythrocytes? Since these drugs are already in clinical use, they might be intriguing candidates as novel antimalarials!

Wallach: This is of interest, but we have no clear evidence yet.

Howard: Since you have demonstrated that one barrier for calcium transport might be in the parasite plasmalemma, could you study synchronous cultures and follow changes in calcium uptake and export during reinvasion? It would be interesting to know if there are drastic fluxes then, especially in relation to the rapid swelling of the erythrocyte at the time when the merozoite apical complex orientates against the red cell membrane.

Wallach: We have thought about this. Unfortunately, in the early stages of invasion we can't detect any abnormality. There is sufficient contamination by uninfected cells for the system to be non-discriminating. We really need to know what happens at the moment of invasion or shortly after, and our techniques don't allow that.

Howard: Are there any fluorescent probes that give a reflection of internal calcium levels?

Wallach: There are, but they are not satisfactory. Fluorescent probes are useful for measuring the association of calcium with cristate mitochondria, which this parasite unfortunately lacks. We have used aequorin to look at the invasive stage, but for some reason it ceases to fluoresce at that point.

Cabantchik: It is well known that a calcium load leads primarily to a massive leakage of potassium from normal red cells—the so-called Gardos effect. This property is certainly retained during the ring stage in infected cells—I don't know about the later stages. This calcium-induced loss of potassium of course changes the membrane potential, making the cells hyperpolarize. I don't know how this could have affected the measurements you have made.

Wallach: Nothing I presented here really relates to this question. We have measured the distribution of other ions, particularly potassium. Remember that we are not seeing an increase in calcium concentration in the red cell cytoplasm, either calmodulin-bound or unbound calcium. (The calmodulin content, incidentally, stays very stable, almost until lysis.) What is happening is that calcium is accumulating inside the parasite. The potassium concentration within the red cell space remains stable until shortly before lysis. I don't see where we would have a calcium-induced change in potassium flux.

Cabantchik: It is enough to have a reduction in pH, to bring about a change in potassium concentration. These two properties are interrelated.

Wallach: Yes, but where does this alter the measurement? We observe an acidification of the red cell cytoplasm, but it apparently is not great enough to cause a massive potassium leakage at that point. When we go one step further, we do get this leakage.

Howard: Would it be technically possible to load erythrocytes with various radioactive anions and cations and then incubate them with merozoites, in order to follow the influxes and effluxes upon invasion? Differential effluxes might suggest selective permeability changes and give some information on the mechanism of invasion.

Wallach: We should be able to do that. It would be a very good experiment.

Sherman: I don't know the situation with *P. chabaudi,* but in a wide variety of malarias the intracellular concentration of sodium in infected red cells shows a marked increase. This occurs from bird malarias to *P. knowlesi.* The work of Dunn (1969) seems to indicate that the sodium pump is impaired in infected red cells.

Wallach: As I mentioned, under the conditions of pH and [ATP] that exist (according to our measurements) in the cytoplasmic space of the infected red cell, the Na^+,K^+-ATPase would work at less than normal efficiency. Certainly the sodium level rises but we do not know the reason for the change in sodium concentration.

Friedman: It seems to me that calcium accumulation by a parasite antiport would require a lower pH (higher H^+ concentration) inside the parasite than outside, since the protons must move out from the parasite to drive calcium in; but you find that the pH is higher in the parasite. A lower internal pH would be necessary if your hypothesis was correct. In other words, I suggest that it is not possible for the proposed mechanism to work. An alternative possibility is that calcium is binding to something when it enters the parasite. This would explain the apparent 'uptake'.

Cabantchik: This is correct; to bring about an up-hill transport of calcium into the parasite one needs a favourable gradient of protons for them to go out of the parasite. According to Dr Wallach the proton source is the red cell cytoplasm, the proton-ATPase of parasite origin pumping protons into the parasite; additional protons could originate of course from glycolysis within the parasite itself. If the calcium is indeed free inside the parasite, and if it is being accumulated against an electrochemical gradient, then according to the proposed scheme, both a favourable H^+ gradient and a $Ca^{2+}-H^+$ antiporter are required in order to build up the Ca^{2+} inside. However, is the Ca^{2+} inside the parasite free or bound? I believe that Dr Wallach has measured total calcium by a chemical method which didn't allow him to distinguish between those two forms of calcium.

Wallach: We certainly agree that an appreciable portion of parasite Ca^{2+} is bound or compartmentalized (perhaps this is a function of the acristate mitochondria). At present we are isolating 'free' parasites that retain a membrane potential, and thus we should be able with existing methods to determine the free Ca^{2+} levels inside parasites.

REFERENCES

Cabantchik ZI, Kutner S, Krugliak M, Ginsburg H 1982 Anion transport inhibitors as suppressors of *P. falciparum* growth in *in vitro* cultures. Mol Pharmacol, in press

Deuticke B, Beyer E, Forst B 1982 Discrimination of three parallel pathways of lactate transport in the human erythrocyte membrane by inhibitors and kinetic properties. Biochim Biophys Acta 684:96-110

Dunn MJ 1969 Alterations of red blood cell sodium transport during malarial infection. J Clin Invest 48:674-684

Ginsburg H, Kutner S, Krugliak M, Cabantchik ZI 1981 Inhibition of *P. falciparum* growth *in vitro* by specific inhibitors of red blood cell anion transport. In: Slutzky GM (ed) Biochemistry of parasites. Pergamon Press, Oxford and New York, p 85-96

The anaemia of *Plasmodium falciparum* malaria

D. J. WEATHERALL, S. ABDALLA and M. J. PIPPARD

Nuffield Department of Clinical Medicine, University of Oxford, John Radcliffe Hospital, Oxford, OX3 9DU, UK

Abstract Anaemia is an important complication of *P. falciparum* malaria infection. This paper describes recent studies that have attempted to define some of the pathophysiological mechanisms involved in different forms of infection and at different stages of the illness.

After an acute infection there is a steady fall in the haemoglobin level with an inappropriate reticulocyte response. Current evidence indicates that this form of anaemia may result from a combination of acute sequestration of iron in the reticuloendothelial system associated with a shortened red cell survival. Recent studies indicate that there may be a dyserythropoietic component as well. The mechanism for the shortened red cell survival is uncertain; although it may be due in part to sequestration of parasitized cells, the haemoglobin level continues to fall for several weeks after the acute episode and other factors must be involved. The role of immune haemolysis appears to be relatively small.

It is becoming apparent that severe dyserythropoiesis with minimal haemolysis plays a major role in the anaemias of *Plasmodium falciparum* infection, particularly in immune individuals. This phenomenon has been studied by both light and electron microscopy and by assessing the *in vitro* kinetics of erythroid precursor proliferation. The results indicate a major defect in erythroid maturation with a significant degree of erythrophagocytosis. Although these studies have provided a clearer picture of the pathophysiology of anaemia at different phases of *P. falciparum* infection, there is still little indication of how the basic changes in red cell production and survival are mediated.

Anaemia is an important cause of morbidity, and probably contributes to mortality, in patients with *Plasmodium falciparum* malaria. It is also the major complication of this form of malaria in children who live in endemic areas (McGregor et al 1956, 1966). However, despite a great deal of work spanning many years the pathogenesis of the anaemia of *P. falciparum* malaria remains uncertain.

Considering the difficulties involved, it is not surprising that progress has been so slow in determining the mechanisms of anaemia in malarial infection.

1983 Malaria and the red cell. Pitman, London (Ciba Foundation symposium 94) p 74-97

Very little is known about the pathogenesis of the anaemia of any form of acute infection. With malaria, the difficulties are compounded by many factors, including the rapidity with which high parasite levels are reached in non-immune individuals and the marked variability of the clinical course of the disorder with respect to racial background and immune status. Furthermore, patients in areas where the condition is common often show multiple pathology, including iron or folate deficiency, bacterial or parasitic infections, genetic diseases of the red cell, and many other complicating factors. In addition, the effects of *P. falciparum* infections are so protean, and involve so many systems, that it is extremely difficult to determine which of a multitude of potential factors are interacting to produce the severe degree of anaemia that often accompanies this condition. The published work on the anaemia of malaria reflects these difficulties and much of it does not include information about the iron or folate status of affected patients or about the presence or absence of associated abnormalities of the red cells, or other forms of infection or infestation.

It is against this unpromising background that we must examine what is known about the pathogenesis of the anaemia of malaria. This subject has been reviewed recently (Esan 1975, Fleming 1981, Weatherall & Abdalla 1982) and much of the experimental work relating to erythrocyte destruction, which is derived from animal studies, has also been analysed recently (Seed & Kreier 1980). In this short account we shall restrict ourselves to a discussion of a few of the mechanisms of anaemia in human malaria which seem to have a reasonably solid basis.

The patterns of anaemia after P. falciparum malaria infection

Surprisingly, there is little published information about the course of anaemia after an attack of *P. falciparum* malaria. Hence, before we attempt to analyse the mechanisms of anaemia it is necessary to try to develop a clear picture of the sequential haematological changes that occur in patients with acute *P. falciparum* malaria infections. The following account is based on the published data of Miller & Reynolds (1972), Woodruff et al (1979) and Abdalla et al (1980) and from some of our unpublished studies of patients admitted to the Infectious Disease Unit in Oxford over the last few years. In addition, we have analysed some unpublished data from the Wellcome Tropical Medicine Unit in Bangkok through the courtesy of Drs D. Warrell and P. Songchai. Although there is remarkable variability in the timing and severity of anaemia between patients, a picture is starting to emerge. Some typical patterns from the study of Abdalla et al (1980) and our unpublished data are shown in Figs. 1 and 2.

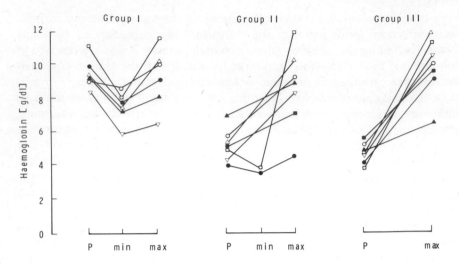

FIG. 1. The patterns of anaemia in different groups of Gambian children with *P. falciparum* malaria. Group I had acute malaria while Group III had chronic malaria with low parasitaemias and grossly dyserythropoietic bone marrows. Group II showed features of both types of illness. (From Abdalla et al 1980.)

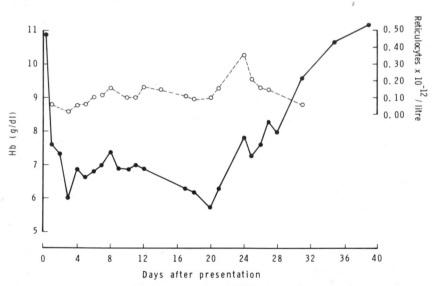

FIG. 2. The haematological changes in a non-immune English male with acute *P. falciparum* malaria. After an initial rapid drop in the haemoglobin level (●——●) there was a progressive, but slower, fall over a period of three weeks. During this period there was an inappropriately low reticulocyte response (○- - -○).

Acute infections

In patients who are not significantly anaemic at presentation there is a rapid fall in the haemoglobin level which corresponds approximately in time with the disappearance of the parasites after treatment. The haemoglobin level then continues to fall for a variable period. Usually, it reaches its lowest level at the end of the first week or ten days, and then there is a reticulocytosis, after which the level gradually returns to normal over the next three or four weeks. However, the anaemia may be more protracted than this. Figure 2 illustrates the course of the haemoglobin level and reticulocyte response in a young, non-immune adult male who was studied in Oxford. After an initial rapid fall the level continued to fall steadily for about 21 days before slowly rising over a period of about 14 days. During the first 21 days of the illness there was a low and inappropriate reticulocyte response, and it was only during the fourth week that the reticulocyte count rose, indicating that the marrow was finally responding to the low haematocrit. This pattern has been observed in several patients whom we have been able to follow without blood transfusion in Oxford.

We have recently attempted to analyse the haematological changes and bone marrow morphology in patients with these forms of anaemia associated with acute *P. falciparum* infection (Abdalla et al 1980; unpublished data). The peripheral blood films do not show any characteristic morphological changes in the red cells and, in particular, spherocytosis is not marked. Features compatible with haemolysis, such as a raised bilirubin level, reduced haptoglobin levels and, in some cases, haemoglobinaemia and haemoglobinuria, are present in some but not all cases. The plasma iron level is reduced despite the presence of stainable iron in the bone marrow. Bone marrow analysis shows that the relative number of erythroid precursors is not increased and that erythropoiesis is normoblastic with minimal dyserythropoietic change. The overall cellularity of the marrow is increased, however, largely due to myeloid hyperplasia; there is also an increase in the lymphoid and monocyte precursor populations. The latter contain ingested malarial pigment and, sometimes, parasitized and non-parasitized red cells.

Chronic P. falciparum malaria

The elegant epidemiological studies of McGregor et al (1956, 1966) indicated that recurrent infection with *P. falciparum* must play a major role in producing the chronic anaemia of children in West Africa. We have attempted to analyse the haematological changes in this form of malaria by studying several groups of severely anaemic Gambian children (Abdalla et al 1980; unpublished data). These children all presented with haemoglobin values of less than 7 g/dl. They appeared to have chronic malaria in that there was no history of acute illness, parasite levels were low, and all had significant splenomegaly. Extensive investigations for other causes of anaemia ruled out iron or folate deficiency, intercurrent bacterial infection or other infestations, and, as far as possible, viral infection. One group of these children showed a reticulocyte response and steady rise in haemoglobin values approximately seven days after commencing antimalarial treatment; a second group were observed without treatment and showed a spontaneous remission of their anaemia with an appropriate reticulocytosis coincident with the disappearance of the parasites from the circulation. These children did not have significant haemolysis and the most consistent and striking findings were marked dyserythropoietic changes in the bone marrow. As might be expected, these studies in The Gambia have revealed many children with haematological findings intermediate between those in the acute and chronic malarial groups—that is, with disorders characterized by variable anaemia, haemolysis and dyserythropoiesis.

Mechanisms of the anaemia of P. falciparum malaria

There is increasing evidence that the anaemia of *P. falciparum* malaria has a complicated and multifactorial basis and that both defective production and increased destruction of red cells are involved. It appears that the relative contributions of each of these mechanisms vary according to the particular clinical form of the infection. However, critical analysis of the work carried out so far indicates that we still have only the flimsiest idea about the basic pathophysiology involved in red cell destruction and in the defective marrow response.

Destruction of parasitized red cells

There is a large body of evidence derived from both animal and human studies that direct damage to the red cells by malarial parasites plays a major role in their premature destruction. The extensive experimental data, derived mainly from the animal malarias, that relates to red cell destruction mechanisms has been reviewed by Seed & Kreier (1980).

It appears that destruction of red cells occurs both intravascularly and by sequestration of parasitized cells in the spleen and in other parts of the microcirculation. Premature lysis of the red cells seems to follow both mechanical disruption, impaired membrane function, and increased rigidity and reduced deformability. Because of its peculiar vascular arrangement, and because red cells become so closely related to macrophages, the spleen is a highly effective filter for damaged or rigid red cells. It is not clear to what extent membrane damage, as compared with increased rigidity, is responsible for the destruction of red cells in *P. falciparum* infections. Rigidity plays an important role in the anaemia of some of the animal malarias. For example, Miller et al (1971, 1972) showed that *P. knowlesi*-infected cells are less able to pass through polycarbonate filter membranes than non-infected cells. The viscosity of infected cells is substantially increased at both low and high shear rates. Attempts at measuring *in vivo* red cell survival, although fraught with difficulties, indicate that in the animal malarias there is a marked shortening during both the acute and recovery phases. The large literature relating to this subject is reviewed in detail by Seed & Kreier (1980).

From observations relating the degree of parasitaemia to the fall in haemoglobin level, it has been a long-held belief that the amount of red cell destruction often exceeds that which would be expected if only parasitized cells were lost from the circulation. It should be remembered that calculations of this type are open to numerous sources of error. Many parasitized cells are sequestered in the microcirculation and hence the relative numbers in the peripheral blood may give little indication of the total parasite load. From animal studies it appears that both endogenous red cell survival, and that of transfused normal erythrocytes, is shortened during the recovery phase of a malarial infection. Studies of this type were reported in human *P. falciparum* malaria by Rosenberg et al (1973). These authors examined the survival of normal red cells transfused into patients who were receiving treatment for *P. falciparum* malaria, so attempting to rule out the possibility that the loss of the normal cells might be a direct effect of parasitization. The results were inconsistent; in some cases the normal cells showed a reduced survival time. Although there seemed to be some correlation between the degree of anaemia and the red cell survival, within the group of non-anaemic patients the ^{51}Cr $t_{\frac{1}{2}}$ ranged from 2.5 to 25.6 days; the ^{51}Cr disappearance curves were not shown. Many of the published survival curves from animal experiments show a biphasic pattern, suggestive of two red cell populations, one with a very short survival and the other with a longer $t_{\frac{1}{2}}$. Unfortunately, this type of information is not available for human malaria infections.

Clearly, more data relating to both endogenous red cell survival patterns and the survival of transfused normal red cells in patients recovering from *P. falciparum* infections are needed. Recently, we have begun to obtain information of this kind. We have analysed the ^{51}Cr survival curves in a young adult with *P. falciparum* malaria. The cells were labelled about ten days after the acute infection had been treated and when an initial phase of abnormal renal function had passed. It was clear that the ^{51}Cr $t_{\frac{1}{2}}$ of the red cells during the subsequent ten days is markedly shortened, and from the shape of the curve it appears that this haemolytic process is starting to decline only after about 21 days. There are two possible interpretations of this result. The first is that a population of cells with a shortened survival remain in the circulation and are gradually removed over two or three weeks; the second is that the shortened red cell survival affects the total cell population and that the underlying mechanism which causes it remains active for two or three weeks after the infection and then gradually resolves. It will be necessary to do cross-transfusion experiments to distinguish unequivocally between these two possibilities.

From the scanty evidence available so far, it is apparent that there is a marked haemolytic component to the anaemia of *P. falciparum* infection. It seems very likely that this does not simply represent the destruction of parasitized red cells but that for some reason part or all the red cell population has a shortened survival for several weeks after an acute infection. So far, we lack the information that would allow a clear distinction between the gradual loss of a cohort of damaged cells or the exposure of the total circulating red cell mass to an exogenous haemolytic system. The next question, therefore, concerns the nature of the haemolytic process that is not related directly to red cell damage by parasites. One possibility that has been raised is immune destruction.

The role of immunity in red cell destruction

Since the work of Zuckerman (1966) there has been considerable interest in the possibility that at least part of the haemolytic component of the anaemia of *P. falciparum* malaria might reflect immune destruction of red cells. Much of the stimulus to this idea has come from reports of the finding of a positive direct Coombs anti-globulin test (DAT) in patients with malaria. A large literature on this subject has appeared and much of it is conflicting (Esan 1975, Facer et al 1979). Studies done over the past two years have partly clarified the position, although many questions remain.

Several large-scale studies attempting to define the significance of a positive DAT in malaria have been done in populations of children in The Gambia (Facer et al 1979, Abdalla et al 1980, Facer 1980, Abdalla & Weatherall 1982) and Kenya (Abdalla et al 1982). In each case the incidence of a positive DAT was significantly higher in children with malaria than in unaffected children, indicating a relationship between the development of a positive DAT and malarial infection. The acquisition of a positive DAT seems to be age-related and is commoner in young children. Using specific antisera it has been found that the most frequent type of red cell sensitization is with C3. Other specificities include IgG alone, IgG plus C3, IgG plus C3 plus C4, and various other combinations of IgG with different complement components. Sensitization with IgA or IgM has not been found. Facer (1980) has shown that the eluted IgG has specific antibody activity against *P. falciparum* schizont antigen, as demonstrated by the indirect fluorescent antibody technique. Thus she has suggested that erythrocyte sensitization results from passive attachment of circulating complement-fixing malaria antigen–antibody complexes. These results are complemented by our recent studies (Abdalla & Weatherall 1982) in which we showed that preincubation with sera from children with a positive DAT, but not from those with a negative DAT, produces phagocytosis of schizonts by peripheral blood mononuclear cells.

These findings leave little doubt that the development of a positive DAT is part of an immune response to *P. falciparum*. Whether it results from passive attachment of complexes or whether, as we have suggested (Abdalla & Weatherall 1982), it reflects the transient development of an autoantibody with both anti-erythrocyte and anti-parasite specificities, remains to be determined.

The question raised by these studies is whether a positive DAT indicates that immune destruction of red cells occurs in *P. falciparum* malaria, as has been suggested by Zuckerman (1966), Woodruff et al (1979) and Facer et al (1979). In the study by Facer et al (1979) one group of children showed a significant correlation between a positive DAT and anaemia but another group from a different village showed no correlation. In both groups there were many patients with a negative DAT who were anaemic, and similarly there were children with a positive DAT who were not anaemic. Interestingly, in the group that appeared to show a correlation between anaemia and a positive DAT, the anaemic children were significantly younger than those who were not anaemic. We have shown a strong correlation between age and both anaemia and a positive DAT (Abdalla & Weatherall 1982) and hence these observations may simply reflect this association. However, Facer et al described four patients who were more severely anaemic and who showed a positive DAT with active C3 components on their red cells. It was possible to demonstrate erythrophagocytosis of non-parasitized erythrocytes by monocytes in the blood films of these patients. This suggests that, occasionally, anaemia in acute *P. falciparum* malaria may result from opsonization and phagocytosis of sensitized red cells.

In a series of studies done in The Gambia on groups of children with *P. falciparum* malaria, we were unable to demonstrate any correlation between a positive DAT due to IgG alone or to IgG plus various complement components and the degree of anaemia, reticulocytosis or any other haematological changes (Abdalla et al 1980) Abdalla & Weatherall 1982). Furthermore, we could find no evidence of spherocytosis or red cell fragmentation, and the osmotic fragility curves of peripheral blood samples taken in the acute phase were either normal or showed increased resistance to osmotic lysis. Certainly there was no evidence of increased osmotic lysis, as has been shown quite clearly in a variety of immune haemolytic anaemias (Dacie 1960). In addition, there was no *in vitro* phagocytosis of erythrocytes from DAT-positive children by normal adult peripheral blood mononuclear cells or by their own monocytes.

In studies of patients in Oxford with severe anaemia and shortened red cell survival following acute *P. falciparum* infection we have been unable to demonstrate any sensitization of the red cells in the weeks after the acute infection. Despite the fall in haemoglobin levels, repeated DAT analyses failed to reveal any immune basis for the haemolysis (unpublished data).

Further information relevant to immunity and the anaemia of *P. falciparum* malaria comes from the work of Facer (1980). She was unable to demonstrate any specificity in eluates prepared from sensitized red cells from children with *P. falciparum* malaria. Thus, using a papain-modified red cell panel she was able to demonstrate that serum, but not eluates, from half of the patients with acute malaria caused agglutination of all panel cells at 37 °C. This was due to increased levels of IgM agglutinins in the sera, as evidenced by loss of activity after treatment by agents which disrupt IgM molecules. It is known, of course, that polyclonal cold agglutinin titres may be elevated in a variety of infections and that in some cases there is associated anaemia. However, it seems unlikely that these antibodies were responsible for red cell sensitization with complement components or that they were in any way related to the anaemia found in the Gambian children. Cold agglutinin titres were always within the normal range and only high titres with a relatively high thermal range seem capable of causing red cell sensitization.

Thus, it appears that about half the children who develop *P. falciparum* malaria in both west and east Africa develop a positive DAT which may be due to passive attachment of circulating malaria antigen–antibody complexes to their red cells or, possibly, to the production of an autoantibody with both red cell and parasite specificities. Although in a few patients additional sensitization with various complement components may cause the cells to be phagocytosed by monocytes in the blood or reticuloendothelial system, in the bulk of cases the haematological changes, taken together with the lack of correlation between the DAT and the degree of anaemia, indicate that immune destruction probably plays a relatively small role in producing the anaemia of acute *P. falciparum* malaria. Certainly, there is no evidence for autoimmune haemolysis in young children or adults with this disorder. Although further work of this type will have to be done in other parts of the world, the evidence for a major immune component in the anaemia of *P. falciparum* malaria is, at the moment, extremely tenuous.

Other haemolytic mechanisms

It is clear from the discussion so far that the reason for the short red cell survival in *P. falciparum* malaria is not understood. Are there any other potential haemolytic mechanisms? It has been suggested that, after damage in the spleen, de-parasitized red cells return to the circulation; these cells have been described as spherocytes and are presumed to have a shortened survival (Conrad 1971, Schnitzer et al 1973). We have done an extensive series of red cell osmotic fragility tests in patients with acute *P. falciparum* malaria. There was no increase in osmotic lysis, which indicates that spherocytes are not present in significant numbers; rather, the osmotic fragility was slightly reduced and returned to normal after two or three weeks (G. Pasvol, unpublished data). Furthermore, sterile incubation of the cells does not result in the appearance of an unusually osmotically active population. More red cell survival data, including the analysis of the fate of donor cells, are required in the acute phase of *P. falciparum* malaria. The fall in haemoglobin level is similar in many ways to that seen after other acute infections, although it appears to be more marked and prolonged in some patients with malaria. It may simply reflect the results of macrophage activation in the spleen and throughout the RE system; as far as we know, there is no good published information on surface counting and analysis of the site of destruction of red cells in malaria. In addition, the haemolysis may, in part, reflect the phase of abnormal renal function which occurs in the acute phase of the illness. Thus, further work is required before the pathogenesis of the haemolytic component of the acute phase of the illness becomes clear.

Defective red cell production

In any haemolytic process a falling haemoglobin level triggers off an increased production of erythropoietin which results in erythroid hyperplasia of the bone marrow and a reticulocytosis. Many workers have observed that there is a relatively poor reticulocyte response to the anaemia in patients with *P. falciparum* malaria. Defective red cell production has been ascribed variably to depression of erythropoiesis (Kuvin et al 1962, Srichaikul et al 1969, 1973, Woodruff et al 1979), and inhibition of reticulocyte release or ineffective erythropoiesis (Hendrickse & King 1958, Srichaikul et al 1967, 1969, 1973, Renricca et al 1974). One of the difficulties in assessing many of these observations is the possibility that factors other than malaria may have been contributing to the poor marrow response, notably iron or folate deficiency, depressed renal function, or the effects of associated illnesses.

Recent studies in The Gambia have thrown further light on the morphological appearances of the bone marrow in different forms of *P. falciparum* infection (Abdalla et al 1980). In children with acute infections the bone marrows contained normal or reduced numbers of erythroid precursors which showed no gross morphological abnormalities. These children had low serum iron concentrations but there was stainable iron in the bone marrow, mainly in the storage compartment rather than in the erythroid precursors. These observations are similar to those described in the anaemia of infection and other chronic disorders (Cartwright & Lee 1971). Further work is needed to determine whether there is acute sequestration of iron in the acute phase of *P. falciparum* malaria. It would be useful to obtain serial serum iron and total iron binding capacity values, together with serum ferritin levels.

Much more impressive changes have been observed in the bone marrows of children who presented with severe anaemia, a low reticulocyte count and low parasitaemia. They showed marked dyserythropoietic changes which included erythroblast multinuclearity, karyorrhexis, incomplete and unequal amitotic nuclear divisions, and cytoplasmic bridging (Fig. 3). These dyserythropoietic changes were confirmed by electron microscopic analysis. There were bi- or multinucleate erythroblasts, bizarre myelinization with loss of parts of the nuclear membrane, and dilatation of the space between the two layers of the nuclear membrane. In addition, there were varying degrees of iron loading of the mitochondria and a reduction of the electron density of the cytoplasmic matrix together with a scarcity of ribosomes. The cytoplasm of the bone marrow macrophages contained erythrocytes or erythroblasts in varying states of degradation.

Erythropoiesis has been studied in the marrows of several Gambian children with this type of dyserythropoiesis, using the technique of combined [^{3}H]thymidine autoradiography and Feulgen microspectrophotometry (Wickramasinghe et al 1982). These studies have confirmed that there is a significant abnormality of red cell proliferation; the most important features include an increased proportion of red cell precursors in G2 and an arrest during the progress of cells through the S phase. These features of dyserythropoiesis are non-specific and similar findings have been observed in a variety of other conditions, including vitamin B$_{12}$ or folate deficiency and in sideroblastic anaemia. Deficiency of B$_{12}$ and folate was ruled out in these children and, as far as possible, so were other associated illnesses. It is always possible, of course, that the children had chronic malaria associated with an intercurrent viral illness, but there was no evidence for this. As the parasites disappeared from the blood, either in response to treatment, or in some cases after a

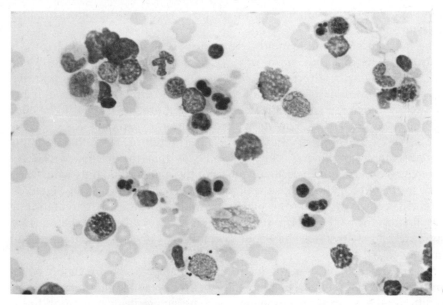

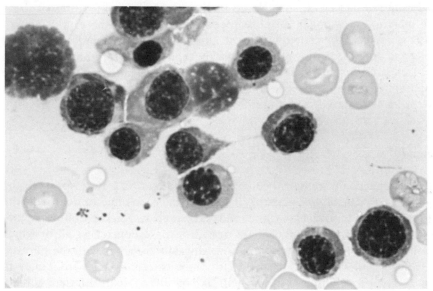

FIG. 3. Morphological changes in the red cell precursors in bone marrow aspirates from Gambian children with severe anaemia and chronic *P. falciparum* malaria. A. A low power view showing marked morphological abnormalities of the red cell precursors, including many multinucleate forms and a bizarre nuclear maturation. B. A higher powered view showing abnormal nuclear maturation and intercytoplasmic bridging. (Abdalla et al 1980.)

period of observation without treatment, there was a reticulocytosis and the dyserythropoietic changes resolved.

The mechanism of the marked dyserythropoiesis in the bone marrows of children with more chronic forms of *P. falciparum* malaria is not clear. There is no evidence for the direct invasion of erythroid precursors by the parasite; parasitized erythroblasts were not observed by either light or electron microscopy. Recent studies indicate that red cell precursors can be invaded directly by *P. falciparum* in *in vitro* culture systems (S. Abdalla & G. Pasvol, unpublished observations). It is not clear, therefore, why they are not invaded commonly *in vivo*. One possibility is that the nucleated red cell precursors lie outside the vascular sinuses of the marrow and only gain access to the latter after maturation as reticulocytes. Hence they may be relatively protected from invasion by the parasites until they enter the circulation as more mature forms. Furthermore, schizogony does not occur in the marrow, making it unlikely that new merozoites would easily invade red cell precursors (Smalley et al 1980).

If the dyserythropoiesis is not due to direct damage to the precursors by the parasite, what is the underlying mechanism? It is possible that under certain conditions, the marrow macrophages become active in damaging and phagocytosing red cell precursors. Some of the morphological features of these bone marrows are similar to those recently described in the erythrophagocytosis syndrome associated with viral illness in immunosuppressed patients (McKenna et al 1981). It is not clear whether the gross dyserythropoiesis seen in *P. falciparum* malaria is unique to malaria or whether it occurs more commonly than has been previously recognized in other infections. Much more work is required in this area.

Summary

In this short account we have been able to touch on only a few aspects of the anaemia of *P. falciparum* malaria. It has not been possible to deal with the various genetic disorders of the red cell such as sickle cell anaemia, thalassaemia or glucose-6-phosphate dehydrogenase deficiency, all of which may modify the anaemia of malaria and whose interactions with the parasite probably provide much of the basis for their extremely high frequency in tropical countries. Similarly, it has been impossible to deal with the problem of tropical splenomegaly and the contributions made to the anaemia of chronic malaria by splenic pooling and hypersplenism.

It is becoming clear that the anaemia of *P. falciparum* malaria results from many different interactions and that shortened red cell survival and dyserythropoiesis all play a major role in different stages of the illness. Many important questions remain. Apart from the intrinsic interest of this subject for haematologists, some of the questions posed by recent studies may be of considerable practical relevance. In particular, it will be important to try to determine the reason for the continued shortened red cell survival after the parasites have been cleared from the circulation and for the marked dyserythropoiesis in children with chronic malaria. These complications of the disease, which may not be due directly to interactions between parasites and the red cell, need fairly urgent study because at the moment, apart from blood transfusion, there is no logical approach to their management.

Acknowledgements

We thank The Rockefeller Foundation and The Wellcome Trust for supporting some of the work reviewed here.

REFERENCES

Abdalla S, Weatherall DJ 1982 The direct antiglobulin test in *P. falciparum* malaria. Br J Haematol 51:415-425

Abdalla S, Weatherall DJ, Wickramasinghe SN, Hughes M 1980 The anaemia of *P falciparum* malaria. Br J Haematol 46:171-183

Abdalla SH, Kasili EG, Weatherall DJ 1982 The Coombs direct antiglobulin test in Kenyans. Submitted for publication

Cartwright GE, Lee GR 1971 The anaemia of chronic disorders. Br J Haematol 21:147-152

Conrad ME 1971 Hematologic manifestations of parasitic infections. Semin Hematol 8:267-303

Dacie JV 1960 The haemolytic anaemias. Part 1: The congenital anaemias. Churchill, London

Esan GJF 1975 Haematological aspects of malaria. Clin Haematol 4:247-256

Facer CA 1980 Direct Coombs antiglobulin reactions in Gambian children with *Plasmodium falciparum* malaria. Clin Exp Immunol 39:279-288

Facer CA, Bray RS, Brown J 1979 Direct Coombs antiglobulin reactions in Gambian children with *Plasmodium falciparum* malaria. 1. Incidence and class specificity. Clin Exp Immunol 35:119-127

Fleming AF 1981 Haematological manifestations of malaria and other parasitic diseases. Clin Haematol 10:983-1011

Hendrickse RG, King MAR 1958 Anaemia of uncertain origin in infancy. Br Med J 2:662-669

Kuvin SF, Baye HK, Stohlman F Jr, Contacos PG, Coatney GR 1962 Malaria in man. Infection by *Plasmodium vivax* and the B strain of *Plasmodium cynomolgi*. JAMA (J Am Med Assoc) 184:1018-1020

McGregor IA, Gilles HM, Walters JH, Davies AH, Pearson FA 1956 Effects of heavy repeated malarial infections on Gambian infants and children. Br Med J 2:686-692

McGregor IA, Williams, K, Biliewicz WZ, Thompson AM 1966 Haemoglobin concentration and anaemia in young West African (Gambian) children. Trans R Soc Trop Med Hyg 60:650-667

McKenna RW, Risdall RJ, Brunning RD 1981 Virus associated hemophagocytic syndrome. Hum Pathol 12:395-398

Miller MB, Reynolds RD 1972 Treatment and complications of malaria in Vietnam. Mil Med 137:267-269

Miller LH, Fremount HN, Luse SA 1971 Deep vascular schizogony of *Plasmodium knowlesi* in *Macaca mulatta*. Distribution in organs and ultrastructure of parasitized cells. Am J Trop Med Hyg 20:816-824

Miller LH, Chien S, Usami S 1972 Decreased deformability of *Plasmodium coatneyi*-infected red cells and its possible relation to cerebral malaria. Am J Trop Med Hyg 21:133-137

Renricca NJ, Stout JP, Coleman RM 1974 Erythropoietin production in virulent malaria. Infect Immun 10:831-833

Rosenberg EB, Strickland GT, Yang S, Whalen GE 1973 IgM antibodies to red cells and autoimmune anemia in patients with malaria. Am J Trop Med Hyg 22:146-152

Schnitzer B, Sodeman TM, Mead ML, Contacos PG 1973 An ultrastructural study of the red pulp of the spleen in malaria. Blood 41:207-218

Seed TM, Kreier JP 1980 Erythrocyte destruction mechanisms in malaria. Malaria 2:1-46

Smalley ME, Abdalla S, Brown J 1980 The distribution of *Plasmodium falciparum* in the peripheral blood and bone marrow of Gambian children. Trans R Soc Trop Med Hyg 75:103-105

Srichaikul T, Panikbutr N, Jeumtrakul P 1967 Bone marrow changes in human malaria. Ann Trop Med Parasitol 61:40-51

Srichaikul T, Wasanosomsithi M, Poshyachinda V, Panikbutr N, Rabieb T 1969 Ferrokinetic studies and erythropoiesis in malaria. Arch Intern Med 124:623-628

Srichaikul T, Siriasawakul T, Poshyachinda M, Poshyachinda V 1973 Ferrokinetics in patients with malaria: normoblasts and iron incorporation in vitro. Am J Clin Pathol 60:166-174

Weatherall DJ, Abdalla S 1982 The anaemia of *P. falciparum* malaria. Br Med Bull 38:147-152

Wickramasinghe SN, Abdalla S, Weatherall DJ 1982 Cell cycle distribution of erythroblasts in *P. falciparum* malaria. Scand J Haematol 29:83-88

Woodruff AW, Ansdell VE, Pettitt LE 1979 Cause of anaemia in malaria. Lancet 1:1055-1057

Zuckerman A 1966 Recent studies on factors involved in malarial anaemia. Mil Med 131:1201-1216

DISCUSSION

Fitch: There is an interesting similarity in the effects on erythropoiesis that you observe in children with chronic *P. falciparum* malaria and the anaemia of vitamin E deficiency in non-human primates and swine (Drake & Fitch 1980). Rhesus monkeys made vitamin E deficient develop severe dyserythropoiesis, with multinucleate erythroid precursors morphologically indistinguishable from those you showed in Fig. 3, erythrophagocytosis, and severe anaemia (haemoglobin concentrations of 2–4 g/dl). When the monkeys are treated with vitamin E there is a prompt response with reticulocyte counts of 30% or more and a complete recovery from the anaemia. Humans do not normally become anaemic when they are vitamin E deficient from malabsorption of fat, and it is difficult to induce vitamin E deficiency in humans by dietary restriction. Nevertheless, it is conceivable that under conditions of stress, such as malnutrition and malaria infection, vitamin E deficiency might cause the haematological picture that you see. It would be interesting to know the plasma vitamin E concentrations in your patients and perhaps to evaluate their responses to vitamin E supplements. It is possible that the patients who show a haematological response despite no malaria chemotherapy are responding to vitamin E provided by the hospital diet.

Weatherall: That is a very interesting suggestion. There is no really clear-cut situation in man in which vitamin E deficiency is known to be important in causing haemolytic anaemia or defective marrow function, except possibly in the newborn. Patients with thalassaemia, whose red cells are subject to oxidative haemolysis, are almost always deficient in vitamin E, however, and when given the vitamin there is some increase in red cell survival (Weatherall & Clegg 1981). This *doesn't* improve their anaemia. The effect of vitamin E deficiency on bone marrow function should certainly be investigated.

Fitch: In connection with your hypothesis that marrow macrophages become activated and cause damage to red cell precursors, activated macrophages generate oxidants such as superoxide or hydrogen peroxide (Nathan 1982). These reactive oxygen intermediates could increase the need for vitamin E locally in the bone marrow.

McGregor: Professor Weatherall's paper offers a new look at a very old problem. As he has pointed out, evidence collected in the field is often difficult to interpret in a coherent way. When one encounters a malarious patient for the first time, it is very difficult to determine whether the attendant anaemia is the result of a single, even primary, attack or whether it represents the end-point of multiple attacks sustained in quick succession. In The Gambia the association of anaemia and malaria in young children is greatest at the time of greatest malaria transmission. At other times of the year the association is much less obvious, despite the fact that the prevalence of parasitaemia shows no great change. It, therefore, appears that parasitaemias which follow inoculations by mosquitoes produce anaemia to a greater extent than do long-persistent, so-called 'chronic' parasitaemias.

How this fits into Christine Facer's observation on red cell sensitization as a cause of blood loss in malaria is not immediately obvious. In young children experiencing acute falciparum parasitaemia a falling haemoglobin level is almost always associated with a virtual absence of reticulocytosis. After eradication of infection by treatment, reticulocytes rapidly increase and gradually the haemoglobin level rises. That, in my experience, is the usual trend of events. I cannot recall instances where the haemoglobin level continues to fall in a persistent fashion after parasitaemia has been eliminated. Sometimes reticulocytosis and haemoglobin recovery may be delayed, but even in this instance the level of haemoglobin does not continue to fall. The rarity of deteriorating haemoglobin levels in the absence of continued parasitaemia raises the question of how frequent and important is the destruction of non-parasitized cells by immunological mechanisms. I would agree with Professor

Weatherall that sensitization of red cells does not *per se* equate with anaemia. Dr Facer's work, showing that the association of anaemia and red cell sensitization occurs in a relatively small group of individuals whose red cells are sensitized in a particular way, is important and could indicate that genetic factors may influence the development of malarial anaemia in some persons.

Professor Weatherall's observations on the occurrence of dyserythropoiesis are of greatest interest. But what is the reason? Could acute-phase proteins play a role by depressing marrow responsiveness? These proteins have been poorly studied in relation to malaria, yet parasitaemia appears to induce great changes in them. C-reactive protein, which is conspicuous in the sera of malarious individuals, is now recognized as an acute-phase reactant which may importantly depress the function of some T cell populations. Could it, or some other acute-phase protein, exert similar depressant action on erythropoiesis? Finally, in the process of parasitization, presumably iron gets immobilized in malaria pigment. How quickly is this iron liberated and reutilized? If this process is prolonged, does the young child who experiences repeated attacks of malaria gradually run into iron deficiency and begin to present an anaemia which bears the stigmata of iron deficiency?

Facer: Perhaps I could clarify the picture as regards anaemia and sensitized erythrocytes in malaria. There are several different categories of sensitization involved and the IgG subclass sensitizing a red cell is an important determinant in the fate of that cell. We know that if red cells are sensitized with IgG1 and/or IgG3 they are likely to be phagocytosed, particularly in the spleen. This is because these two subclasses of IgG fix complement and also because phagocytic cells have Fc receptors for IgG1 and IgG3 and not for IgG2 or IgG4. So when one is discussing the relevance of red cell sensitization with IgG and malaria, it is important to define the subclass of IgG present on those cells and then make a statistical analysis to define correlations (Facer 1980). This may explain why Professor Weatherall was unable to demonstrate an association between anaemia and erythrocyte sensitization in the study just mentioned.

Turning now to complement sensitization, we found that a small proportion of Gambian children had active C3b on their red cells and were very anaemic. Their peripheral blood films demonstrated erythrophagocytosis of non-infected red cells by monocytes which carry C3b receptors (Facer et al 1979, Facer & Brown 1981). There was no doubt that red cell sensitization and extravascular haemolysis here was contributing to the anaemia. However, phagocytosis *per se* is not a necessary prerequisite for cell damage, since monocytes will also express cytotoxicity for C3b-coated red cells with lysosomal enzyme release following contact with the sensitized cell (Engelfriet et al 1980). This could be yet another mechanism of red cell destruction in malaria.

To conclude, when an immune reaction takes place on the red cell membrane with C3 activation, I believe that, at that stage, immune adherence, phagocytosis and monocyte cytotoxicity are contributing to the patients' anaemia. The immune reaction in the Gambian children we believe was a result of attachment of malaria antigen–antibody complexes to the red cell via the C3b receptor. Recently, Siegal et al (1981) have suggested that the red cell, in addition to its respiratory function, also acts as an immunocyte, in that 95% of C3b receptors within the circulation are located on red cells. He estimated that an antigen–antibody complex has a 500–1000 times greater chance of being removed from the circulation by a red cell than by a white cell. He feels that immune complexes, produced both physiologically and pathologically, are disposed of largely by this mechanism. In fact, Peter Lachmann suggested this some years ago (unpublished). Siegal's hypothesis substantiates our theory that immune complexes in malaria are adhering to the red cells at the cost of a proportion of those red cells. However, I agree that red cell sensitization with immune complexes does not adequately explain the shortened red cell survival over a period of 20 days in your non-immune patient.

Weatherall: Are you arguing that this type of sensitization will be active in destroying red cells for only a short period, and hence that the affected cohort will be rapidly removed from the circulation?

Facer: Not the entire cohort, but a certain proportion of it. Immune complex formation and complement fixation (involving malaria antigens) might be expected to be a rapid phenomenon after antimalarial chemotherapy, rather than a prolonged phenomenon. In addition, the half-life of C3b is relatively short; for example, the half-life of immune adherence activity of a C3b-coated red cell is about 30 minutes. Serum C3b inactivator then converts the C3b to C3d which remains membrane-bound. Since red cells sensitized with C3d have a normal survival (Frank 1977), they represent the 'survivors' of an immune reaction on the surface of that cell. It would be relevant to know the percentage of red cells that do not survive!

Friedman: Are you convinced that the reticuloendothelial system is working during malaria infection?

Facer: It is probably functional in a non-immune subject with a first infection, but I am less sure about the situation for example in children in endemic areas exposed to continuous malaria infections.

Cohen: The persistence of immune complexes after the disappearance of parasitaemia has been studied by Philip Shepherd in a simian model in our laboratory (Shepherd et al 1982). The complexes may persist for long periods (weeks) after clearance of parasites. By the methods used to measure these complexes they occur in two waves, the first during and immediately after parasitaemia and the second two or three weeks later. The constitution of these (second-wave) complexes is unclear, but one possibility is that they are anti-idiotype complexes appearing late in the infection. So there is a possible mechanism for complexes persisting for several weeks at least.

Facer: These were complement-fixing immune complexes?

Cohen: Yes.

Facer: One doesn't know what the malarial antigen component of the soluble complexes is.

Cohen: No; one doesn't even know whether there is antigen there, but the complexes are still capable of activating complement.

McGregor: Wilson et al (1975) observed that in humans malarial antigen could persist for many weeks after an episode of parasitaemia and then suddenly disappear with the occurrence in serum of homologous antibody. Presumably, in such instances, immune complexes are formed remote from the acute episode of parasitaemia and after a prolonged period of antigen circulation.

Jarra: Is it possible to have sensitization but to be unable to detect it by the Coombs' test?

Facer: Yes, but what significance that has in terms of red cell destruction is another matter. The DAT is unable to detect fewer than 150–300 molecules of IgG per red cell (Dupuy et al 1964), so a more sensitive technique such as radioimmunoassay may detect IgG on red cells in Coombs-negative patients.

Brown: Is it possible that the shortened red cell survival that you see is an enhanced immunological removal of aged red cells, which might derive from the fact that parasites alter red cells? In such circumstances, erythrocytes may be removed earlier in their lifespan by a more sensitive primed immune mechanism. You wouldn't detect this unless you were using aged red cells. There is some evidence that the removal of aged red cells has an immunological basis, in that it is a response to antigens that are exposed during ageing (Lutz & Kay 1981).

Weatherall: That is possible.

Wyler: Along a similar line, what is the relative osmotic fragility of uninfected erythrocytes in the malaria patients?

Weatherall: This is an important question. If a red cell is damaged and loses membrane it becomes spherical. This change is well documented in hereditary spherocytosis but also occurs in acquired disorders, notably the immune haemolytic anaemias. There is very good evidence (Dacie 1962) that individuals with immune haemolysis have populations of spherocytes in the peripheral blood. The osmotic fragility curve is shifted to the right; that is, there is a population of cells with increased osmotic activity. If, as has been suggested, there is a major immune basis for the anaemia of *P. falciparum* malaria, or if deparasitized spherocytes are returned into the circulation, this should be reflected by an increased osmotic fragility of the peripheral blood cells. Either the entire cell population should have increased fragility or at least there should be a small population of cells showing increased lysis and appearing as a 'tail' on the standard osmotic fragility curve. In fact, we have done detailed osmotic fragility tests in patients with *P. falciparum* malaria, in both the acute and convalescent phases, and have found no evidence for increased osmotic lysis. It is difficult to reconcile these findings with any significant immune haemolysis, or damage to red cells with the return of spherocytes to the circulation. Perhaps Dr Pasvol, who has done a lot of these experiments in The Gambia and in Oxford, might like to enlarge on this topic.

Pasvol: There has always been thought to be a population of very fragile red cells in malaria infections in experimental animals (Fogel et al 1966, George et al 1967). There is also Conrad's idea of the pitting of parasitized red cells and their return as parasite-free spherocytes to the circulation (Conrad & Dennis 1968). I have always been interested to find fragile cells in human infections. In acutely infected children in The Gambia we found no evidence of fragile cells but in fact the opposite— cells with increased resistance to osmotic stress. At no time did we find a subpopulation of fragile cells which would indicate sphero-cytes, or any sign of cells being deparasitized and returned to the circulation. In our studies in Oxford, in patients exposed to malaria for the first time, we have found cells with increased osmotic resistance, which return to normal after recovery (unpublished results). The return to normal osmotic fragility seems to correlate with the reticulocyte response.

Facer: Professor Weatherall, you said you thought that the dyserythropoiesis described in Gambian children might not be due to their malaria infection; was this because you didn't find it in your non-immune patients with malaria?

Weatherall: We are being cautious about this, because the dyserythropoiesis is so unexpected and so gross. For example, we considered intercurrent viral infections as an explanation, because of evidence that in certain virus illnesses in immunosuppressed individuals an acute erythrophagocytosis syndrome de-velops (McKenna et al 1981). The marrow becomes filled with phagocytosed red cell precursors. Our children did not have an acute systemic illness, but that doesn't mean they didn't have a viral illness. But we never found these dysery-thropoietic changes in marrows of the non-immune cases of malaria studied in Oxford.

Luzzatto: Are these non-immune cases the same patients in whom you found persistent haemolysis?

Weatherall: Yes.

Luzzatto: And you are saying that this dyserythropoiesis is probably not due to an immune mechanism in the conventional sense, and it is probably not due to macrophages either. I think you have some ideas about the basis of this?

Weatherall: I wish I had! It may be due to macrophage activity, but there is no evidence that it is.

Greenwood: A significant proportion of the anaemic children with dysery-thropoiesis have an associated *Salmonella* septicaemia, suggesting that these children are immunosuppressed. It would therefore not be surprising if they had other infections as well, as you suggest. These children are often kept in the ward for several days during which time they receive good food and vitamins, which may contribute to their haematological recovery.

Weatherall: Yes. It is difficult to rule out nutritional deficiencies in these children. Certainly they were not iron, folate or vitamin B_{12} deficient.

Bannister: Would the treatment used have an effect on bone marrow function?

Weatherall: I don't think so. Chloroquine or quinine were given. We plan to study the effect of the antimalarial drugs on the bone marrow in Thailand; there is no evidence so far of marrow suppression.

Facer: Are you planning to transfuse compatible chromium-labelled red cells into your non-immune patients to see whether an exogenous factor(s) is involved in the decreased red cell survival? Rosenberg et al (1973) have described a shorter than normal half-life of normal red cells transfused into *P. falciparum*-infected patients under treatment with antimalarials.

Weatherall: That is the next step, if we can find the right patients. It was attempted in Thailand, as you say, but the results were equivocal (Rosenberg et al 1973). That would answer the question of whether there is an 'endogenous' or 'exogenous' haemolytic system—that is, whether the red cells had been damaged during the phase of parasitaemia and are being removed over a period of a few weeks, or whether the reticuloendothelial system is capable of prematurely removing normal cells for some time after a malarial infection.

Facer: We have incubated normal red cells with compatible immune malaria serum, compatible normal serum as a source of complement, and antigen from a culture of *P. falciparum*. A positive Coombs' test was obtained after incubation at 37 °C. Incubation with the addition of trypan blue (which inhibits C3 activation) did not give Coombs-positive red cells (unpublished observations). This clearly demonstrates that red cells take up immune complexes, presumably via the C3b receptor.

McGregor: I would like to counsel caution in the use of the term 'chronic malaria', for I really do not know what it means. Very often it is used to describe a fairly profound anaemia in a person with low-grade parasitaemia. Often in African children this state is reached after immunological recovery in the absence of chemotherapy. What we see in this instance is not an ongoing, long-continued chronic process but the tail end of an acute process and the beginning of convalescence. Such an individual may have many acute-phase reactants circulating in his plasma at the time and may be acutely immunosuppressed. I prefer to avoid use of the term 'chronic' in relation to malaria.

Much recent work has drawn attention to the fact that *in vitro* studies have shown that the young red cell is particularly susceptible to invasion by *P. falciparum*. To what extent does this young cell susceptibility influence the course of parasitaemia in the host and what is its epidemiological significance? A non-immune person given an adequate dose of *P. falciparum* parasites will develop a massive and fulminating infection. Is this because his red cells are predominantly young, or is it because this parasite remains a very competent invader of mature erythrocytes? Were the merozoite an obligate parasite of the young erythrocyte one would expect malaria to be a relatively mild and self-limiting infection in persons other than those possessing abnormally immature erythrocyte populations. Its role as an important anaemia-producing disease throughout the developing world would also be reduced. Do you think that red cell age influences either the clinical or the epidemiological manifestations of malaria?

Pasvol: On the first point, about the use of the term 'chronic', one can only get round that by taking a history. If there is no story of an acute febrile illness within the past 10 days, then one might assume that this is not acute malaria. But as you say, it is unreliable. Our interest in the invasion of young and old cells came about for non-clinical reasons. In children under six months with both haemoglobins A and F present and with malarial infections, we found more parasites in the cells containing haemoglobin A. This was found to have nothing to do with the haemoglobin type but was related to cell age, the haemoglobin A-containing cells being younger (Pasvol et al 1980). The only possible clinical relevance of this is during the first three months of life where erythropoiesis is switched off and malarial infections are rare. We have seen this preference for young cells consistently *in vitro* and in acute infections *in vivo*. What I have never commented on is the age susceptibility during prolonged infection where immune or other mechanisms might alter that predilection. In the 1930s, Kitchen (1939) found that the preference for invasion of reticulocytes over non-reticulocytes could change within the same patient during the course of prolonged infections.

McGregor: Is it possible that young erythrocytes have a special role in helping merozoites emerging from liver schizonts to adapt to the problems of invading and living within erythrocytes? If the young red cell somehow transiently facilitated the establishment of the erythrocytic cycle of development, I can see how red cell age could be an important factor in pathogenesis. However, if it does not operate at that sort of level, I have difficulty in understanding how erythrocyte age effectively influences the course of malaria in humans.

Pasvol: In the studies in which children were re-fed and their free iron levels suddenly rose, that correlated for example with an increase in young red cells (Murray et al 1978a). I'm not sure whether the recrudescence of malaria resulted from the availability of iron or availability of young cells.

McGregor: I don't know either. The observations that iron repletion exacerbates latent malaria infections are interesting but difficult to explain. I have treated many individuals with iron for iron deficiency anaemia. Many of these persons have exhibited asymptomatic malaria infections, but I have never seen therapeutic iron exacerbate parasitaemia or induce episodes of clinical malaria.

That experience is clearly very different from that reported by the Murrays (1975, 1978b). It may be that the Gambian population with whom I worked and the nomadic tribesmen with whom the Murrays worked differed greatly in respect of acquired immunity to malaria. In the former, any tendency to increased parasite replication might have been checked by effective immunity; in the latter, immunity may not have been solid enough to curtail the parasite replication induced by iron or by an increase in young red cells.

Pasvol: There you are getting into the question of iron and infection, a subject in its own right (Bullen 1981).

McGregor: Yes, it is a complex subject, but the phenomenon of iron activating latent malaria is by no means widespread. I think Brian Greenwood would agree that exacerbation of malaria is not a noticeable consequence of iron supplementation in highly malarious regions of West Africa.

Greenwood: Clinically I haven't noticed that giving iron treatment, for example to patients with iron deficiency anaemia caused by hookworm, precipitates exacerbations of malaria; but one might not notice this unless one undertook a formal study.

Weatherall: There are some extremely interesting results from Papua New Guinea suggesting that babies who have been iron-repleted at birth probably have much higher parasitaemias at 3–6 months than babies who have not, in an iron-deficient population (S. Oppenheimer, personal communication). This observation may be of considerable practical importance.

REFERENCES

Bullen J J 1981 The significance of iron in infection. Rev Infect Dis 3:127-1138
Conrad ME, Dennis LH 1968 Splenic function in experimental malaria. Am J Trop Med Hyg 17: 170-172
Dacie J V 1962 Haemolytic anaemia, 2nd edn. Part 2: autoimmune anaemias. Churchill, London, p 361-363
Drake JR, Fitch CD 1980 Status of vitamin E as an erythropoietic factor. Am J Clin Nutr 33: 2386-2393
Dupuy ME, Elliot M, Masouredis SP 1964 Relationship between red cell bound antibody and agglutination in the antiglobulin reaction. Vox Sang 9:40
Engelfriet CP, von dem Borne AEG, Fleer A, van der Meulen FW, Roos D 1980 In vivo destruction of erythrocytes by complement-binding and non-complement-binding antibodies. Prog Clin Biol Res 43:213-226
Facer CA 1980 Direct antiglobulin reactions in Gambian children with *P. falciparum* malaria. III. Expression of IgG sub-class determinants and genetic markers and association with anaemia. Clin Exp Immunol 41:81-90
Facer CA, Brown J 1981 Monocyte erythrophagocytosis in falciparum malaria. Lancet 1: 897-898
Facer CA, Bray RS, Brown J 1979 Direct anti-globulin reactions in Gambian children with *P. falciparum* malaria. I. Incidence and class specificity. Clin Exp Immunol 35:119-127

Fogel B, Shields C, Von Doenhoff A 1966 The osmotic fragility of erythrocytes in experimental malaria. Am J Trop Med Hyg 15:269-275

Frank M 1977 Pathophysiology of immune haemolytic anaemia. Ann Intern Med 87:210-222

George JN, Wicker DJ, Fogel BJ, Shields CE, Conrad ME 1967 Erythrocytic abnormalities in experimental malaria. Proc Soc Exp Biol Med 124:1086-1089

Kitchen SF 1939 The infection of mature and immature erythrocytes by *P. falciparum* and *P. malaria*. Am J Trop Med 19:47-62

Lutz HU, Kay MMB 1981 An age-specific cell antigen is present on senescent human red blood cell membranes. Mech Ageing Dev 15:65-75

McKenna RW, Risdall RJ, Brunning RD 1981 Virus associated hemophagocytic syndrome. Hum Pathol 12:395-398

Murray MJ, Murray AB, Murray NJ, Murray MB 1975 Refeeding malaria and hyperferraemia. Lancet 1:653-654

Murray MJ, Murray AB, Murray MB, Murray CJ 1978a The adverse effect of iron repletion on the course of certain infections. Br Med J 2:1113-1115

Murray MJ, Murray AB, Murray NJ, Murray MB 1978b Diet and cerebral malaria: the effect of famine and refeeding. Am J Clin Nutr 31:57-61

Nathan CF 1982 Secretion of oxygen intermediates: role in effector functions of activated macrophages. Fed Proc 41:2206-2211

Pasvol G, Weatherall DJ, Wilson RJM 1980 The increased susceptibility of young red cells to invasion by the malarial parasite *Plasmodium falciparum*. Br J Haematol 45:285-295

Rosenberg EB, Strickland GT, Yang S, Whalen GE 1973 IgM antibodies to red cells and autoimmune anemia in patients with malaria. Am J Trop Med Hyg 22:146-152

Shepherd PS, Burke P, Thomas A, Mitchell GH, Cohen S 1982 Circulating immune complexes in Plasmodium-knowlesi infected kra, and merozoite vaccinated rhesus monkeys. Clin Exp Immunol 48:315-320

Siegal I, Liu TL, Gleicher N 1981 The red-cell immune system. Lancet 2:556-559

Weatherall DJ, Clegg JB 1981 The thalassaemia syndromes, 3rd edn. Blackwell Scientific Publications, Oxford

Wilson RJM, McGregor IA, Hall PJ 1975 Persistence and recurrence of S-antigens in plasmodium falciparum infections in man. Trans R Soc Trop Med Hyg 69:460-467

The spleen in malaria

DAVID J. WYLER

Division of Geographic Medicine, Department of Medicine, Tufts University School of Medicine, 136 Harrison Avenue, Boston, MA 02111, USA

Abstract The mechanisms underlying splenic host defence in malaria have not been precisely defined but they include both immunological and non-immunological interactions with parasitized erythrocytes. Studies of the intravascular clearance of ^{51}Cr-labelled *Plasmodium berghei*-infected erythrocytes in the rat show that these cells are cleared predominantly by the spleen, and to a greater extent in immune than non-immune animals. Transfer of hyperimmune rat serum imparted protection to challenge with *P. berghei*-infected red cells but did not alter the magnitude or rate of clearance of the infected cells. Rising parasitaemia during acute infection was associated with diminished splenic clearance of the infected cells as well as of rigid, uninfected red cells (heated or Heinz body-containing). Just before the onset of spontaneous resolution (crisis) a marked increase in splenic clearance was observed. These changes could be related to alterations in the splenic microcirculation. From these studies it is concluded that opsonization of *P. berghei*-infected erythrocytes is not an important mechanism of protection in the rat. Rather, the altered rheological properties of these cells may result in their trapping within the spleen. Presumably, these rheological changes occur in malarias caused by different *Plasmodium* species. On the other hand, opsonization of parasitized erythrocytes, although not found in rodent malaria, might yet prove to be an important defence mechanism in primate malaria.

The spleen plays a central role in the immune response and host defence to intravascular pathogens, and is also endowed with the ability to remove damaged and effete erythrocytes. It is therefore not surprising that the spleen is of such importance in host defence in malaria (Wyler et al 1979). Alterations in the metabolism and antigenic composition of infected erythrocytes are undoubtedly important determinants of the ability of the spleen to remove infected red cells. Evidence to be presented here also suggests that the altered rheological properties of infected erythrocytes profoundly affect their removal by the spleen. A brief summary of current knowledge of the role of the spleen in host defence against malarial infection will serve to place the newer information in an appropriate clinical context.

1983 Malaria and the red cell. Pitman, London (Ciba Foundation symposium 94) p 98-116

Immunological aspects

Although the induction of immune responses to plasmodial antigens has received little attention, it is reasonable to extrapolate to malaria the conclusions derived from studies of immune responses to uninfected heterologous erythrocytes. Observations in rats sensitized to sheep erythrocytes (Rowley 1950) indicated that the spleen is critically important in the induction of primary responses to intravenously injected antigens. After the induction of anti-malarial immune responses the spleen remains a repository of immunocompetent cells which, when adoptively transferred to syngeneic rodent recipients, impart protection against homologous parasite challenge (Brown et al 1976). It appears that this protection depends largely on T lymphocytes (Brown et al 1976). Whether these are exclusively helper subpopulations, which promote protective antibody synthesis and secretion, or include T-dependent, antibody-independent mechanisms as well (Grun & Weidanz 1981), remains to be elucidated.

A curious paradox exists in the case of quartan malaria, as exemplified by *Plasmodium inui* infection in rhesus monkeys (Wyler et al 1977). On the one hand, splenectomized monkeys uniformly experience significantly higher peak parasitaemias and mortality than intact monkeys when infected with this parasite, which emphasizes the importance of the spleen in the initial response of the host to infection. Surviving splenectomized recipients, on the other hand, are able to achieve rapid self-cure of their infection, whereas intact monkeys characteristically experience several years of chronic infection. The deleterious function of the spleen in late host defence, as revealed by these observations, may involve active immunosuppressive pathways, perhaps mediated through humoral or cellular mechanisms.

Macrophages

A role for splenic macrophages in the attrition of asexual parasitized erythrocytes or free merozoites from circulation is more implied than established. Splenic macrophages laden with pigment and other debris were observed in the malaria patients studied by Golgi nearly a century ago. This finding has led to the present-day notion that phagocytosis of parasitized erythrocytes is an important defence mechanism (Taliaferro & Mulligan 1937). Direct support for this concept was gained from *in vitro* studies which demonstrated that macrophages could ingest opsonized *P. knowlesi* (Brown 1971) or *P. berghei*-parasitized erythrocytes (Hunter et al 1979). Our studies in *P. berghei* in the rat, which were designed to test this concept *in vivo*, failed however to corroborate the *in vitro* observations (see below). This discrepancy may be accounted for by the possibility that in the unphysiological conditions prevailing in the *in vitro* cultures, alterations in the erythrocyte plasma membrane led to exposure of surface (? parasite) antigens not normally expressed *in vivo*. Indeed, when parasite antigens are expressed, opsonization can occur. This has been demonstrated *in vivo* for trophozoites mechanically freed from erythrocytes (Hamburger & Kreier 1975) and *in vitro* for free merozoites (Khusmith et al 1982).

In contrast to the lack of convincing evidence for the opsonization of infected erythrocytes *in vivo*, indirect *in vivo* evidence for the opsonization of free merozoites has been reported. Monkeys immunized with *P. knowlesi* merozoites in Freund's complete adjuvant developed antibody which prevented merozoite invasion of erythrocytes *in vitro* and also protected the monkeys from homologous challenge (Butcher et al 1978). Splenectomy had no effect on the presence of circulating invasion-blocking antibody, but rendered the monkeys once more susceptible to challenge. One explanation for these observations is that in addition to blocking invasion, anti-merozoite antibody opsonized free parasites for phagocytosis by splenic macrophages. The unique importance of splenic macrophages, in contrast to hepatic macrophages, may possibly relate to the specific isotype and density of antibody on the merozoite and the relation of these determinants to complement activation. These features have been shown to be critically important in determining whether antibody-coated red cells are cleared by splenic or hepatic macrophages (Frank et al 1977). Additional support for this notion derives from our studies in rats (Quinn & Wyler 1979b). On challenge with 10^9 *P. berghei*-infected erythrocytes, intact non-immune recipients of normal rat serum experienced rapidly rising parasitaemia (to 4.5% in 24 h), whereas parasitaemia rapidly fell in the recipients of hyperimmune serum (smear-negative in 24 h). Splenectomized recipients of hyperimmune serum experienced persistent but constant levels of parasitaemia (1.5%). Analysis of differential counts of ring forms and trophozoites at various times after challenge in these animals suggested that hyperimmune serum may have effectively interfered with reinvasion after schizont rupture in intact rats, but only partially so in splenectomized rats. Perhaps a subpopulation of merozoites which escaped opsonization was available for infecting erythrocytes in splenectomized but not intact rats. Direct confirmation of this hypothesis must await further investigation, however. Collectively, these observations emphasize that the host indeed makes opsonizing antibody but that the expression of parasite antigen on the infected erythrocyte is the critical determinant of immune clearance by the spleen.

In addition to their ability to phagocytose and kill pathogens by intracellular microbicidal mechanisms, macrophages can secrete a number of soluble products that exert cytostatic or cytocidal effects in the extracellular milieu. These products include a number of molecular species of reduced oxygen, such as hydrogen peroxide and superoxide, and biochemically less well-characterized molecules that can inhibit tumour growth (tumour necrosis factor). The possibility that these or related macrophage products might interfere with the intraerythrocytic development of some *Plasmodia* and *Babesia* species has been suggested as an explanation for the occurrence of 'crisis' (Allison & Clark 1977). This is the sudden decrease in parasitaemia observed in certain acute experimental malarias (e.g. *P. berghei* in the rat); it may also occur in selected (albeit poorly documented) cases of human malaria. Crisis is characterized by the appearance in the circulation of stunted intracellular trophozoites ('crisis forms') which characteristically possess scant cytoplasm and pyknotic nuclei. The fact that crisis is reversible and spleen-dependent has been suggested by our finding in *P. berghei* infection in rats that splenectomy during crisis resulted in the rapid disappearance of crisis forms and a rise in parasitaemia (Quinn & Wyler 1980). It is therefore possible that during their sojourn in the spleen, intraerythrocytic trophozoites encounter macrophage-derived soluble factors which interfere with their intracellular maturation.

In an effort to quantitatively assess the role of the spleen in malarial host defence, my colleague Dr Thomas C. Quinn and I have examined the clearance of *P. berghei*-infected erythrocytes in rats. The results of these studies, summarized here, provided evidence that splenic trapping of parasitized erythrocytes is an important defence mechanism. Furthermore, the ability of the spleen to trap erythrocytes alters dramatically during the course of infection. Our studies have led us to the conclusion that the altered rheological properties of infected erythrocytes—specifically, their decreased deformability—rather than their surface antigenic composition may be particularly important determinants of splenic clearance in this rodent malaria model.

Materials and methods

Malaria infection

P. berghei infection was initiated in adult Wistar rats by the intravenous inoculation of 10^7 parasitized rat erythrocytes suspended in saline solution. Infection was generally non-lethal (10% mortality) and asynchronous (i.e. different stages of parasite maturation were represented in the circulation at any given time during the infection). Parasitaemia rose to a peak of 40–60% infected erythrocytes over a two-week period, and then suddenly declined to less than 1% during the crisis period of 48–72 h. When the acute infection had resolved, the rats were resistant to challenge with the homologous parasite (immune rats). After repeated challenges, their serum (hyperimmune serum) contained IgG antibody which, upon transfer, could protect a non-immune recipient from homologous challenge (Diggs & Osler 1969).

Clearance studies

To quantify the magnitude and rate of removal of an inoculum of parasitized erythrocytes from circulation, we labelled infected rat erythrocytes with ^{51}Cr using standard techniques (Quinn & Wyler 1979a). Briefly, a population of cells highly enriched for *P. berghei*-infected erythrocytes (85–90%) was obtained by low speed centrifugation of donor rat blood suspended in citrate-phosphate-dextrose solution. Erythrocytes were labelled by incubating red cells in $Na_2{}^{51}CrO_4$ (200 μCi/ml packed cells) for 30 min at 20 °C and then washing them extensively in phosphate-buffered saline. Labelled erythrocytes (10^9) in saline were injected into the tail vein of recipient rats, and blood was obtained from the retro-orbital plexus at different intervals. The amount of radiolabel present in a standard volume of these blood samples was determined in a gamma counter and the percentage of label remaining in circulation at each time point was calculated from these determinations. In addition, organ uptake of ^{51}Cr-tagged erythrocytes was determined by measuring the gamma emission from specimens of spleen, liver, lung, bone marrow, kidney and intestines of sacrificed rats.

Results and discussion

Clearance of ^{51}Cr-tagged erythrocytes in non-immune and immune rats

Uninfected rat erythrocytes disappeared gradually from circulation in a monophasic pattern and at the same rate in immune and non-immune rats ($t_\frac{1}{2} = 16.1 \pm 1.2$ days). Parasitized erythrocytes, in contrast, were cleared more rapidly and in a biphasic manner in both groups of rats (Fig. 1). During a rapid initial phase lasting about an hour, infected erythrocytes were cleared predominantly by the spleen, and to a lesser extent by the liver. After the first hour, a more gradual but constant disappearance of ^{51}Cr from circulation was observed and, we believe, resulted primarily from the asynchronous rupture of the erythrocytes containing mature schizonts with renal excretion of the radionuclide.

Relatively little of the ^{51}Cr accumulated in any of the reticuloendothelial organs during this second phase (shown for liver and spleen in Fig. 1). The

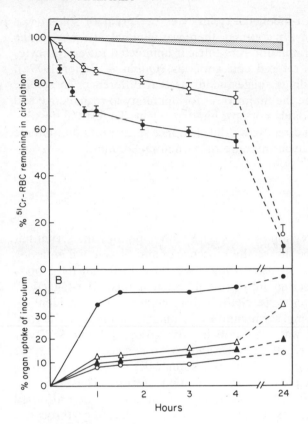

FIG. 1. Clearance of ^{51}Cr-labelled *P. berghei*-infected erythrocytes (RBC) in immune (closed symbols) and non-immune (open symbols) rats. A. Disappearance of labelled red cells from circulation. Stippled area is 95% confidence interval for clearance of uninfected cells. Mean + SEM, 15 experiments. B. Uptake of labelled parasitized red cells by spleen (circles) or liver (triangles) during clearance. Mean of five experiments shown; SEM ≤ 1% of mean. (Adapted from Quinn & Wyler 1979a by permission of The Rockefeller University Press.)

only difference between immune and non-immune rats in their ability to clear tagged infected erythrocytes was observed during the first phase, at which time non-immune rats cleared 11.5 ± 1.5% of the inoculum, whereas immune rats cleared 32.0 ± 2.2%. These differences could be readily explained by the splenomegaly which developed in the immune rats (2.8 ± 0.9 g *vs.* 1.1 ± 2 g in non-immune rats; $P < 0.005$) and the greater ability of their enlarged spleens to remove the infected erythrocytes. In related experiments we observed that the splenic uptake of these cells was directly related to spleen weight (correlation coefficient, $r = 0.92$), irrespective of whether splenomegaly was induced by malaria or non-specifically by treatment with methylcellulose.

Indeed, the uptake of ^{51}Cr-labelled erythrocytes per gram of spleen was constant under all conditions. In contrast, there was minimal difference in the ability of immune and non-immune rats to clear uninfected rat erythrocytes sensitized with rabbit anti-rat red cell antibody (Quinn & Wyler 1979a). Taken together, these findings suggested to us that differences in splenic trapping were unlikely to be the major basis for immunity to rechallenge and that this immunity was probably not opsonin-dependent. To test the possible role of *in vivo* opsonization directly, we did clearance studies on non-immune rats which received either hyperimmune or normal rat serum.

Serum transfer studies

The ability to transfer protection to *P. berghei* with hyperimmune serum has been previously shown to be due to the presence of anti-plasmodial antibody of the IgG isotype (Diggs & Osler 1969). We injected 0.5 ml/100 g body weight of unfractionated serum into normal recipient rats. ^{51}Cr-tagged *P. berghei*-infected erythrocytes were cleared from circulation in an identical manner in recipients of normal serum and hyperimmune serum, and the total reticuloendothelial uptake was the same in both groups (Quinn & Wyler 1979b). In contrast, the resulting parasitaemia rose steadily during the 24-hour study period in recipients of normal serum, but fell progressively to undetectable levels in recipients of hyperimmune serum. These *in vivo* observations thus suggested that the antibody-mediated protection afforded by hyperimmune serum was not due to opsonization of infected erythrocytes.

   Since these studies had focused exclusively on the rechallenge of actively or passively immunized rats, we could not be sure that our conclusions also pertained to the events responsible for resolving the acute infection during crisis. Indeed, there is reason to believe that different mechanisms of host defence might be responsible for the resolution of acute infection and for resistance to rechallenge in previously infected immune subjects (Wyler et al 1979). Accordingly, we examined the clearance of ^{51}Cr-tagged infected erythrocytes in rats at different times during their infection.

Clearance during acute infection

We observed that during an ongoing infection, as splenomegaly was developing, splenic uptake of an inoculum of ^{51}Cr-tagged parasitized erythrocytes per gram actually *decreased* to subnormal (below uninfected control) levels. At the onset of crisis, however, splenic clearance suddenly became supernormal.

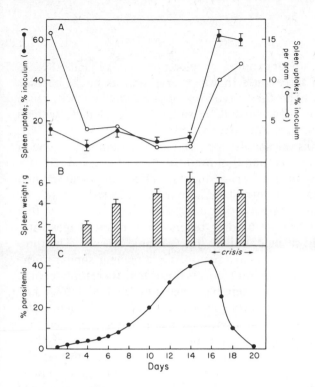

FIG. 2. Splenic clearance (24 h) of ^{51}Cr-labelled *P. berghei*-infected cells during *P. berghei* malaria in the rat. A. Splenic uptake in rats at different times of infection; mean ± SEM, five experiments. B. Spleen weight; mean ± SEM, five experiments. C. Parasitaemia, mean of 15 experiments; SEM ≤ 1% of mean. (Adapted from Quinn & Wyler 1979a by permission of The Rockefeller University Press.)

This was not due to a sudden enlargement of the spleen (Fig. 2). Thus, we could conclude that during the pre-crisis period of rising parasitaemia, the trapping efficiency of the spleen was actually impaired. Presumably this reduction in splenic function permitted the parasitaemia to rise. Since the onset of crisis corresponded to a dramatic increase in trapping function (Fig. 2), it seemed likely that this played a causal role in the removal of parasites from the circulation during resolution of the acute infection. Our observation that crisis was spleen-dependent (Quinn & Wyler 1980) supported this hypothesis. These considerations stimulated us to investigate the possible mechanisms by which the splenic trapping of infected erythrocytes is regulated.

Mechanism of trapping

In the light of our present understanding of spleen physiology generally, we considered that there are three ways in which erythrocytes might become sequestered in the spleen. The first, involving opsonin-mediated clearance whereby cells are actually phagocytosed by splenic macrophages, seemed unlikely, from our previous serum transfer studies (Quinn & Wyler 1979b). The possibility that opsonins transiently appeared in the serum at the time of crisis was excluded by the observation that preincubation of infected red cells in serum obtained at the time of crisis did not affect their subsequent clearance when inoculated into normal or immune uninfected rats (T. C. Quinn & D. J. Wyler, unpublished observations). The second possibility, that serum factors promote erythrocyte binding reversibly to macrophages without phagocytosis occurring, seemed unlikely for the same reasons. The third possibility, that infected erythrocytes are removed in a manner similar to the removal of poorly deformable, uninfected erythrocytes, therefore seemed attractive. Such a concept seemed tenable since Miller et al (1971) had already shown that parasitized erythrocytes are less deformable than uninfected erythrocytes. This non-immunological splenic function has been proposed as an important mechanism for removing effete and damaged erythrocytes in both normal and pathological conditions. Of relevance to malaria, this filtering function increases in the setting of splenomegaly, and is presumably responsible for certain haematological abnormalities associated with an enlarged spleen.

To understand splenic filtration it is necessary to consider the major defined microcirculatory routes available to erythrocytes percolating through the spleen. Blood entering the spleen can pass directly into the cords—a matrix comprised of various cells, including macrophages, and connective tissue. This channel lacks an endothelial lining and is thus referred to as the 'open pathway', through which erythrocytes slowly percolate. After traversing the cords they re-enter the endothelially lined sinuses by squeezing through narrow interendothelial slits and then drain from the sinuses to tributaries of the splenic veins. It is at the interendothelial slits that the erythrocyte membranes must suffer marked deformation in order to squeeze through spaces that are in the range of 0.5–2.5 μm (Chen & Weiss 1973). Since poorly deformable erythrocytes are unable to undergo the necessary membrane contortions to pass into the sinuses, they become trapped in the cords and are phagocytosed by resident macrophages. It is postulated that trapping at this site is increased in splenomegaly because the interendothelial slits become effectively narrower. Erythrocytes can bypass the cordal obstacle by remaining within endothelially lined channels (thus, 'closed pathway') which empty directly into the sinuses. Rigid erythrocytes circulating through the closed pathways are therefore not filtered out by the spleen and can re-enter the systemic circulation.

We reasoned that if parasitized erythrocytes were filtered in the spleen on the basis of their decreased deformability, alterations in the clearance pattern observed during acute infection should be similar for parasitized erythrocytes and rigid but uninfected erythrocytes. We therefore compared the clearance of *P. berghei*-infected erythrocytes with that of (1) uninfected rat erythrocytes containing Heinz bodies, induced by phenylhydrazine treatment, and (2) uninfected erythrocytes heated to 50 °C for 30 min. These treatments alter the erythrocytes in several ways and result in their decreased deformability. The comparison was made in rats at different stages of malarial infection (Table 1). Splenic uptake of rigid uninfected erythrocytes progressively decreased

TABLE 1 Effect of malaria on clearance and 24-hour splenic uptake of P. berghei-infected, heated and Heinz body-containing red blood cells (RBC)

Parasitaemia (%)	$T_{\frac{1}{2}}(min)$			Splenic uptake (% inoculum)		
	Infected RBC	Heated RBC	RBC with Heinz bodies	Infected RBC	Heated RBC	RBC with Heinz bodies
Uninfected	540	45	20	19	75	62
10	600	90	70	10	40	40
20	660	130	95	7	20	40
40	720	>500	150	5	10	10
Crisis	180	10	10	70	78	80

(Adapted from Quinn & Wyler 1979a and Wyler et al 1981 by permission of The Rockefeller University Press.)

during the pre-crisis period as parasitaemia rose, but reverted to normal or even supernormal levels just before crisis—the same pattern as we had earlier noted for parasitized red cells (see p 104-105 and Fig. 2).

These observations thus provided strong circumstantial evidence supporting the concept of filtration as the basis for the splenic trapping of parasitized erythrocytes. From these findings we suggested that alterations in clearance during infection are a function of changes in splenic microcirculatory patterns. We reasoned that the ability of the spleen to remove the three different populations of rigid erythrocytes might reflect a decrease in cordal blood flow and a shunting of blood directly into the sinuses via the closed pathways. To test this, we undertook studies (Wyler et al 1981) with Dr Li-Tsun Chen (then of Johns Hopkins University School of Medicine), who had recently described a method for quantifying the relative distribution of splenic blood flow through the open and closed pathways (Chen 1978).

We injected carbonized plastic microspheres of 3–4μm diameter intravenously into rats. Five to six seconds later, the blood flow was stopped by transthoracic transection with a guillotine. The distribution of the microspheres in the splenic cords and sinuses was then assessed by examining histological preparations of fixed spleen tissue. Since the size of the particles permitted their entry into, but not exit from, the cords, and since particle distribution is directly proportional to microcirculatory flow rate, we could use the results to assess alterations in relative flow patterns during infection with *P. berghei*. In normal rats, splenic flow was predominantly through the open pathways, since over 98% of the microspheres in the spleen were found in the cords (Table 2). In rats with rising parasitaemias, cordal circulation was

TABLE 2 Effect of P. berghei infection in rats on the relative blood flow via splenic cords (open pathway) and directly to sinuses (closed pathway), as determined by microsphere distribution

		% flow	
State of infection	*Parasitaemia*	*Cords*	*Sinus*
Uninfected rats	0	98.3 ± 0.3	1.7 ± 0.3
Pre-crisis	24–50	61.8 ± 2.6	38.2 ± 2.6
Crisis	0–10	89.4 ± 1.9	10.6 ± 1.9

(Adapted from Wyler et al 1981 by permission of The Rockefeller University Press.)

markedly reduced and flow via the closed pathways was increased. This pattern reverted toward normal with the onset of crisis. These results clearly indicated that the splenic microcirculation underwent substantial changes during infection and did so in a manner which could explain the alterations in erythrocyte clearance patterns observed. The supernormal clearance of parasitized erythrocytes during crisis could be explained by the restoration of cordal blood flow in the setting of splenomegaly, a condition we had found to increase the clearance of these cells (Quinn & Wyler 1979a). The superior trapping ability of the enlarged spleens clearly required normal circulation through the open cordal pathway. Splenomegaly in the setting of reduced cordal flow did not result in supernormal trapping.

An important unanswered question is what regulates the alterations in splenic microcirculation in malaria. One possibility is that the infected erythrocytes rapidly obstruct the interendothelial spaces and thereby cause stasis in the cords. Although this seems a reasonable possibility and may constitute one form of 'splenic blockade', it fails to provide an explanation for the subsequent restoration of cordal flow just before crisis. Regional hyperplasia of erythroid and lymphoid elements might also physically obstruct the open pathways; cordal flow might then be restored when these cells migrate out of the spleen. Alternatively, alterations in splenic flow might be under pharmacological control, although too little is known about this generally to make such speculation compelling.

We can attempt to integrate the concept of a mechanism for spleen macrophage-mediated inhibition of parasite maturation in crisis with our observations on spleen blood flow by means of the following hypothesis. During rising parasitaemia in an acute infection, antigen-specific immune responses are initiated in the spleen. These include the local elaboration of macrophage-activating factors as a result of the interaction of plasmodial antigens with specifically sensitized splenic lymphocytes. As a result, cordal macrophages become armed and, on close contact with infected erythrocytes, secrete mediators that inhibit parasite maturation. The exclusion of parasitized erythrocytes from the cords in the pre-crisis period prevents the expression of this potential defence mechanism. At crisis, some parasitized erythrocytes are removed from the circulation by trapping. Those which escape back into circulation are imparted the crisis 'kiss of death' by activated macrophages.

We do not know why the events of crisis, so prominent in rodent malarias, are so infrequently recognized in human and other primate malarias. Possibly crisis-like events do occur in acute human malaria but go undetected. Alternatively, in malarias in which the expression of antigens on the surface of infected erythrocytes is more prominent, opsonization may be a more important defence mechanism. Thus, the spleen may have the potential for exerting a variety of defences against *Plasmodia*. The relative importance of any of these mechanisms may vary for different malarial parasites.

Conclusions

The spleen is a complex organ endowed with a multiplicity of functions, many of which remain mysterious. Although it is clear that the spleen plays a critical role in host defence in malaria, the precise mechanisms involved are still obscure. Since the parasitization of erythrocytes markedly alters their metabolic, antigenic and rheological characteristics, it is likely that many of these changes have important consequences for the interaction of erythrocytes with the spleen. Understanding these interactions is complicated by the likelihood that different *Plasmodia* species induce different alterations in the erythrocytes of their hosts, so that conclusions obtained in one experimental model may not be broadly applicable to all malarias. Nonetheless, we are slowly dissecting out the *principles* of splenic host defence in malaria. There can be no doubt that the application of these principles to new knowledge about the infected erythrocyte will greatly enhance our understanding of host–parasite biology in malaria.

Acknowledgement

This work was done while the author was a Senior Investigator in the Laboratory of Parasitic Diseases, NIAID, at the National Institutes of Health, Bethesda.

REFERENCES

Allison AC, Clark IA 1977 Specific and non-specific immunity to hemoprotozoa. Am J Trop Med Hyg 26:216-222

Brown KN 1971 Protective immunity to malaria provides a model for the survival of cells in an immunologically hostile environment. Nature (Lond) 230:763-767

Brown KN, Jarra W, Hills LA 1976 T cells and protective immunity to *Plasmodium berghei* in rats. Infect Immun 14:858-871

Butcher GA, Mitchell GH, Cohen S 1978 Antibody mediated mechanisms of immunity to malaria induced by vaccination with *Plasmodium knowlesi* merozoites. Immunology 34:77-86

Chen LT 1978 Microcirculation of the spleen: an open or closed circulation? Science (Wash DC) 201:157-159

Chen LT, Weiss L 1973 The role of the sinus wall in the passage of erythrocytes through the spleen. Blood 41:529-537

Diggs CL, Osler AG 1969 Humoral immunity in rodent malaria. II. Inhibition of parasitemia by serum antibody. J Immunol 102:298-305

Frank MM, Schreiber AD, Atkinson JP, Jaffe CJ 1977 Pathophysiology of immune hemolytic anemia. Ann Intern Med 87:210-222

Grun JL, Weidanz WP 1981 Immunity to *Plasmodium chabaudi adami* in the B-cell deficient mouse. Nature (Lond) 290:143-145

Hamburger J, Kreier JP 1975 Antibody-mediated elimination of malaria parasites (*Plasmodium berghei*) *in vivo*. Infect Immun 12:339-345

Hunter KW Jr, Winkelstein JA, Simpson TW 1979 Serum opsonic activity in rodent malaria: functional and immunochemical characteristics *in vitro*. J Immunol 123:2582-2587

Khusmith S, Druilhe P, Gentili M 1982 Enhanced *Plasmodium falciparum* merozoite phagocytosis by monocytes from immune individuals. Infect Immun 35:874-879

Miller LH, Usami S, Chen S 1971 Alteration in the rheologic properties of *Plasmodium knowlesi*-infected red cells. A possible mechanism for capillary obstruction. J Clin Invest 50:1451-1455

Quinn TC, Wyler DJ 1979a Intravascular clearance of parasitized erythrocytes in rodent malaria. J Clin Invest 63:1187-1194

Quinn TC, Wyler DJ 1979b Mechanisms of action of hyperimmune serum in mediating protective immunity to rodent malaria (*Plasmodium berghei*). J Immunol 123:2245-2249

Quinn TC, Wyler DJ 1980 Resolution of acute malaria (*Plasmodium berghei* in the rat); reversibility and spleen dependence. Am J Trop Med Hyg 29:1-4

Rowley DA 1950 The effect of splenectomy on the formation of circulating antibody in the adult male albino rat. J Immunol 64:289-295

Taliaferro WH, Mulligan HW 1937 The histopathology of malaria with special reference to the function and origin of the macrophages in defense. Indian Med Res Mem 29:1-138

Wyler DJ, Miller LH, Schmidt LH 1977 Spleen function in quartan malaria (due to *Plasmodium inui*): evidence for both protective and suppressive roles in host defense. J Infect Dis 135:86-93

Wyler DJ, Oster CN, Quinn TC 1979 The role of the spleen in malaria infections. In: UNDP/World Bank/WHO Special Programme for Research in Tropical Diseases. The role of the spleen in the immunology of parasitic diseases. Schwabe & Co, Basel (Trop Dis Res Ser no 1) p 183-204
Wyler DJ, Quinn TC, Chen LT 1981 Relationship of alterations in splenic clearance function and microcirculation to host defense in acute rodent malaria. J Clin Invest 67:1400-1404

DISCUSSION

Howard: What do you see as the mechanism for the changes in splenic microcirculation?

Wyler: The decrease in clearance during the rising parasitaemia might be a simple clogging-up of the splenic cords by parasitized erythrocytes. The shunting of blood to the closed pathways might therefore be simply a matter of microcirculatory haemodynamics. But why the cordal pathway opens up at crisis is harder to understand. Very little is known about the normal regulation of splenic flow generally. Perhaps there is some kind of regulation of effective interendothelial slit width which has escaped the physiologists. Another possibility is that blockade is due in part to localized but transient cellular hyperplasia (? extramedullary erythropoiesis) in the spleen. Perhaps these splenic cells are released at the time of crisis, thereby opening up the cordal channels. We really have no clear explanation at present.

Howard: Can you simulate the change in the splenic microcirculation seen during malaria using any drugs? Is it possible that the changed microcirculation reflects a pharmacological mechanism induced by the pathology of malaria infection?

Wyler: We have considered this idea, but are stymied by the fact that one can't effectively target vasoactive drugs to act selectively on the spleen. Since these agents would undoubtedly also produce alterations in other vascular beds, it would be very hard to interpret the results.

Howard: Could you study this in perfused spleens in organ culture?

Wyler: That's an intriguing idea and one which we have thought about. There are some considerable technical problems involved, such as providing perfusion through the several splenic arteries and selecting the appropriately physiological perfusion media. I don't think these are insurmountable challenges, and this approach could be well worth the effort.

Brown: It is interesting that you found no opsonization of parasitized reticulocytes. Zweig & Singer (1979) recently showed that reticulocytes can aggregate and endocytose ligands like concanavalin A over areas of their surface where there is no spectrin network. We also showed that parasitized reticulocytes will aggregate (and possibly cap) bound antibody and shed it (Brown et al 1982). A reticulocyte thus differs from a mature red cell in this respect and might be able to get rid of antibody binding to its surface by capping; hence the parasitized reticulocyte might not be susceptible to opsonization, unlike the mature red cell.

Wyler: That is an excellent point. In support of your idea are our preliminary observations on clearance of chromium-tagged *P. knowlesi*-infected erythrocytes in rhesus monkeys (T.C. Quinn & D.J. Wyler, unpublished results). These observations are consistent with the idea that schizonts may in fact be opsonized *in vivo*, but more work needs to be done before this conclusion is on solid ground. I certainly hold to the view that opsonization *in vivo* of parasitized erythrocytes depends upon the *stable* expression of antigens on the extracellular merozoite or parasitized erythrocytes. The topographical distribution of these antigens might well influence whether antibodies directed against them can effect clearance.

Brown: They are apparently expressed on the surface of reticulocytes in *P. berghei*; the difference is that they appear to be shed as aggregates in the presence of specific antibody. Although we haven't demonstrated unequivocally antigen coded by the parasite on the reticulocyte surface, we have shown antigens that can be absorbed only with parasitized erythrocytes.

Secondly, the splenic removal of parasites appears to be T cell-dependent, because in hosts deprived of their T cells you don't see the 'crisis'. How would that fit into your concept of the crisis phenomenon?

Wyler: First, we need to distinguish the T-dependence of 'crisis' from clearance. I know of no data which suggest that clearance *per se* is in any way modulated by T cell function. Furthermore, although 'crisis' is clearly spleen-dependent (Quinn & Wyler 1980), it is not simply due to enhanced clearance. For one thing, we see the 'crisis forms' in the peripheral circulation, so they haven't been removed by the spleen. My concept of how crisis fits into the clearance story is that cordal macrophages, when activated through T-dependent mechanisms, can impart a 'kiss of death' to the intracellular parasite. That is, they may through soluble mediators or direct contact somehow affect the ability of the parasite to undergo normal maturation. If the macrophages are not 'activated' (for example, in T-deprived animals) or if the parasitized erythrocytes are excluded from the cords (as occurs during the pre-crisis period of rising parasitaemia) crisis cannot occur. Only when both features are operative will crisis occur. Resolution of acute rodent malaria depends, in my mind, on more than just trapping of parasitized erythrocytes in the spleen.

Brown: I tend to see it from a different angle, with the infection giving a massive T cell stimulation, by a whole range of parasite antigens. But the host is also synthesizing specific antibody to exposed surface antigens. This antibody begins to reduce the parasitaemia somewhat. This in turn increases the amount of antigen going to the spleen, which there stimulates the sensitized T cells.

Then you get the Allison effect, a cascade of products released from T cells and macrophages which now begin to destroy the parasites. But I think it likely that the important initial event is synthesis of a specific antibody.

Wyler: I don't agree with your concept. I think there is little to suggest that antibody is involved in resolution of the acute infection (in rodent malaria), but it is the key to protection upon rechallenge. We found that incubating parasitized erythrocytes in serum from rats undergoing crisis did not affect their clearance (T.C. Quinn & D.J. Wyler, unublished results). Clearly, parasitized erythrocytes are 'damaged', in the sense that they are cleared more rapidly than uninfected cells. But the qualitative changes in clearance during infection are similar to those of rigid uninfected erythrocytes. This argues that we don't have to involve antibody-mediated mechanisms in this model. Furthermore, if we use chromium-tagged *P. berghei*-infected erythrocytes from rats with only 24 or 48 hours of infection, we get the same results as those I presented. Obviously, the donor rats in this case have not yet produced specific antibody.

Phillips: Most of our recent work has been with the mouse and *P. chabaudi*. Your clearance studies were done in rats recently recovered from a primary infection. It is necessary to distinguish between an animal that has been reinfected and is controlling this or subsequent challenge infections, and one that has recently controlled a primary infection. At what stage in the infection in your immune rats were you doing the clearance studies? In *P. chabaudi* in the mouse, the spleen is also important at crisis in the control of the falling parasitaemia. If the spleen is removed at that stage, the parasitaemia continues to fall for one or two days and then rises again. With *P. chabaudi* we are dealing with a synchronous infection and because of this we have been able to identify the schizont-infected cell or the merozoite as the vulnerable stage. In a mouse that has recovered from a *P. chabaudi* infection and is then reinfected, so that it has a high level of immunity, a large intravenous challenge dose of parasites given 7–14 days later is rapidly cleared equally well, with or without the spleen. In these conditions the spleen seems to play no part in removing infected cells. As I understand it, you are talking about rats that have recently removed their primary infection?

Wyler: We have done clearance studies on rats at many different times after resolution of their primary infection. The only factor which seemed to be important in accelerating clearance in these rats was spleen size. The time from the resolution of acute infection to the clearance study was not a variable which influenced clearance rates independent of spleen size. Our contention is that the immune rats are resistant to rechallenge because they have antibody, which probably exerts its effects on the terminal maturation of schizonts or on merozoites. As I mentioned, the only role of the spleen in these animals might be to clear a small subpopulation of merozoites. So your findings with *P.*

chabaudi are compatible with our observations in rats that upon rechallenge the situation is very different from the resolution of an acute infection.

Phillips: We have done lymphocyte migration studies using ^{51}Cr as a marker in *P. chabaudi*-infected mice at different stages during the primary parasitaemia, studying migration of peripheral lymph node cells from both infected and uninfected mice (Kumararatne, Phillips, Sinclair, Parrott & Forrester, unpublished). Just after crisis, around Day 11, the localization of normal peripheral lymph node cells into the spleen is markedly reduced and is markedly increased in the liver. This is true for both T and B cells. One possible explanation of the reduced localization of lymphocytes in the spleen is that the microcirculation in the spleen is altered just after peak parasitaemia. We shall use the microsphere technique which you describe to see whether the microcirculation is altered in the spleen and whether this accounts for the changed migration patterns of lymphocytes in these infected mice.

Wyler: I think that's an interesting finding. The blockade in the cordal circulatory pathways may also occur in human malaria. Perhaps this is an explanation for the overwhelming bacterial sepsis observed in some malaria patients. Perhaps the bacteria are not being cleared normally by the spleen, since they may be shunted away from the cords, where most of the macrophages are located.

McGregor: It is always difficult to extrapolate from animal studies to man, and the role of the spleen in malaria infections in man is far from clear. Epidemiological evidence indicates a role of considerable immunological importance. You, Dr Wyler, consider that rheological factors, such as the reduced deformability of the parasitized red cell and the special architecture of the spleen, are important in the killing of parasites, perhaps even more important than mechanisms involving immunological sensitization. Perhaps the study of malaria in pregnancy may shed some light on this point. Where malaria is highly endemic, the young female develops and maintains an effective protective immunity. When she first becomes pregnant, however, she shows increased levels of peripheral parasitaemia, enhanced frequency of pyrexial illness and anaemia, and extremely dense parasite colonization of maternal placental blood. Often, at delivery, the infant is found to be of low birth weight. In short, the first pregnancy appears to induce a breakdown of immunity which has adverse effects on both mother and child. However, in subsequent pregnancies the adverse effects are less obvious. Parasite rates and densities in both peripheral and placental blood fall; there is much less maternal illness and infant birth weights are less depressed (McGregor 1978). It could be argued that the exacerbation of parasitaemia that occurs in first pregnancies is the consequence of sequestration of the parasites in a new blood reservoir, the placenta, which obviates the rheological hazards of passage through the spleen. On the other hand, the progressive improvement in host well-being that occurs in subsequent pregnancies perhaps argues that an immunological effector mechanism, which is probably not rheologically assisted, develops within the uterus and placenta and becomes capable of controlling parasite replication in the vascular spaces of these organs. My own working hypothesis of naturally acquired malarial immunity is that it is spleen centred, requiring sensitized, immobilized parasites or parasitized cells to be conveyed by the blood flow to the spleen for killing by splenic effector cells. The killing process may be assisted by rheological factors, but the time taken for the human host to develop effective immunity suggests that the main killing mechanism has a specific, immunological basis.

Wallach: Regarding the possible mechanism of non-immune clearance, as I mentioned earlier, the parasitized red cell can probably sustain the export of calcium from the cytoplasm to maintain normal intracytoplasmic calcium levels under quiescent conditions, but not in conditions of high shear. Then the intracytoplasmic calcium level will increase, and the cells become less deformable and therefore are cleared more readily. The possible significance of these mechanisms could be tested by loading normal red cells with calcium up to a five times normal concentration and monitoring their clearance.

Cohen: Dr Wyler, the enhanced clearance of parasites in your immune rats seems to affect only about 20% of parasites. From the ability of parasites to pass through small pore filters, it appears that the diminished deformability is found from about the stage of the trophozoite onwards. It would be interesting to know whether the initial rapid filtration out of the circulation involves only the more mature parasites.

Wyler: We didn't look at this directly, but I suspect you're correct. Dr Ken Hunter has repeated these kinds of studies in mice with *P. yoelii* and has fractionated the parasites into late trophozoites plus schizonts, and ring forms. It is predominantly the trophozoites and schizonts that are being cleared, which would support your point (K.W. Hunter Jr, personal communication). An important aspect of the *in vivo* studies was demonstrated by Dr Hunter's experience. He was able to demonstrate opsonization of the *P. yoelii* -infected red cells by mouse macrophages *in vitro* (Hunter et al 1979), but was not able to show opsonization *in vivo* (K.W. Hunter Jr, personal communication). In interpreting *in vitro* phagocytosis and opsonization studies, we should take into account the unphysiological conditions which prevail in their cultures. Leaching of erythrocyte plasma membrane components *in vitro* may expose antigens that are not normally expressed *in vivo*. This may explain why Dr Hunter found opsonization *in vitro* but not *in vivo*.

Anders: You mentioned that splenectomy of rhesus monkeys abolished the recrudescences of *P. inui*. Is anything more known about that?

Wyler: We first speculated that this might be due to an immunosuppressive role of the spleen (Wyler et al 1977). I now wonder whether we were seeing something along the lines of Dr Barnwell's findings—that is, of alterations in the virulence of the parasite for reasons other than immunological ones.

REFERENCES

Brown KN, McLaren DJ, Hills LA, Jarra W 1982 The binding of antibodies from *Plasmodium berghei*-infected rats to isoantigenic and parasite-specific antigenic sites on the surfaces of infected reticulocytes. Parasite Immunol (Oxf) 4:21-31

Hunter KW Jr, Winkelstein JA, Simpson TW 1979 Serum opsonic activity in rodent malaria: characteristics *in vitro*. J Immunol 123:2582-2587

McGregor IA 1978 Topical aspects of the epidemiology of malaria. Isr J Med Sci 14:523-533

Quinn TC, Wyler DJ 1980 Resolution of acute malaria (*Plasmodium berghei* in the rat); reversibility and spleen dependence. Am J Trop Med Hyg 29:1-4

Wyler DJ, Miller LH, Schmidt LH 1977 Spleen function in quartan malaria (due to *Plasmodium nui*): protective and suppressive roles in host defense. J Infect Dis 135:86-93

Zweig S, Singer SJ 1979 Con A induced endocytosis in rabbit reticulocytes and its decrease with reticulocyte maturation. J Cell Biol 80:487-491

Influence of the spleen on the expression of surface antigens on parasitized erythrocytes

JOHN W. BARNWELL, RUSSELL J. HOWARD and LOUIS H. MILLER

Laboratory of Parasitic Diseases, NIAID, National Institutes of Health, Bethesda, Md 20205, USA

Abstract Two malaria parasites, *Plasmodium knowlesi* and *P. falciparum*, when passaged in splenectomized hosts alter or fail to express parasite-dependent antigens on the surface membrane of erythrocytes infected with mature parasites. Experiments with cloned populations of *P. knowlesi* show this change to be phenotypic and to be modulated by the spleen of the host. In addition, the induction of antigen variation in *P. knowlesi* malaria apparently requires two factors: specific antibody and the spleen. Along with the altered expression of *P. knowlesi* variant antigen on the infected erythrocyte surface, there is a decrease in parasite virulence in non-splenectomized monkeys. It is suggested that the spleen-dependent expression of malarial antigens on the parasitized erythrocyte may be an adaptation of the malaria parasite for survival in the presence of a potentially destructive spleen-mediated host immunity.

The spleen is of prime importance to man's survival in malarious areas of the world. Although the mechanisms by which the spleen kills malaria parasites are not completely understood, this organ is the primary defence of the host against the erythrocytic stage of the malaria parasite and its removal frequently results in the resurgence of barely detectable parasitaemias to high levels that are often fatal for the host. However, there is yet another aspect to the interaction between the spleen and the intraerythrocytic malaria parasite. This additional aspect is the modulation of antigen expression on the surface of malaria-infected erythrocytes by the spleen and the ability of malaria parasites to evade this organ of host defence.

The plasma membrane of erythrocytes infected with malaria parasites undergoes profound changes as the intraerythrocytic parasite matures. With certain species of *Plasmodium* it has been found that neoantigens are expressed on the surface membrane of the parasitized host cell. Erythrocytes infected with the primate malaria parasite, *Plasmodium knowlesi*, were first shown to express parasite-dependent antigens on their surface when Eaton (1938) demonstrated that immune sera from infected rhesus monkeys (*Macaca mulatta*) would

1983 Malaria and the red cell. Pitman, London (Ciba Foundation symposium 94) p 117-136

agglutinate erythrocytes containing mature parasites (schizonts). Primary infections of *P. knowlesi* are usually fatal in rhesus monkeys unless early in infection the high parasitaemias are suppressed by antimalarial drugs. The infections then follow a chronic course with repeated waves of parasitaemia. The studies of K.N. Brown & I.N. Brown (1965), using the schizont-infected cell agglutination (SICA) assay, revealed that *P. knowlesi* undergoes antigenic variation and during each recurrent parasitaemia a new variant antigen (= SICA antigen) appears on the surface of parasitized erythrocytes (Fig.1). Antigenic variation occurs at frequent intervals during the many months that the infection can persist chronically (I.N. Brown et al 1968).

The human malaria parasite, *P. falciparum*, induces visually dramatic alterations in the membrane of the infected erythrocyte. As the intraerythrocytic parasite matures to the trophozoite stage, electron-dense excrescences, commonly known as 'knobs', appear. At the time when these knobs appear on the membrane of the parasitized erythrocyte, the trophozoite-infected cells retreat from the peripheral circulation to become sequestered along the venules and capillaries in certain organs such as the heart (Fig.1). The very close apposition

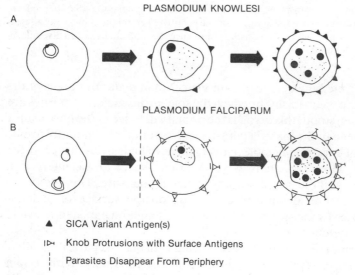

PLASMODIUM KNOWLESI

PLASMODIUM FALCIPARUM

▲ SICA Variant Antigen(s)

ID▷ Knob Protrusions with Surface Antigens

Parasites Disappear From Periphery

FIG. 1. Expression of parasite-induced antigens and alterations on erythrocytes parasitized by *Plasmodium knowlesi* and *P. falciparum*.

of these knob-like structures to the capillary endothelium *in vivo* (Luse & Miller 1971) and to endothelial cells *in vitro* (Udeinya et al 1981), as seen by electron microscopy, suggests that these structures mediate the specific attachment of *P. falciparum*-infected erythrocytes to these host cells. Immunoelectron microscopy has shown the area of the erythrocyte membrane over these electron-dense structures to be antigenic (Kilejian et al 1977, Langreth & Reese 1979).

Malaria parasites have necessarily evolved mechanisms to evade the spleen. The capacity of *P. knowlesi* to express variant antigens on the surface of parasitized erythrocytes is thought to be one mechanism whereby this parasite evades a host antibody response. Additionally, evidence from our research suggests that the parasite may also suppress, or otherwise evade, a spleen-dependent immune response. The attachment of *P. falciparum*-parasitized erythrocytes in sites away from the spleen may also be a protective adaptation of this malaria parasite, since the mature schizont-infected cells that are seques-tered would be more likely to suffer splenic clearance if they were to circulate, even in the absence of specific immune responses, simply as a consequence of the large size of the parasite inclusion at this stage.

Although there are hints in the literature that changes in malaria parasite biology might occur in splenectomized hosts (Garnham 1966, 1970), the first direct evidence of this was found with the Malaysian H strain of *P. knowlesi* (Barnwell et al 1982) and the Palo Alto strain of *P. falciparum* (David et al 1982). Our studies on modulation of the expression of parasite-induced surface antigens on parasitized erythrocytes by the spleen have used primarily two malarial species, *P. knowlesi* and *P. falciparum*. However, we believe that indirect evidence accumulated for other primate malarias and even for other haemosporidial parasites (e.g. *Babesia*) suggests that the phenomena we des-cribe here for *P. knowlesi* and *P. falciparum* may be of wide applicability.

Splenectomy and erythrocyte surface antigen expression in P. knowlesi malaria

Two lines of the Malaysian H strain of *P. knowlesi* had been carried in our laboratory for several years in rhesus monkeys. Both lines originated from a single infection of a rhesus monkey but one line had been passaged only in non-splenectomized (intact) monkeys (Line-I), while the other line was routinely passaged in splenectomized monkeys (Line-S).

When the parasitized erythrocytes from these two lines of *P. knowlesi* were screened with a battery of immune sera from chronically infected monkeys in the SICA test, a remarkable difference was noted. The Line-I infected erythro-cytes were agglutinated while the parasitized erythrocytes of Line-S were not. Such immune sera were known to be cross-reactive and will agglutinate many different parasite variant types of a given strain (Brown et al 1968). The lack of agglutination with the Line-S parasites was not due to their possession of a variant antigen other than those recognized by antibodies in the chronic im-mune sera. Antisera raised by twice infecting two monkeys with parasites of Line-S would also not agglutinate the parasitized erythrocytes of Line-S. *P.*

knowlesi parasites that had been passaged only in non-splenectomized monkeys (Line-I) were serially passaged in splenectomized animals. The parasitized cells from an intact monkey were strongly agglutinated by the immune sera. A SICA test on infected erythrocytes collected from the first passage in a splenectomized monkey revealed that the schizont-infected erythrocytes were still agglutinated by immune sera, but the titres were significantly reduced (four- to eight-fold). When these parasites were subpassaged to another splenectomized monkey and the parasitized erythrocytes again collected, the infected cells could not be agglutinated (see summary of results in Table 1).

The phenotype of *P. knowlesi* parasites that can be agglutinated by immune sera has been designated as SICA[+]. The phenotype of parasites that cannot be agglutinated by immune sera that are derived by passage of SICA[+] parasites in splenectomized monkeys has been designated SICA[−].

The fact that SICA[−] parasites are non-agglutinable and that this phenotype became evident only after passage in splenectomized monkeys suggested two important points. First, that in SICA[−] parasites the variant antigen normally expressed on the infected erythrocyte membrane is altered or absent and, second, that the spleen maintains the SICA[+] phenotype.

Altered expression of variant antigen is phenotypic

In the experimental conditions described above, the replacement of the SICA[+] phenotype of *P. knowlesi* by SICA[−] parasites in splenectomized monkeys could conceivably have resulted from the *selection* and *expansion* of a genotypically distinct population within a mixed population that was predominantly SICA[+]. Alternatively, the SICA[+] parasites could have *altered* their phenotype to SICA[−] when transferred to a splenectomized host.

To test these alternative possibilities, we cloned SICA[+] parasites in the following way. Individual schizont-infected erythrocytes were micromanipulated and cultured *in vitro* briefly, to allow rupture and reinvasion of fresh erythrocytes, which were injected intravenously into non-splenectomized monkeys. Several SICA[+] clones were derived in this way. Two such cloned SICA[+] parasite lines (Pk 1(A)+ and Pk 1(B)1+) were then passaged serially in splenectomized monkeys in the same way as for the uncloned line of SICA[+] parasites.

The kinetics and characteristics of the conversion of SICA[+] parasites to the SICA[−] phenotype were studied by the SICA test (agglutination) and also by surface-specific immunofluorescence of the parasitized erythrocytes (Table 2). Schizont-infected erythrocytes from intact monkeys were agglutinated to high titres with variant-specific or chronic immune sera. On passage in splenectomized monkeys the agglutination titres initially decreased steadily, as

TABLE 1 Summary of agglutinating activity of P. knowlesi parasites passaged in intact (Line-I) or splenectomized monkeys (Line-S)

Parasite line	Monkey status	Antisera for schizont-infected cell agglutination (SICA) test				
		Chronic cross-reactive	Anti-I(A) specific	Anti-I(B) specific	Anti-S One infection	Anti-S Two infections
S	Spx	-	-	-	-	-
I(A)	Intact	+++	+++	-	-	
I(B)	Intact	+++	-	+++	-	
I(A)	1st spx[a]	+	+	-		
I(A)	2nd spx[a]	-	-	-		

+, positive agglutination; number of +'s, relative titre of agglutination.
-, no agglutination at 1 : 10 dilution of sera.
(A) or (B) refers to two different variant populations of Line-I.
[a] Serial passage of Line-I in splenectomized monkeys (spx).

previously seen with uncloned parasites, and then became negative for agglutination. The percentage of parasitized erythrocytes reacting by immunofluorescence in non-splenectomized monkeys was > 99% at this time. On first
passage of the SICA[+] parasites in a splenectomized monkey the percentage
of fluorescence-reactive parasitized cells remained the same (> 99%), even
though agglutination titres had fallen 4–16-fold. However, the intensity of the
fluorescence was less than that seen with the parasitized erythrocytes from an
intact animal. When infected cells were negative for agglutination, the parasitized cells were also negative by immunofluorescence (Table 2).

These results show that the switch from the SICA[+] phenotype to a
SICA[−] phenotype in splenectomized hosts is an alteration of expression by
the total SICA[+] population rather than the result of selection of genotypically distinct SICA[−] parasites in the original population. Furthermore, the
transition from SICA[+] to SICA[−] is characterized by a decrease in the
quantity of SICA antigen expressed on the erythrocyte membrane. The results
do not suggest that there is a change in the equilibrium of alternating SICA[+]/
SICA[−] phenotypes; if this were so we should have seen some parasitized
erythrocytes becoming SICA[−] with others remaining SICA[+] and strongly
fluorescence-reactive. The latter situation of alternating phenotypes of a stable
genotype is common to bacterial phase variation—for example, the switch
between H1 and H2 flagellar antigens in *Salmonella* (Zieg et al 1977) and the
piliated and non-piliated states of *Escherichia coli* (Swaney et al 1977),
although it should be noted that piliation in *E. coli* may also show a quantitative
regulation of expression. Whether the regulation of the expression of the
surface antigens on *P. knowlesi*-parasitized erythrocytes is by mechanisms
similar to those regulating bacterial phase variation is not known.

Antigenic variation in P. knowlesi and the spleen

The evidence of K.N. Brown (1973) using non-cloned *P. knowlesi* parasites led
to the postulate that antigenic variation in *P. knowlesi* malaria was an antibody-
induced phenotypic change rather than immunoselection of spontaneously
occurring mutations in the variant population. With cloned *P. knowlesi* parasites of different variant antigen specificities we have been able to re-examine
the nature of the antigenic variation in *P. knowlesi* (Table 3). When infected
monkeys were challenged with the same cloned variant with which they had
been previously infected, and drug-cured, there was a switch in variant type
(homologous challenge). Although the parasitized erythrocytes of the infection which resulted from the challenge were not agglutinated by prechallenge
sera, the parasitized erythrocytes were agglutinated by chronic immune sera,

TABLE 2 Expression of variant antigen by P. knowlesi clones in intact monkeys and after passage in splenectomized monkeys

Parasite clone	Sera	Intact monkey	Agglutination titres and (% + fluorescence) after passage in splenectomized monkeys		
			1st passage	2nd passage	3rd passage
1(A)+	anti-1(A)+	+++(>99.0)	+(>99.0)	−(0.0)	−(0.0)
	anti-1(B)1+	−(0.0)	−(0.0)	−(0.0)	−(0.0)
	chronic	+++(99.0)	+(>99.0)	−(0.0)	−(0.0)
1(B)1+	anti-1(A)+	−(0.0)	−(0.0)	−(0.0)	−(0.0)
	anti-1(B)1+	++++(>99.0)	++(>99.0)	+(98.0)	−(0.0)
	chronic	+++(>99.0)	++(>99.0)	+(89.0)	−(0.0)

showing that the parasites were SICA[+] but of a different variant specificity not recognized by the antibody present in prechallenge sera. Challenge of monkeys with a variant type different to the one used for the initial infection (heterologous challenge) did not result in a change of variant type in the infection produced by the challenge, as judged by agglutination with sera specific for the challenge variant type. Prechallenge sera from the two monkeys did agglutinate the parasitized cells of the variant type used to sensitize the monkeys (not shown in Table 3), but not the parasitized erythrocytes of the challenge inocula or of the infection resulting from the challenge inocula. This has provided the first evidence that cloned SICA[+] parasites can alter their variant type, indicating that parasites of a particular phenotype have a geno-type which codes for more than one variant phenotype. Furthermore, in non-splenectomized monkeys antigenic change appears to depend on the presence of the appropriate (homologous) anti-variant antibody. Taken together, our evidence suggests that antigenic variation in *P. knowlesi* is an antibody-induced alteration of gene expression.

We have also used splenectomized monkeys with circulating variant-specific agglutinating antibodies to test for the parasites' capacity to display antigenic variation in this host environment (Table 3). In these experiments intact monkeys were first infected with a clone of known variant specificity, the infection was cured, and the animals were immunized with killed schizont-infected cells of the same variant type in Freund's incomplete adjuvant to boost the agglutination titres. The monkeys were then splenectomized and three to six weeks later challenged with parasites of the same variant type used for sensitizing the animal. The post-splenectomy but prechallenge sera agglutin-ated not only the parasitized erythrocytes of the challenge inocula, but also the parasitized erythrocytes of the infection resulting from challenge, albeit at much lower titres. Although specific antibody was present at the time of challenge, the parasites did not switch their variant type, as would have occur-red in non-splenectomized monkeys, suggesting that antigenic variation re-quires the spleen, in addition to variant-specific agglutinating antibodies. Why this is so is unknown, but it does seem that the spleen modulates molecular expression in *P. knowlesi* in two ways. In the first, the spleen regulates the expression of variant antigen on the erythrocyte surface. The failure to express parasite-induced antigens on the erythrocyte membrane in splenectomized hosts may involve either a failure in the transport to and insertion of variant antigen into the host cell membrane, or a failure in expression (transcription) or synthesis (translation) at the gene level. Either way would result in a decreased level of variant antigen expressed on the erythrocyte membrane. The second modulating influence of the spleen involves an all-or-none mechan-ism, such that in splenectomized hosts alternative genes for variant antigen are not expressed even when variant-specific antibody is present.

TABLE 3 Antigenic variation of cloned P. knowlesi in non-splenectomized and splenectomized monkeys

Monkey status	Variant used for challenge[a]	Parasites from:	Antisera for agglutination		
			Prechallenge	Variant-specific	chronic
Intact	Homologous	Challenge inocula	+++	+++	+++
		Infection after challenge	−	−	+++
Intact	Heterologous	Challenge inocula	−[b]	+++	+++
		Infection after challenge	−	+++	+++
Splenectomized	Homologous	Challenge inocula	+++	+++	+++
		Infection after challenge	+	+	+

[a] Homologous variant challenge refers to the inoculation of monkeys with the same variant type of parasite to which the monkeys had been previously sensitized by infection and drug cure. Heterologous challenges are initiated with variant types initially different from the variant types with which the monkeys had originally been sensitized.

[b] The prechallenge sera from these monkeys did agglutinate erythrocytes parasitized with the variant type to which they were initially sensitized by primary infection and drug cure.

Surface antigen expression in P. falciparum malaria

P. falciparum trophozoite- and schizont-infected erythrocytes have knob-like excrescences in their surface membranes which mediate the attachment of these cells to endothelial cells *in vivo* (Luse & Miller 1971) and *in vitro* (Udeinya et al 1981), probably via a specific receptor molecule on the erythrocyte membrane surface. These parasitized erythrocytes also bind by the same mechanism to cultured human melanoma cells (Schmidt et al 1982). Parasite-dependent antigens on the *P. falciparum*-infected erythrocyte surface have been demonstrated by immunoelectron microscopy (Kilejian et al 1977, Langreth & Reese 1979) and by the binding of infected erythrocytes to antibody-coated protein A–Sepharose beads, as well as by surface immunofluorescence (Hommel et al 1982).

Observations of schizont-infected cells in the circulation (schizontaemia) of splenectomized chimpanzees and humans with falciparum malaria (Garnham 1966) contrast dramatically with the almost complete absence of these cells from the peripheral circulation of intact hosts. These results suggest that changes in membrane antigens might also occur with *P. falciparum*. David et al (1982), using squirrel monkeys (*Saimiri sciureus*) infected with *P. falciparum*, found differences in the expression of antigens on the surface of parasitized erythrocytes from intact and splenectomized monkeys. Parasitized erythrocytes from intact monkeys bound *in vitro* to melanoma cells and were sequestered *in vivo*. *P. falciparum*-infected erythrocytes from splenectomized monkeys were not sequestered *in vivo* and did not bind to melanoma cells *in vitro*. With surface immunofluorescence methods it was found that immune sera from intact monkeys reacted only with the parasitized erythrocytes from intact monkeys, and immune sera raised against parasites passaged in splenectomized animals reacted only with parasitized erythrocytes from splenectomized monkeys. These results suggest that *P. falciparum* may exist in alternative antigenic stages, depending on whether the host is splenectomized or not.

Our experiments along similar lines with *P. falciparum* in non-splenectomized and splenectomized owl monkeys (*Aotus trivergatus griseimembra*) are summarized in Table 4.

Briefly, an isolate of *P. falciparum* (St. Lucia strain from El Salvador, a gift of W. E. Collins, CDC), previously passaged in three splenectomized owl monkeys, was inoculated into a fourth splenectomized monkey. The infection was characterized by peripheral schizontaemia. Furthermore, parasitized erythrocytes taken from the animal when parasites were at the ring stage, and grown *in vitro* to the trophozoite stage, failed to bind to cultured endothelial cells, suggesting that some alteration had occurred in the nature of the knobs on the surface of these parasitized erythrocytes. In fact, electron microscopy revealed

TABLE 4 Summary of results with P. falciparum in intact and splenectomized owl monkeys

Monkey status	Knobs (% K+)	In vivo sequestration	In vitro binding (B)
Intact	K+(100)	++	++
Spx[a] (1st passage)	K+(100)	+	+
Spx (2nd passage)	K+(100)	−	−
Spx (4th passage)	K+/K−(43)	−	−
Spx (chronic)	K−(0)	−	−
Spx (4th passage) → intact	K+/K−(88)	+	+

[a]Splenectomized.

a mixed population of knobby (K+) and knobless (K−) parasitized erythrocytes from this splenectomized animal. This infection was allowed to become chronic, and exhibited several recrudescences (five) over a nine-month period. Parasitized erythrocytes from the fourth recrudescence were all K− and failed to bind (symbolized as [B−]) to cultured endothelial or melanoma cells. The K+/K− mixed population from the initial parasitaemia of the fourth splenectomized passage was inoculated into a non-splenectomized monkey. The parasites from this intact monkey bound to cultured endothelial and melanoma cells. Although some of the infected erythrocytes were K−, the percentage of K+ infected erythrocytes was greater than that found in the splenectomized monkey (88% vs. 43%). After further passage in intact monkeys the parasitized erythrocytes were all K+ and continued to bind (symbolized as [B+]) to melanoma cells *in vitro* and to be sequestered *in vivo*. A fascinating additional change in the parasite phenotype resulted from passage of this population serially in two splenectomized monkeys. The resultant parasites possessed knobs (100% K+) but did *not* become sequestered *in vivo* and did *not* bind *in vitro* to melanoma cells. No significant difference in knob density was found in the K+ parasitized erythrocytes from intact or splenectomized monkeys.

These results suggest that the morphological alterations of the outer membrane of *P. falciparum*-infected cells known as knobs result from more than one altered membrane component. There are components responsible for the morphological alteration itself, and others responsible for the capacity of the parasitized cells to bind to endothelium. Clearly, several antigens of different functions may contribute to this membrane alteration and *P. falciparum*, like *P. knowlesi*, shows changes in the expression of one or both of these knob components when passaged in an asplenic host.

These changes can develop rapidly, as in the change from the K+/B+ to the K+/B− phenotype or vice versa; or slowly, as in the transition from K+/B− to a K−/B− phenotype; or changes can be virtually non-existent, as we have noted for one strain of *P. falciparum*. The Malayan-Camp CH/Q strain remains

as the K+/B+ phenotype, even after multiple serial passages in splenectomized animals. *P. fragile,* a falciparum-like parasite of macaque monkeys, also
switches very rapidly from a non-sequestering parasite to a sequestering parasite when passaged from a splenectomized to a non-splenectomized monkey. In
contrast, *P. coatneyi,* another falciparum-like parasite of macaques, does not
become non-sequestering when passaged in splenectomized monkeys (J.
Leech, unpublished data).

The spleen as a modulator of parasite antigen expression

The existence of the SICA[+] phenotype in non-splenectomized monkeys and
the conversion to the SICA[−] phenotype in splenectomized monkeys suggests
that the spleen maintains the SICA[+] phenotype. That the alteration from
SICA[+] to SICA[−] and the reverse (SICA[−] to SICA[+]) is phenotypic,
and not the result of the selection of genotypes, also supports the idea that the
spleen modulates the expression of parasite-dependent antigens on the
erythrocyte membrane. It could be argued that the spleen functions as a
'conditioner' of the erythrocyte membrane which is required for the expression
of antigens as the erythrocytes pass through the splenic architecture (Cooper et
al 1974). However, this is probably not the case, since SICA[+] parasites
passaged through splenectomized monkeys for the first time still express
variant antigen, although at reduced levels. In addition, SICA[−] parasites
inoculated into non-splenectomized monkeys initially do not always express
variant antigen.

The alternative hypothesis that we favour at present supposes that *P. knowlesi, P. falciparum* and other malaria parasites are capable of responding to
certain environmental conditions in the spleen, or to other stimuli such as
soluble factors or mediators released in the spleen, in such a way that certain
parasite antigens such as the SICA variant antigen are only then expressed.

Environmental and physiological factors are known to influence bacterial
phase variation. Culture conditions influence whether or not *E. coli* strains
exhibit pili (Swaney et al 1977), and different opacity variants of *Neisseria
gonorrhoeae* are associated with the menstrual cycle in women (Salit et al
1980). A spleen cell factor is also known to inhibit the transformation *in vitro* of
Leishmania from the amastigote to the promastigote stage (Brun et al 1976).

Surface antigen expression, virulence and the spleen

In addition to a loss of agglutinability in the SICA assay, we have preliminary
results to suggest that *P. knowlesi* parasites passaged in splenectomized monk-

eys (SICA[−]) are less virulent than normal in intact monkeys. *P. knowlesi* is normally highly virulent in non-splenectomized rhesus monkeys and usually kills this host (Garnham 1966). We have also found this to be the case with SICA[+] parasites, but not always with SICA[−] parasites. In four examples of intact monkeys infected with SICA[+] parasites, parasitaemias rose 8–10-fold daily and would have killed the animals if antimalarial drugs had not been administered. The peak parasitaemias were 16%, 19%, 21% and 25% at the time of treatment (Fig. 2A).

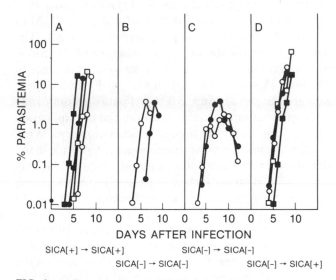

FIG. 2. A. Parasitaemias of SICA[+] *P. knowlesi* in four intact rhesus monkeys. B–C. Parasitaemias of SICA[−] parasites in intact monkeys where parasites remained SICA[−] (see text). D. Parasitaemias of SICA[−] parasites in intact monkeys which converted to SICA[+]. The different symbols indicate the individual monkeys.

Infection of intact rhesus monkeys with SICA[−] parasites also resulted in 8- to 10-fold daily increases in parasitaemia at low parasitaemias (< 1%). However, the parasitaemias in four monkeys began to decline after reaching peaks of 1–6%. Two monkeys were given chloroquine after the initial decline in parasitaemia (Fig. 2B). In two additional monkeys the infections were followed for several days during the parasitaemic decline before antimalarial therapy was given (Fig. 2C). In four other monkeys, parasitaemias continued to rise to 21%, 25%, 27% and 60% before the initiation of drug therapy (Fig. 2D). SICA tests were done on the parasitized erythrocytes at the time of peak parasitaemia. In those cases where infections were controlled the parasites remained SICA[−], whereas in the monkeys which did not control their infections the parasites were found to have converted from SICA[−] to the

SICA[+] phenotype. Splenectomized rhesus monkeys, in contrast, do not control infections with SICA[−] or SICA[+] parasites.

Decreased virulence to intact animals has been produced in other haemo-protozoans by passage in splenectomized hosts— for example, *Plasmodium cynomolgi* in rhesus monkeys (L.H. Schmidt, unpublished data) and *Babesia bovis* in cattle (Callow 1977).

An intriguing aspect of our results is the correlation of virulence and expression of the SICA phenotype. If the loss of agglutinability (SICA[−] phenotype) and not some other unidentified change was the cause of the decreased virulence of *P. knowlesi*, then parasites that express variant antigen (SICA[+] phenotype) may have a survival advantage when the spleen is present. The ability of SICA[+] *P. knowlesi* to vary the antigenic structure of the SICA determinant of itself suggests that this is important to its survival in the face of an immune response by the host. However, the variant antigen does not appear to be required for parasite growth *per se*, since SICA[−] parasites uniformly reach high parasitaemias in splenectomized animals and initial multiplication rates for SICA[+] and SICA[−] parasites are similar in intact monkeys. Why, indeed, does the SICA[+] parasite insert a highly immunogenic molecule in the erythrocyte membrane that it must vary to escape an antibody response? It may be that the variant antigen expressed on the surface of parasitized erythrocytes functions additionally to depress a spleen-dependent immune response to another target of parasiticidal immunity (variant or strain transcending?), or to prevent access of the immune response to the parasite. The ability of parasitized erythrocytes to avoid passage through the spleen would be one way in which a spleen-mediated immune response would not be able to act against the malaria-parasitized erythrocyte. *P. knowlesi* is sequestered to some extent, primarily in the liver, during the early parasitaemic rise (Miller et al 1971). Sequestration in *P. falciparum* malaria is much more evident, though. The expression of a receptor molecule on the surface of parasitized erythrocytes that serves to attach these cells to endothelium clearly would prevent their passage through a hostile spleen. This does not preclude the possibility that *P. falciparum* may also produce a molecule that depresses a spleen-dependent immune response.

P. inui, a quartan malaria parasite of macaques, survives as a chronic infection for many years and is analogous to *P. malariae* in humans. It has been observed that in splenectomized rhesus monkeys infected with *P. inui* the duration of the chronic infection is much shorter than chronic infections of this parasite in intact monkeys, even though in the splenectomized rhesus monkeys there was a much higher mortality rate during each peak of parasitaemia (Wyler et al 1977). It was suggested that the spleen had both protective and suppressive roles in host defence, acting at different stages of the infection. There may be a parallel between our observations with *P. knowlesi* on the role of the spleen in modulating antigenic expression and parasite virulence and these studies with *P. inui*. In the splenectomized monkeys the *P. inui* parasites may have failed to express antigens that function in parasite survival, and as a consequence they were more easily eliminated by host immunity.

The ability of malaria parasites to express molecules on the surface membrane of the infected erythrocyte in response to the spleen may be an adaptation of malaria parasites that enhances their survival in the presence of a potentially lethal, spleen-mediated host immunity.

Acknowledgements

We thank Dr Hayden Coon for the micromanipulation in cloning *P. knowlesi* and Drs Masamichi Aikawa and Yoshihiro Ito for the electron microscopy on *P. falciparum*.

REFERENCES

Barnwell JW, Howard RJ, Miller LH 1982 Altered expression of *Plasmodium knowlesi* variant antigen on the erythrocyte membrane in splenectomized rhesus monkeys. J Immunol 128:224-226

Brown IN, Brown KN, Hills LA 1968 Immunity to malaria: the antibody response to antigenic variation by *Plasmodium knowlesi*. Immunology 14:127-138

Brown KN 1973 Antibody induced variation in malaria parasites. Nature (Lond) 242:49-50

Brown KN, Brown IN 1965 Immunity to malaria: antigenic variation in chronic infections of *Plasmodium knowlesi*. Nature (Lond) 208:1286-1288

Brun R, Berens, RL, Krassner SM 1976 Inhibition of *Leishmania donovani* transformation by hamster spleen homogenates and active human lymphocytes. Nature (Lond) 262: 689-691

Callow LL 1977 Vaccination against bovine babesiosis. Adv Exp Med Biol 93:121-149

Cooper RA, Kimball DB, Durocher JR 1974 Role of the spleen in membrane conditioning and hemolysis of spur cells in liver disease. N Engl J Med 290:1279-1284

David PH, Hommel M, Udeinya IJ, Miller LH 1982 *Plasmodium falciparum* malaria in the squirrel monkey: surface modifications of infected erythrocytes are modulated by the spleen. Fed Proc 41:483 (abstr 1243)

Eaton MD 1938 The agglutination of *Plasmodium knowlesi* by immune serum. J Exp Med 67:857

Garnham PCC 1966 Malaria parasites and other haemosporidia. Blackwell Scientific Publications, Oxford, p 287, 383

Garnham PCC 1970 The role of the spleen in protozoal infections with special reference to splenectomy. Acta Trop (Basel) 27:1

Hommel M, David PH, Oligino LD, David JR 1982 Expression of strain specific surface antigens on *Plasmodium falciparum*-infected erythrocytes. Parasite Immunol (Oxf), in press

Kilejian A, Abati A, Trager W 1977 *Plasmodium falciparum* and *Plasmodium coatneyi*: immunogenicity of 'knob- like protrusions' on infected erythrocyte membranes. Exp Parasitol 42:157-164

Langreth SG, Reese RT 1979 Antigenicity of the infected erythrocyte and merozoite surfaces in *falciparum* malaria. J Exp Med 150: 1241-1254

Luse SA, Miller LH 1971. *Plasmodium falciparum* malaria: ultrastructure of parasitized erythro-
    cytes in cardiac vessels. Am J Trop Med Hyg 20:655-660
Miller LH, Fremount HN, Luse SA 1971 Deep vascular schizogony of *Plasmodium knowlesi* in
    Macaca mulatta. Am J Trop Med Hyg 20:816-824
Salit IE, Balake M, Gotschlich EC 1980 Intra-strain heterogeneity of gonococcal pili is related to
    opacity colony variance. J Exp Med 151:716-725
Schmidt JA, Udeinya IJ, Leech JH, Hay RJ, Aikawa M, Barnwell JW, Green I, Miller LH 1982
    Plasmodium falciparum malaria: an amelanotic melanoma cell line bears receptors for the knob
    ligand on infected erythrocytes. J Clin Invest, in press
Swaney LM, Liu YP, To CM, To CC, Ippen-Ihler K, Brinton CC Jr 1977 Isolation and character-
    ization of *Escherichia coli* phase variants and mutants deficient in type 1 pilus production. J
    Bacteriol 130:495-505
Udeinya IJ, Schmidt JA, Aikawa M, Miller LH, Green I 1981 Falciparum malaria-infected
    erythrocytes specifically bind to cultured human endothelial cells. Science (Wash DC) 213:555-
    557
Wyler DJ, Miller LH, Schmidt LH 1977 Spleen function in quartan malaria (due to *Plasmodium
    inui*): evidence for both protective and suppressive roles in host defense. J Infect Dis 135:86-93
Zieg J, Silverman M, Hilmen M, Simon M 1977 Recombinational switch for gene expression.
    Science (Wash DC) 196:170-172

DISCUSSION

Brown: Have you looked at *P. knowlesi* in *Macaca irus*, the natural host?

Barnwell: I have tried to do that, but unfortunately most of the cynomolgus monkeys that we get have already been naturally infected, and reinfecting them is not always possible. In one test we found that in *M. irus* we could get agglutination of *P. knowlesi* -infected cells that was variant-specific. We would need laboratory-raised cynomolgus monkeys to do this type of comparative study.

Brown: The rhesus monkey system has many advantages, but one disadvantage is that the induction of protection is so prolonged. That can be an advantage in some ways, of course.

Barnwell: At least you can get enough parasites to test and do biochemical studies on. If you manipulate the system, it reveals certain biological differ-ences that might not be seen in a system where there are only low-grade infections, as in the natural host for *P. knowlesi*, namely *M. irus*.

Brown: Have you looked at protein synthesis in the SICA[−] parasites?

Barnwell: We are doing that now, trying to see whether there is a failure to express this antigen on the surface of the infected red cell, or a complete cessation in the production of the variant antigen, and if there are any other major differences, besides lacking variant antigen, between SICA[−] and SICA[+] parasites.

Howard: We see over 500 malarial proteins on a two-dimensional gel after biosynthetic radiolabelling with amino acids. In order to see differences in proteins synthesized by SICA[+] and SICA[−] parasites it has been necessary to use computer-assisted analysis. Only a small number of proteins that are quantitatively minor malarial proteins are actually different (R.J. Howard, S.B. Aley & P. Lemkin, unpublished results).

Brown: So you see nothing comparable to Kilejian's K− parasites (*P. falciparum*), which are apparently not synthesizing one particular protein?

Howard: There are no *gross* changes in the proteins of SICA[−] and SICA[+] parasites. The knob-related protein identified by Kilejian was a major biosynthetic component readily identified on a one-dimensional gel. We haven't identified an analogous difference with SICA[+] and [−] parasites.

Barnwell: In an intact or a splenectomized host, at least initially the growth rates for the SICA[+] and SICA[−] parasites are virtually identical. There is no inhibition of the parasite growth as a result of lack of some metabolic function.

Sherman: In *P. falciparum*, you found 100% K+ parasitized erythrocytes after the second passage in a splenectomized host, and these cells did not bind to melanoma cells *in vitro* (Table 4). You concluded that having knobs is not directly correlated with ability to bind to host cells. As Dr Brown says, Kilejian (1979) has reported a protein band that seems to be associated with K positivity (presence of knobs). We (J. Gruenberg & I.S. Sherman, unpublished results) attempted to repeat her work, comparing K− and K+ strains and employing metabolic labelling with a mixture of ^{14}C-labelled amino acids and electrophoretic separation on one-dimensional gels. We could not find a distinct 80 000 M_r protein that characteristically appeared in K+ and was absent in K− parasitized cells. The strain used is the Gambian FCR3, originally derived from William Trager's laboratory, sent to Ted Green and later obtained from NIH.

Howard: We have also looked for the knob-related protein of Kilejian with Dr Terry Hadley at NIH. In two experiments we have so far not found this protein, so we are hoping to repeat this work in close collaboration with Dr Kilejian. It is possible that the parasites used by us and by Dr Kilejian are different or that our conditions of culture affect synthesis of the knob-related protein. We also believe that it will be necessary to compare the proteins synthesized by several K+ and K− lines of different origin to define knob-related components.

Sherman: Of course, the protein identified by Dr Kilejian may not be localized in the knob.

Howard: True; it may be related to knob synthesis or expression, but within the parasite. We expect that several components are involved in the knob structure on infected cells. In *P. brasilianum*, knobs appear at high density on the surface of infected erythrocytes but these cells are not sequestered. The knobs of *P. brasilianum* presumably have some function other than the function identified for knobs of *P. falciparum*-type parasites (namely, containing endothelial cell-binding components). Knobs may also function as localized zones of altered membrane permeability where transport proteins are situated. Antigens may be released from knobs to function as modulators of host immune responses. They should also have structural components which create the membrane shape change and electron-dense material below the membrane. Knobs may have a complex structure, involving more than one new protein.

Sherman: You discussed the role of the spleen as a 'modulator' of antigenic expression by the parasite. What does 'modulation' mean in this context?

Barnwell: To me it means that the parasite is reacting to the host, probably in response to a specific splenic function. One can postulate that there is something different about the erythrocytes of the splenectomized host that does not allow expression of the SICA antigen on the surface of the parasitized erythrocyte. However, on first passage of SICA[+] cells in splenectomized monkeys, when all the parasites are in the splenectomized host cells the antigen is still expressed, though to a decreased extent. Also, when you pass SICA[−] parasites from splenectomized to intact animals, they do not always immediately re-express the antigen. Perhaps, like other organisms, the parasite can respond to conditions in its environment, whatever those conditions may be. Smaller molecular weight compounds might be released at certain times, or continuously, by the spleen; or perhaps splenic factors are produced as part of the early development of an immune response to which a parasite may react.

Sherman: Do you see this as a turning on of a gene or genes in the parasite, the gene product(s) then being transported to the surface of the erythrocyte?

Barnwell: Yes, that is one possibility.

Anders: There are interesting parallels with the *Babesia bovis* system, although that is not so well worked out. The vaccine for tick fever of cattle in Australia is an attenuated parasite produced by passaging a virulent isolate of *B. bovis* through splenectomized calves (Callow & Mellors 1966). Lesley Kahl in our group, in collaboration with colleagues at the Tick Fever Research Station, Wacol, Queensland, has been looking at the pattern of antigens in various strains of *B. bovis* (L.P. Kahl et al, unpublished work). There are major biosynthetically labelled proteins which are dominant antigens unique to different strains of *B. bovis*. The avirulent form of one strain (used for vaccination) has two dominant antigens not present as dominant antigens in the virulent strain from which it was derived. Changes in the expression of one or the other of these antigens occur when the avirulent *B. bovis* is passaged through the tick vector or through intact cattle. Dr Barnwell, what happens when you put your SICA[−] parasite back through a mosquito?

Barnwell: We have fed mosquitoes on splenectomized monkeys containing SICA[−] parasites. These infected mosquitoes were then fed again on intact (non-splenectomized) monkeys. The parasites from the infection that resulted in the intact monkeys remained SICA[−].

Cohen: I would like to make another suggestion about the mechanism underlying loss of virulence. This concerns the expression on the merozoite-infected cell of the variable antigen. When you test antibodies *in vitro* against *P. knowlesi,* they seem to act predominantly against merozoites and inhibit their reinvasion. If you test sera derived either by infection or by vaccination with defined variants, that inhibition is predominantly variant-specific but not entirely so; there is cross-variant inhibition at a lower titre. Presumably this is why you see rapid protective responses against new variants in immune monkeys. One then asks whether the variant-specific antigen on the schizont-infected red cell is the same as the variant antigen on the merozoite-infected cell. Apparently it is not, because using SICA-specific antisera one cannot visualize the SICA antigen on the surface of the merozoite. Evidently, the merozoite surface includes a specific variant antigen which, although not identical to the antigen on the surface of the schizont, is related to it, and some other antigens which are common to different variants. An interesting question is whether, in *P. knowlesi* from splenectomized monkeys, the variant-specific antigen is present on merozoites. Loss of that antigen (concomitantly with loss of SICA[−] antigen) may lead to loss of virulence. For example, in the natural host (*Macaca fascicularis*), born in the UK and hence not previously exposed, infection leads to the expected pre-patent period followed by a rising parasitaemia for five days that is identical to that in the rhesus monkey, but is followed by control of the infection. Those early sera, 5–7 days after infection, when tested *in vitro,* inhibit merozoites of several different variants. The natural host (*M. fascicularis*), unlike the rhesus monkey, has the capacity to 'look' chiefly at those antigens that are common to all variants, and rapidly controls the infection. If the merozoites released from your SICA[−] schizonts lack the dominant variant-specific antigen, then the rhesus monkey may also react predominantly against common antigens, which would explain the loss of virulence. Have you thought along those lines?

Barnwell: Yes. We are trying now to set up such studies with the Central Drug Research Institute in India, to be able to develop more sound statistical and immunobiological information on this difference in virulence between SICA[+] and SICA[−] parasites. One project is to use *Macaca radiata,* which has a similar pattern of *P. knowlesi* infection as *M. irus,* and see what happens there. So we are thinking along these lines. The other possibility is that SICA[+] parasites may depress certain immune responses and that SICA[−] parasites don't.

Phillips: We (McLean et al 1982) have been looking at antigenic variation in the erythrocytic parasites of *P. chabaudi* in the mouse. Starting with a cloned and mosquito-passaged population, our preliminary results suggest that recrudescent populations are usually antigenically different from the infecting population. After the recrudescent parasites have gone through the mosquito they revert to the original population in their antigenic type. One difficulty in all this work is that we can't identify the variant type of a single infected red cell; for this and other reasons we have been cloning recrudescent populations, because we had an indication that the recrudescent populations are antigenically heterogeneous. The initial results indicate that they are in fact heterogeneous populations. Do you find that the populations of *P. knowlesi* that you have cloned are heterogeneous in the antigenic types present?

Barnwell: There is some antigenic heterogeneity between cloned populations derived from one uncloned infection. But we don't know whether it's because there is heterogeneity in the original, uncloned population, or because, as the clone is growing up in the monkey, changes in antigenicity are occurring over the 10–11 day period. Some rhesus monkeys develop immune responses in that time and antigenic variation may occur.

Wyler: I believe Dr Leon Schmidt has made similar (unpublished) observations on virulence in *P. cynomolgi,* which suggest that your findings might also be extended to vivax types of malaria. Thinking of the role of the spleen, a similarity between the spleen and deep vascular beds is the low oxygen tension there. Have you any thoughts about the interaction of parasitized red cells with vascular endothelium and whether the fact that they are sequestered in deep vascular beds, and the necessary adaptation to low oxygen tension, might be related to a similar experience of these cells in the spleen?

Barnwell: This is an interesting possibility. I have cultured *P. knowlesi* under a range of physiological conditions. When we culture parasitized cells we use a low oxygen tension (3%). We culture for one to six days and then test for SICA antigen. Under this low oxygen tension, and a higher CO_2 tension (6%), there is no change in SICA phenotype. I don't know whether this situation is similar to what happens *in vivo.* I have recently, in a preliminary trial, co-cultured spleen cells from an *Aotus* monkey with *P. falciparum* -infected red cells *in vitro* and converted a K$^-$ parasite to a K$^+$ phenotype. Supernatants from *in vitro* cultured spleen cells also had a similar effect (J. W. Barnwell, unpublished observations).

REFERENCES

Callow LL, Mellors LT 1966 A new vaccine for *Babesia argentina* infection prepared in splenectomised calves. Aust Vet J 42:464
Kilejian A 1979 Characterization of a protein correlated with the production of knob-like protrusions on membranes of erythrocytes infected with *Plasmodium falciparum.* Proc Natl Acad Sci USA 76:4650-4653
McLean SA, Pearson CD, Phillips RS 1982 *Plasmodium chabaudi* : evidence of antigenic variation by the parasite during recrudescent parasitaemias in mice. Exp Parasitol, in press

Protective immunity to malaria and anti-erythrocyte autoimmunity

W. JARRA

Division of Parasitology, National Institute for Medical Research, Mill Hill, London NW7 1AA, UK

Abstract The intraerythrocytic development of malaria parasites results in considerable modification and destruction of erythrocytes. This may lead to the breaking of tolerance such that immune recognition of 'self' or 'modified self' erythrocyte antigens by B or T lymphocytes occurs. Such recognition may be a vital factor in the induction of protective immunity even though it may also cause immunopathology. Serological and immunocytochemical assays have been used to demonstrate, in the serum of *Plasmodium berghei*-infected or immune rats, antibodies to isoantigenic determinants on infected erythrocytes. Absorption studies indicated that antigens specifically associated with parasitized erythrocytes and erythrocyte isoantigens were closely associated at the surface membrane.

Extensive erythrocyte modification and destruction, artificially generated by phenylhydrazine treatment, significantly enhanced immunity against rodent malaria. In contrast, the generation of an incomplete anti-erythrocyte autoantibody response in mice by the injection of cross-reacting rat erythrocytes failed to augment protective responses to *P. chabaudi*. The reinjection of rat erythrocytes into mice previously injected with rat erythrocytes suppresses further autoantibody synthesis and the mice revert to the normal (Coombs-negative) state. Spleen cells from rat erythrocyte-treated mice transfer this suppression when injected into syngeneic recipients. Coombs-negative mice reinjected with rat erythrocytes failed to show enhanced protective responses to *P. chabaudi*. Spleen cells from such Coombs-negative mice, injected into sublethally irradiated recipients, increased the protective effects of concurrently transferred spleen cells from malaria-immune donors when the recipients were challenged with *P. chabaudi*.

Protective immunity to malaria

Protective immunity to erythrocytic malaria in man initially results in a decrease in the numbers or frequency of fevers and a reduction of parasitaemia to subpathogenic levels. Depending on the parasite species, subsequent recrudescences or relapses may then occur, which may be either acute and run a clinical course, or asymptomatic. Attacks then decrease in severity

1983 Malaria and the red cell. Pitman, London (Ciba Foundation symposium 94) p 137-158

with time, and infections with even the most virulent species tend towards chronicity. In inhabitants of regions where almost uninterrupted transmission and thus continual reinfection occur, consistent patterns of susceptibility and resistance are observed. A high incidence of often severe erythrocytic infection occurs in children, while comparatively few parasites are detected in adults (I. N. Brown 1969). Protective immunity develops slowly and apparently requires prolonged, often clinically significant attacks for its generation. Individuals able to survive this period become semi-immune, yet parasites persist in their blood in low numbers. This persistence may reflect the parasite's ability to evade the host's immune response. From studies in experimental animals infected with malaria, a number of possible evasion mechanisms have been proposed (reviewed by Cohen 1980), of which the most pertinent to this paper is intrastrain antigenic variation. Host immunity must be capable of transcending such variation, so that parasitaemias are maintained at low levels. With the possible exception of *Plasmodium malariae* infections, parasites may eventually be eradicated, after which immunity may be rapidly lost.

Protective immunity is species- and strain-specific and primarily antibody-mediated in man (Cohen 1979) and in experimental animals such as rodents (Nussenzweig et al 1978). The *in vitro* parasite-neutralizing effects of antibody can be demonstrated only in assays for opsonizing antibodies (K. N. Brown & Hills 1974, Shear et al 1979), merozoite reinvasion inhibition (Cohen 1979), or antibody-dependent cellular cytotoxicity (J. Brown & Smalley 1980), although activity detected by such tests does not invariably correlate with protection *in vivo* (Wilson & Phillips 1976). Protective immunity is also thymus- and T lymphocyte-dependent (reviewed by K. N. Brown et al 1976, Nussenzweig et al 1978).

Attempts to artificially generate protective immunity by vaccination with blood preparations enriched for asexual erythrocytic parasite stages (see Desowitz & Miller 1980) are usually only partially successful. In most instances such preparations require the additional immunopotentiating properties of, for example, Freund's complete adjuvant, to produce the variation-transcending immunity characteristic of chronic infection. In some cases vaccinated animals generate considerable amounts of antibody with potent *in vitro* parasite-neutralizing properties in the apparent absence of protection. Often the parasites observed in this situation constitute a different antigenic variant.

The possibility that B lymphocyte recognition of antigens of asexual erythrocytic parasites does not invariably lead to variation-transcending immunity implies that immune recognition of, and responses to some other component of the parasite or parasitized erythrocyte may be required. Protective immunity is often labile; that is, it is rapidly lost after infections are resolved immunologically or cured by means of drugs. This, together with the difficulties encountered in successfully generating protection either naturally or artificially, suggests that this second response may itself be difficult to induce or maintain, perhaps because it is (anti-erythrocyte) autoimmune and thus normally suppressed.

Parasite-induced erythrocyte modification

The intraerythrocytic maturation and replication of malaria parasites produces extensive modification and destruction of erythrocytes during considerable periods of chronic infection, resulting in a massive antigenic stimulus to the host. To elucidate the definitive roles of different leucocyte and lymphocyte subsets responding to this stimulus we need to examine, at the cellular, ultrastructural and ultimately molecular level, the interaction between parasite and erythrocyte, and between this complex and the host immune system. Modification of the erythrocyte and its surface membrane in parasitized erythrocytes has been studied at the cellular (Bodammer & Bahr 1973) and ultrastructural levels (McLaren et al 1979), and appears to be most extensive in mature parasite stages (Aikawa 1977, Langreth & Reese 1979). At the molecular level, changes may be induced in the erythrocyte membrane either through the activity of parasite-derived enzymes on membrane components (Sherman & Jones 1979, Howard & Day 1981), possibly leading to the exposure of previously cryptic isoantigens, or by the insertion of parasite-coded proteins or glycoproteins (Wallach 1979, Newbold et al 1982). The infected host may thus be exposed to erythrocyte components, parasite-modified erythrocyte components, parasite-specific constituents or complexes between erythrocyte and parasite components. In the manner and on the scale they are presented to the host immune system, these could lead to both immune and, if tolerance to 'self' erythrocyte antigens is broken, autoimmune responses.

Immune and autoimmune recognition of parasitized erythrocytes

Agglutination by isoantibodies

Results from some of the antigen characterization studies indicate that recognition of parasite antigens by B lymphocytes may occur. In some cases, antibodies synthesized by B lymphocytes recognize antigens of merozoites or of mature intraerythrocytic parasites (Newbold et al 1982); monoclonal antibodies have been used to identify and isolate antigens subsequently used to actively immunize mice (Holder & Freeman 1981, D. B. Boyle & C. I. Newbold, unpublished results). It is not yet known which antigens of parasites or parasitized erythrocytes are recognized by T lymphocytes. A possibility raised by K. N. Brown is based on findings that when August rat reticulocytes are parasitized by *P. berghei* KSP 11, there is considerable

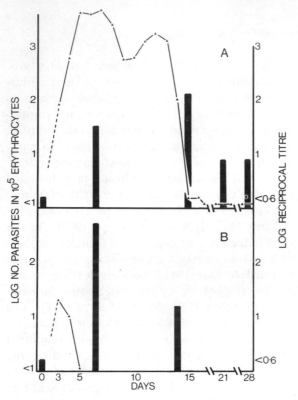

FIG. 1. Groups of five inbred August rats infected (A) with 1×10^6 *P. berghei* KSP 11-parasitized erythrocytes and (B) reinfected with 4×10^6 parasitized erythrocytes after resolution of a primary infection (above). ▲——▲, log geometric mean blood parasitaemia of a representative group. The solid bars show the log reciprocal titres against fresh *P. berghei*-parasitized reticulocytes of serum samples taken at the times indicated. (From K. N. Brown et al 1980.)

modification of erythrocyte surface membrane antigens, or the cyclical expression of normally cryptic isoantigens (K. N. Brown et al 1980). In this model, in which protective immunity had already been shown to be T lymphocyte-dependent (K. N. Brown et al 1976), antibodies that bound to the surface of, and agglutinated, infected reticulocytes were found in the serum of normal, infected or immune (reinfected) rats. Agglutination occur-

red only at low titres with normal serum, while immune serum also agglutinated uninfected reticulocytes only at low titres; these reactions were most
evident at +4 °C (K. N. Brown et al 1980). In contrast, serum from infected
and particularly immune (rechallenged) rats had much higher titres against
infected reticulocytes at both +4 °C and +20 °C (Fig. 1). The agglutination of
infected reticulocytes was partially reduced by heat inactivation, mercaptoethanol treatment or the preabsorption of immune serum with high
concentrations of sonicated infected or uninfected reticulocytes (Table 1).

TABLE 1 Agglutination of unfixed P. berghei KSP 11-infected August rat reticulocytes by
preabsorbed normal or hyperimmune sera

| Serum | Preabsorbed with: | Reciprocal titres | |
		+4°C	+20°C
Normal	Sonicated P. berghei KSP 11-infected reticulocytes	<4	<4
Normal	Sonicated uninfected reticulocytes	<4	<4
Normal	Sham (no cells)	8	<4
Immune	Sonicated P. berghei KSP 11-infected reticulocytes	<4	<4
Immune	Sonicated uninfected reticulocytes	<4	<4
Immune	Sham (no cells)	>512	512

(From K. N. Brown et al 1980.)

This indicated that antigen(s) recognized by the agglutinins were usually
expressed on reticulocytes and that the agglutination reaction, unlike that
seen in P. knowlesi-infected rhesus monkey cells (I. N. Brown et al 1968), was
not specific for determinants of components of parasitized erythrocytes. The
antigen(s) were reticulocyte-coded and expressed, but normally mainly
hidden, and were more readily exposed by the intracellular growth of the
parasite. The antibodies detected appeared to have the characteristics of
predominantly cold-reacting IgM isohaemagglutinins.

Immunocytochemistry

Further investigations of antibody binding by immunocytochemistry, using
ferritin-conjugated goat anti-rat IgG antiserum (K. N. Brown et al 1982),
showed that antibody in serum from rats hyperimmune to P. berghei KSP 11
bound to the surface of both glutaraldehyde-fixed and unfixed infected
reticulocytes, but not uninfected cells; normal serum did not label infected

reticulocytes (Fig. 2). Energy-dependent aggregation, shedding and endo-cytosis of labelled material was observed at the surface of unfixed infected reticulocytes. Membrane-associated labelled material also appeared to be dissociating from the surface of pre-fixed infected reticulocytes (Fig. 3). Absorption of hyperimmune serum with infected reticulocytes reduced the surface ferritin labelling, while preabsorption with uninfected reticulocytes or heat inactivation resulted in increased labelling (Fig. 3). These findings

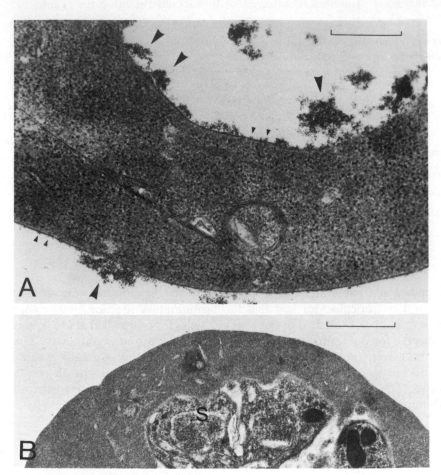

FIG. 2. A. At +4 °C, *P. berghei* KSP 11-infected reticulocytes were pre-fixed with 1.2% glutaraldehyde, incubated with serum from rats hyperimmune to *P. berghei* KSP 11 and then exposed to ferritin-conjugated goat anti-rat IgG antiserum. Ferritin particles showing sites of antibody binding are present in large aggregates (▲) or small clusters (▲) over most of the cell surface. Bar, 0.5 μm. B. Cells as in A but incubated with normal rat serum. No labelling is seen. S, schizont. Bar, 1 μm. (From K. N. Brown et al 1982.)

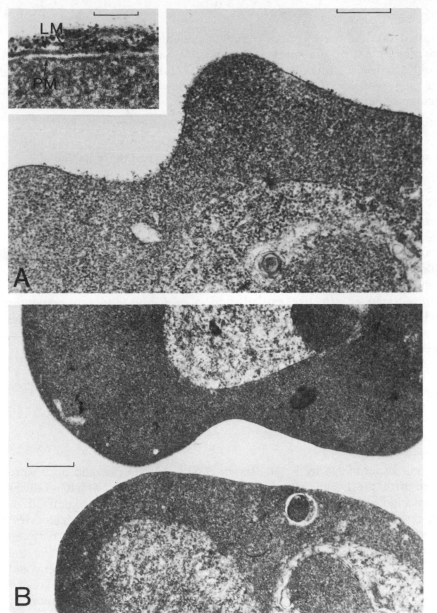

FIG. 3. A. At +4 °C, *P. berghei* KSP 11-infected reticulocytes were incubated with serum from rats hyperimmune to *P. berghei* KSP 11. This serum had been preabsorbed with sonicated uninfected reticulocytes. The cells were then exposed to ferritin-conjugated goat anti-rat IgG antiserum. Ferritin particles are evenly distributed over the cell surface. Bar, 0.2 μm. *Insert:* sloughing of labelled membrane (LM) from the surface of plasma membrane (PM). Bar, 0.1 μm. B. Cells as in A, but incubated with hyperimmune serum preabsorbed with sonicated *P. berghei*-infected reticulocytes. Note absence of ferritin labelling. Bar, 0.5 μm. (From K. N. Brown et al 1982.)

indicated that antibodies specific for components of infected reticulocytes were present in such sera, but that their binding was normally blocked by that of cold-reactive isoantibodies (agglutinins?). This blocking effect suggested a close juxtaposition of such components and isoantigens in the infected reticulocyte surface membrane.

T lymphocyte recognition of parasitized erythrocytes and the induction of protective immunity

K. N. Brown & Hills (1981) have proposed that T lymphocytes may recognize determinants of the isoantigenic component of a combined variable parasite antigen–isoantigen complex or, alternatively, determinants of modified erythrocyte components closely or spatially related to parasite antigens. This would allow for a degree of common T cell recognition between variants which, if it increased in effectiveness as the infection proceeded, might result in more rapid or effective variant-specific protective antibody responses which could transcend variation, control, and eventually eliminate, the infection (K. N. Brown et al 1976).

Erythrocyte modification: an analysis of the breaking of tolerance to 'self' erythrocyte antigens and immunity to malaria

The use of phenylhydrazine

In recent experiments by K. N. Brown & Hills (1981) rats and mice were treated with the haemocytotoxic agent, phenylhydrazine, which produces anaemia and reticulocytosis, and immunized with either sonicated unfixed, or formalin- or glutaraldehyde-fixed *P. berghei* KSP 11-infected reticulocytes. On challenge with live *P. berghei* KSP 11, a synergistic interaction between the immunostimulatory properties of these antigen preparations and the effects of phenylhydrazine was observed (see Fig. 4). The haemopoietic and erythrocyte modification resulting from treatment with phenylhydrazine appeared to stimulate a recognition event with an immune basis. Memory of the event was retained, was transferable to normal syngeneic recipients with spleen cells from treated donors, and had either enhancing or suppressive effects on the induction of protection, depending on the experimental design (K. N. Brown & Hills 1981).

   If autoimmune anti-erythrocyte recognition occurs during malaria infec-tions, this may also affect uninfected erythrocytes, and to some extent explain

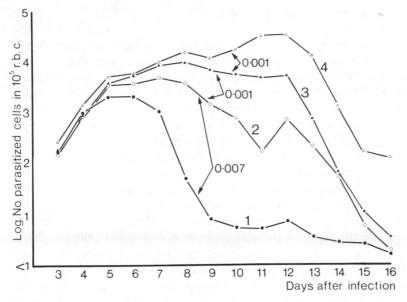

FIG. 4. Groups of five August rats injected with (1) sonicated *P. berghei* KSP 11-infected reticulocytes and 0.25% phenylhydrazine (●); (2) sonicated infected reticulocytes (○); (3) phenylhydrazine (▲); (4) untreated control (△). Antigen injected Days −14 and −7, and phenylhydrazine, Days −14, −11, −10, −9, before challenge. Lines show log geometric mean parasitaemias resulting from challenge with 1×10^6 *P. berghei* KSP 11-parasitized erythrocytes on Day 0. Arrows indicate probability values for differences in median values between Days 3 and 16. (From K. N. Brown & Hills 1981.)

the high levels of infection-associated anaemia and reticulocytosis frequently observed. This is often not commensurate with the degree of parasitaemia, and appears to have both specific and non-specific, as well as immunological and non-immunological, causes (Abdalla et al 1980). Of these, probably the most relevant in the context of this paper relates to the production of anti-erythrocyte autoantibodies in the infected host (Strickland & Hunter 1980). That such responses occur at all stems from the concept that in some cases specific acquired immunity against 'self', rather than being functionally deleted, is normally actively suppressed (reviewed by Teale & Mackay 1979). In this situation and during malaria infections, these lymphocytes may then be activated non-specifically by parasite-derived mitogens or polyclonal lymphocyte activators. Alternatively, some negative feedback control system normally operative may be bypassed, because of presentation to the host's immune system of altered 'self'—that is, foreign (parasite) antigens closely associated with 'self' (erythrocyte or modified erythrocyte components) (see reviews by Allison et al 1971, Elson et al 1979).

Use of the Playfair & Marshall-Clarke model

The relevance of anti-erythrocyte autoimmune recognition to protection in malaria-infected mice was further investigated using a well-characterized model for the experimental induction of anti-erythrocyte autoimmunity (Playfair & Marshall-Clarke 1973, and see review by Naysmith et al 1981). These authors showed that mice injected with rat erythrocytes synthesized complete agglutinins to rat erythrocytes and (in a thymus-dependent manner) incomplete IgG antibodies to cross-reacting determinants on both rat and mouse erythrocytes. These antibodies were detected by a Direct Coombs' test (DCT). The reinjection of rat erythrocytes evoked a secondary autoantibody response which was rapidly suppressed, and mice reverted to the Coombs-negative state. Spleen and lymph node cells taken from such rat erythrocyte-treated mice could adoptively transfer to normal syngeneic recipients the ability to specifically suppress the autoantibody component of the recipients' subsequent response to rat erythrocytes. Suppressor activity was found mainly in the T lymphocyte population (Cooke et al 1978).

Under normal circumstances the anti-erythrocyte autoantibody is not produced because the T helper lymphocytes required for its synthesis are either suppressed or perhaps deleted. To explain their original findings, Playfair & Marshall-Clarke (1973) hypothesized that a subset of T lymphocytes stimulated by determinants specific to rat erythrocytes were able to bypass this normal deficiency in 'self'-reactive T helper lymphocytes. B lymphocyte recognition of the cross-reacting erythrocyte antigen then occurs within the context of this T helper activity and results in autoantibody synthesis.

My studies (W. Jarra, unpublished observations) have shown that CBA/Ca mice, infected with or immune to *P. chabaudi*, do not become Coombs-positive, suggesting that humoral anti-erythrocyte autoimmune recognition does not occur in these mice, although the Coombs' agglutination test is not the most sensitive assay for surface-bound Ig. The Playfair & Marshall-Clarke model has thus been used to determine whether:

(i) A progressive, artificially induced anti-erythrocyte autoantibody response affects the course of a concurrent *P. chabaudi* infection;

(ii) Active suppression of such a response *in situ* could affect a *P. chabaudi* infection; and

(iii) Spleen cells from mice actively suppressing autoantibody formation interact synergistically with spleen cells from *P. chabaudi*-immune mice when injected into irradiated syngeneic recipients.

In mice rendered Coombs-positive by the preinjection of rat erythrocytes and challenged with *P. chabaudi* at the peak of the autoantibody response, parasitaemias were only slightly different from those in the controls (Fig. 5).

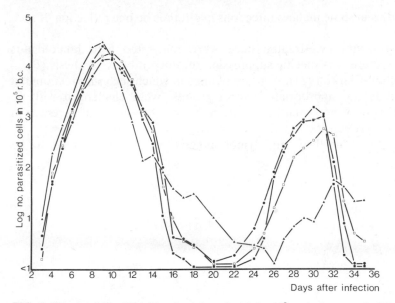

FIG. 5. Groups of five CBA/Ca mice injected with 2×10^8 washed syngeneic (■), rabbit (□) or rat (●) erythrocytes or diluent (▲) on Days −56, −49, −42, −35. Lines show log geometric mean parasitaemias resulting from challenge with 5×10^4 *P. chabaudi*-parasitized erythrocytes on Day 0. Rat erythrocyte recipients were Coombs-positive on day of challenge.

The parasitaemia in mice pretreated with syngeneic erythrocytes was also modified. Statistically, these differences were significant, although it is possible that they resulted from changes in the overall age distribution of erythrocytes in the treated mice. Such changes might arise from the injection of large numbers of syngeneic and predominantly mature erythrocytes, or from the anaemia and reticulocytosis which may accompany autoantibody formation in mice injected with rat erythrocytes (Naysmith et al 1981). When such mice were injected with *P. berghei* KSP 11, parasitaemias were enhanced over those of control groups (data not shown). In contrast to the results of these experiments, a small proportion of C3H/He mice pretreated with rat erythrocytes were protected against a lethal *Plasmodium* infection— species not given (unpublished results of G. F. Mitchell, D. A. Cunliffe & N. F. Gare, cited in Knopf et al 1979).

We used the Playfair & Marshall-Clarke model in this study on the supposition that the mouse erythrocyte autoantigen may be modified in *P. chabaudi*-parasitized erythrocytes. T lymphocyte recognition of epitopes of this molecule might be central in the synthesis of antibodies against erythrocyte determinants, either normally expressed or cryptic, or against epitopes of parasite-specific membrane components. The appearance of anti-erythrocyte autoantibodies in some malaria infections might thus be one reflection of such responses.

When rat erythrocyte-treated mice were reinjected with homologous erythrocytes there was specific suppression of autoantibody synthesis (Playfair & Marshall-Clarke 1973). A group of mice in which such suppression had been induced, and appropriate control groups, were challenged with *P. chabaudi*. Figure 6 shows that, as in the previous experiment, differences in parasitaemia between the individual groups were only marginal.

Events such as erythro- and lymphopoiesis might be expected to be

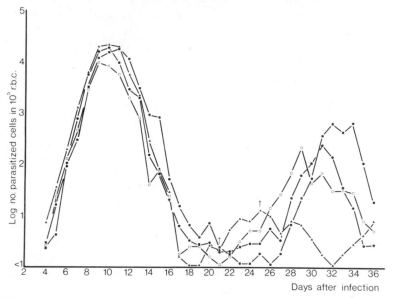

FIG. 6. Groups of five CBA/Ca mice first injected with 2×10^8 washed syngeneic (■), rabbit (□), or rat (●) erythrocytes or diluent (▲) on Days −355, −341, −334, −329 and reinjected on Days −28, −21, −16, −7. Lines show log geometric mean parasitaemias resulting from challenge with 5×10^4 *P. chabaudi*-parasitized erythrocytes on Day 0. Rat erythrocyte recipients were Coombs-negative on day of challenge. †, deaths.

severely affected (either enhanced or suppressed) during the different phases of a progressive erythrocytic malaria infection. Such changes would almost certainly have extensive repercussions on immune responsiveness. Infected mice would still attempt to maintain homeostasis even while trying to control and eliminate the infection. A potentially immunopathological anti-erythrocyte autoimmune response occurring as a consequence of, or a component of, immunity to parasitized erythrocytes might be quickly suppressed. At the same time, if such recognition was a prerequisite for the induction of protective antibody synthesis, its suppression would have to be partially counteracted; only then could the host protect itself against potentially irreversible and fatal haemolysis resulting from uncontrolled parasite multiplication. The situation overall may thus be dynamic, yet finely balanced. It should be emphasized here that attempts to manipulate such a system, even by grossly altering one of the variables, may be difficult to quantify in the intact host, which can rapidly compensate for such alterations. We therefore examined the role of anti-erythrocyte autoimmune recognition in protection in a situation where the potential contribution of the host was reduced.

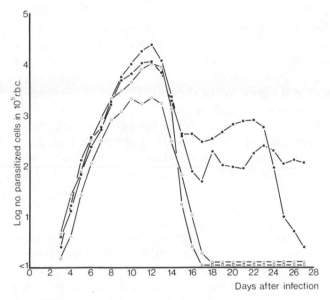

FIG. 7. On Day −1, spleen cells were taken from groups of CBA/Ca mice previously injected with syngeneic or rat erythrocytes, or with diluent on Days −317, −310, −303, −296 and on Days −15, −8. Cells were also taken from mice previously infected with *P. chabaudi* on Day −143, and from age, weight, sex-matched normal controls. Groups of syngeneic recipients pre-irradiated with 450 rads were injected with 2.8×10^7 *P. chabaudi* immune or normal spleen cells $+2.3 \times 10^7$ cells from either mouse or rat erythrocyte-treated donors in the following combinations: immune + mouse, □; normal + mouse, ■; immune + rat, ○; normal + rat, ● (immune or normal + diluent-treated—data not shown). Lines show log geometric mean parasitaemias resulting from challenge with 5×10^4 *P. chabaudi*-parasitized erythrocytes on Day 0.

In the autoimmunity model, suppression of autoantibody formation was transferable with spleen cells (see above). Suppression was predominantly mediated by transferred T lymphocytes (Cooke et al 1978), which stimulated T suppressor cell activity in the recipients rather than directly affecting T helper or B lymphocytes (Hutchings & Cooke 1981). Spleen cells from mice suppressing autoantibody formation were mixed with *P. chabaudi*-immune spleen cells and transferred to sublethally irradiated syngeneic recipients. These two cell populations interacted synergistically and considerably modified the course of a challenge parasitaemia, compared with the control groups (Fig. 7). This interaction was specific, as spleen cells containing suppressor activity had no effect when transferred with cells from any of the control groups for erythrocyte treatment.

Summary and conclusions

The relevance of anti-erythrocyte autoimmune recognition events in the immunopathology of erythrocytic malaria, or in the induction of protective immunity, is at present unclear. The studies described here have demonstrated that serum of *P. berghei*-infected rats contained cold-reactive antibodies to cryptic erythrocyte antigens. While they may have little relevance *in vivo*, these isoantibodies blocked the binding of antibody specific for components of parasitized erythrocytes. This indicates a close association between autoantigen and such components at the surface of parasitized erythrocytes. It has been suggested that this association may represent a structural basis for possible differential B and T lymphocyte recognition events leading to the synthesis of protective antibody.

The induction of protection in *P. chabaudi*- or *P. berghei*-infected mice did not correlate with Coombs' positivity artificially induced by the injection of cross-reacting rat erythrocyte antigen. Although the relevance of suppression of such autoimmune recognition to protection was difficult to demonstrate in intact animals, cell transfers into immunocompromised recipients showed interaction between spleen cells containing suppressor activity and at least a subset of *P. chabaudi*-immune spleen cells. This implied that autoimmune recognition of 'self' or modified 'self' determinants of the surface membrane of parasitized erythrocytes might be relevant in protection.

A more precise view of such recognition events awaits more sophisticated experimentation, both *in vivo* and *in vitro*, using defined antigen preparations and lymphocyte subpopulations.

Acknowledgements

I am grateful to World Health Organization Publications, Blackwell Scientific Publications and Georg Thieme Verlag for permission to reproduce in part Fig. 1 and Table 1, Figs. 2 and 3, and Fig. 4 respectively. My thanks are also due to Drs S. R. Smithers and D. B. Boyle for helpful advice and critical evaluation of the text, and to Dr D. J. McLaren and Mr C. R. Witherington for preparations of Figs. 2 and 3. Part of the work reviewed here was originally supported by grants from the World Health Organization.

REFERENCES

Abdalla S, Weatherall DJ, Wickramasinghe SN, Hughes M 1980 The anaemia of *P. falciparum* malaria. Br J Haematol 46:171-183

Aikawa M 1977 Variation in structure and function during the life cycle of malaria parasites. Bull WHO 55:139-156

Allison AC, Denman AM, Barnes RD 1971 Cooperating and controlling functions of thymus-derived lymphocytes in relation to autoimmunity. Lancet 2:135-140

Bodammer JE, Bahr GF 1973 The initiation of a 'metabolic window' in the surface of host erythrocytes by *Plasmodium berghei* NYU-2. Lab Invest 28:708-718

Brown IN 1969 Immunological aspects of malaria infection. Adv Immunol 11:267-367

Brown IN, Brown KN, Hills LA 1968 Immunity to malaria: the antibody response to antigenic variation by *Plasmodium knowlesi*. Immunology 14:127-138

Brown J, Smalley ME 1980 Specific antibody-dependent cellular cytotoxicity in human malaria. Clin Exp Immunol 41:423-429

Brown KN, Hills LA 1974 Antigenic variation and immunity to *Plasmodium knowlesi*: antibodies which induce antigenic variation and antibodies which destroy parasites. Trans R Soc Trop Med Hyg 68:139-142

Brown KN, Hills LA 1981 Erythrocyte destruction and protective immunity to malaria: enhancement of the immune response by phenylhydrazine treatment. Tropenmed Parasitol 32:67-72

Brown KN, Jarra W, Hills LA 1976 T cells and protective immunity to *Plasmodium berghei* in the rat. Infect Immun 14:858-871

Brown KN, Grundy MS, Hills LA, Jarra W 1980 Cold isohaemagglutinins in *Plasmodium berghei*-infected rats reacting with parasitized reticulocytes. Bull WHO 58:449-457

Brown KN, McLaren DJ, Hills LA, Jarra W 1982 The binding of antibodies from *Plasmodium berghei*-infected rats to isoantigens and parasite-specific antigenic sites on the surfaces of infected erythrocytes. Parasite Immunol (Oxf) 4:21-31

Cohen S 1979 Immunity to malaria. Proc R Soc Lond B Biol Sci 203:323-345

Cohen S 1980 *Plasmodium*—mechanisms of survival. In: Van den Bossche H (ed) The host–invader interplay. Elsevier/North-Holland Biomedical Press, Amsterdam, p 191-203

Cooke A, Hutchings PR, Playfair JHL 1978 Suppressor T cells in experimental autoimmune haemolytic anaemia. Nature (Lond) 273:154-155

Desowitz RS, Miller LH 1980 A perspective on malaria vaccines. Bull WHO 58:897-908

Elson CJ, Naysmith JD, Taylor RB 1979 B cell tolerance and autoimmunity. Int Rev Exp Pathol 19:137-203

Holder AA, Freeman RR 1981 Immunization against blood stage rodent malaria using purified parasite antigens. Nature (Lond) 294:361-364

Howard RJ, Day KP 1981 *Plasmodium berghei*: modification of sialic acid on red cells from infected mouse blood. Exp Parasitol 51:95-103

Hutchings P, Cooke A 1981 Analysis of the cellular interactions involved in the regulation of induced erythrocyte autoantibodies. Cell Immunol 63:221-227

Knopf PM, Brown GV, Howard RJ, Mitchell GF 1979 Immunoprecipitation of biosynthetically-labelled products in the identification of antigens of murine red cells infected with the protozoan parasite *Plasmodium berghei*. Aust J Exp Biol Med Sci 56:553-559

Langreth SG, Reese RT 1979 Antigenicity of the infected erythrocyte and merozoite surfaces in *falciparum* malaria. J Exp Med 150:1241-1254

McLaren DJ, Bannister LH, Trigg PI, Butcher GA 1979 Freeze fracture studies on the interaction between the malaria parasite and the host erythrocyte in *Plasmodium knowlesi* infection. Parasitology 79:125-139

Naysmith JD, Ortega-Pierres MG, Elson CJ 1981 Rat erythrocyte-induced anti-erythrocyte autoantibody production and control in normal mice. Immunol Rev 55:55-87

Newbold CI, Boyle DB, Smith CC, Brown KN 1982 Identification of a schizont-infected and species-specific surface glycoprotein on erythrocytes infected with rodent malarias. Mol Biochem Parasitol 5:45-54

Nussenzweig RS, Cochrane AH, Lustig HJ 1978 Immunological responses. In: Killick-Kendrick R, Peters W (eds) Rodent malaria. Academic Press, London, p 247-307

Playfair JHL, Marshall-Clarke S 1973 Induction of red cell autoantibodies in normal mice. Nat New Biol 243:213-214

Shear HJ, Nussenzweig RS, Bianco C 1979 Immune phagocytosis in murine malaria. J Exp Med 149:1288-1298

Sherman IW, Jones LA 1979 *Plasmodium lophurae:* membrane proteins of erythrocyte-free plasmodia and malaria-infected red cells. J Protozool 26:489-501

Strickland GT, Hunter KW 1980 Red cell antibodies in malaria: immunity or autoimmunity? In: Van den Bossche H (ed) The host–invader interplay. Elsevier/North-Holland Biomedical Press, Amsterdam, p 357-370

Teale, JM, Mackay IR 1979 Autoimmune disease and the theory of clonal abortion. Is it still relevant? Lancet 2:284-287

Wallach DFH 1979 Membrane pathobiology of malaria. Cell Biol Int Rep 3:395-408

Wilson RJM, Phillips RS 1976 Method to test inhibitory antibodies in human sera to wild populations of *Plasmodium falciparum*. Nature (Lond) 263:132-134

DISCUSSION

Howard: Our recent studies on the plasma membrane of reticulocytes and normal erythrocytes in the mouse may be relevant to Dr Jarra's very interesting paper. We have labelled the glycoproteins of acetyl phenylhydrazine-induced mouse reticulocytes, reticulocytes from hyper-bled mice, and normal BALB/c mouse erythrocytes (Howard et al 1982). We saw no quantitative or qualitative differences in the patterns of glycoproteins on one-dimensional sodium dodecyl sulphate gels. However, in collaboration with Dr R. Schauer, I have shown, and Fabia et al (1979) have also shown, that the sialic acid content of mouse reticulocytes is significantly higher than that of erythrocytes. Furthermore, we found no alteration in the ratio of the two types of sialic acid (*N*-acetylneuraminic acid and 9-*O*-acetyl-*N*-acetylneuraminic acid) in erythrocytes from infected mice, although there is an increase in the total amount of sialic acid of malaria-infected erythrocytes. You studied reticulocytes induced by phenylhydrazine. It would be interesting, in the light of your results and our knowledge of sialic acid content, to continue the studies of Poels et al (1978), who showed that infected reticulocytes were better immunogens for protective immunity in mice than infected erythrocytes. Before immunization you could treat the infected reticulocytes with neuraminidase and see whether presentation of parasite antigens to the immune system on the surface of reticulocytes with reduced sialic acid content removes the enhanced protection obtained by immunizing with reticulocytes.

Jarra: I have attempted to do a similar experiment to those of Poels et al (1978) who used *P. berghei,* which preferentially invades reticulocytes (see Carter & Diggs 1977). In my experiments (Jarra & Brown 1980) I used CBA/Ca mice infected with *P. chabaudi,* which is believed to have a preference for normocytes. When examining blood films stained with brilliant cresyl blue and Giemsa's stain, using the technique described by Zuckerman (1957), I found that around crisis and resolution of the parasitaemia, up to 25% of the parasites were inside reticulocytes. Admittedly, this staining technique is not perhaps the most sensitive assay for reticulocytes. By inducing anaemia and subsequently erythropoiesis by injecting mice with phenylhydrazine, it was possible to produce animals whose erythrocytes were 50% reticulocytes. When these mice were injected with large numbers of *P. chabaudi* -parasitized erythrocytes and blood films were examined, 50% of the parasites observed were inside reticulocytes at the time of peak parasitaemia. Blood preparations from such mice, when rendered non-infective by γ-irradiation and injected into normal mice challenged with *P. chabaudi,* proved to induce slightly more protective immunity than infected blood containing low numbers of parasitized reticulocytes. So there may be a similar situation with *P. chabaudi* to the experiment of Dr Poels and his colleagues, although this parasite is not normally regarded as having a reticulocyte preference. We have not looked at enzyme-treated parasitized reticulocytes, but it certainly seems to be an interesting idea.

Howard: I am wondering whether there are some parasite membrane antigens that are closely associated with host sialoglycoproteins such that they are presented together to the immune system. This could explain the more potent immunization resulting from use of infected reticulocytes of high sialic acid content, as compared to infected erythrocytes of lower sialic acid content. Ashwell has shown that removing sialic acid from serum glycoproteins results in their rapid clearance (Morell et al 1971). The sialic acid content of host membrane sialoglycoproteins that are tightly associated with parasite membrane antigens might therefore determine the rate and route of antigen clearance and consequently affect the nature of the anti-parasite immunity elicited. The experiment that I suggested with neuraminidase-treated reticulocytes might begin to answer this question. It would also be interesting to follow the clearance rates *in vivo* of infected erythrocytes and reticulocytes that have been treated with neuraminidase for various times and to attempt to relate clearance rate to sialic acid content.

We have also shown that acetyl phenylhydrazine (APH) oxidizes components of the erythrocyte membrane such that treatment with NaB^3H_4 alone labels many proteins and lipids. Perhaps the malaria parasite within a reticulocyte induces membrane oxidation similar to that induced by APH. Proteins may then be cross-linked covalently to each other and to lipids, resulting in the creation of new antigens. The degree and nature of cross-linking of membrane proteins could be investigated, if purified membranes from infected cells could be obtained, by electrophoresis on agarose–acrylamide gels, and Western blotting using antibodies to malarial proteins and to proteins of normal erythrocyte membranes.

And, finally, I would like to clarify my understanding of your results. Is it true that by immunoelectron microscopy you have demonstrated a group of isohaemagglutinins that also agglutinate infected reticulocytes, and that when these are adsorbed out, antibodies remaining can be shown to bind to the infected cell surface but do not agglutinate?

Jarra: No; there are two different things here, and it may be difficult to relate them. The serum from immune rats agglutinates infected reticulocytes. If we preabsorb this serum with uninfected or infected reticulocytes, that agglutination is removed. At the same time, if we look at antibody binding by electron microscopy using ferritin-conjugated anti-rat IgG, immune serum preabsorbed with uninfected cells still produces labelling. If we preabsorb the immune serum with infected cells, we don't see labelling. From the experiments we have done, we cannot directly relate what we observe at the EM level with the results from the agglutination assay.

Friedman: As a non-immunologist, I am not clear what the significance of a cold-reacting antibody is. I don't really know what it is, or whether it has *in vivo* significance at normal body temperature. So are the antibodies which block parasite-specific binding dependent on temperature? And finally, you said that your mice that had been treated with rat red cells were not significantly different from controls, but in fact they consistently did *worse* than controls in the second peak of infection. Did that have something to do with this blockage? That is, did the presence of isoantibodies prevent the development of a response to parasite-specific antigen, *in vivo* ?

Jarra: Cold agglutinins are agglutinating antibodies of either IgM or IgG class which are detected at maximum titres at temperatures below 37 °C. They are usually directed against epitopes of the erythrocyte surface. As to their significance in relation to malaria, this could be quite different in experimental models and in man. Certainly in rodent malarias, Lustig et al (1977), Hunter et al (1980) and Ronai et al (1981) have shown that predominantly cold-reacting antibodies can be found on infected and uninfected red cells at both agglutinating and sub-agglutinating levels, as detectable by the Coombs' test, radioimmunoassay, or the use of the fluorescence-activated cell sorter. Hunter et al (1980) have suggested that such antibodies may be one cause of the excessive haemolytic anaemia often observed in these infections.

Friedman: Do the antibodies bind at 37 °C?

Jarra: In our hands with *P. berghei*-infected reticulocytes and serum from immune rats, there is minimal binding at 37 °C. Lustig et al (1977) using *P. berghei*-infected mice detected the binding of such antibodies to erythrocytes at both low temperature and 37 °C. We haven't been able to look at the question of whether blockage is temperature-dependent. All our experiments with electron microscopy were done at +4 °C. That is an aspect to be looked at. On your last question, I don't think our experiments do show that isoantibodies prevent the recognition of parasite-specific antigens *in vivo*, because they may not bind *in vivo*. This is only an *in vitro* system at present.

Brown: You think this may happen because of the heightened recrudescence, Dr Friedman?

Friedman: Yes.

Brown: Isn't it just possible that immune recognition might be reduced if there is a blocking effect *in vivo*, and that may be why you get the heightened parasitaemia?

Jarra: It is possible, but I don't think the experiments with *P. chabaudi* indicate that. In those parasitaemias the effect on the recrudescence is not specific for the rat erythrocyte treatment. The recipients of rabbit red cells also suffered a recrudescence that was modified, and they were relatively speaking Coombs-negative. It is perhaps a non-specific effect, possibly due to reticuloendothelial system blockade. In some cases the mice received their last injection of red cells only a week before challenge with *P. chabaudi*.

Wyler: Dr Brown referred earlier to the possibility that reticulocyte surface antigens can aggregate. You are doing agglutination in the cold, so perhaps you are preventing capping. On the other hand, the blocking of the interaction between the parasite and isohaemagglutinins with anti-parasite antibodies could be by steric hindrance or by the creation of rigidity in the red cell membrane.

Jarra: The electron micrographs were prepared using prefixed cells. We have also looked at agglutination with glutaraldehyde-fixed and formalin-fixed infected and uninfected reticulocytes, but the patterns of agglutination seen then with normal or immune, untreated or heat-inactivated serum, are quite different from those seen with unfixed cells. In the electron microscope study we attempted to block capping with 4 mM-sodium azide. Although the results don't suggest that capping is occurring, they indicate that azide inhibited the aggregation, or perhaps patching, of some surface membrane component that appears to be labelled by the antibody.

Phillips: Are effects obtained with phenylhydrazine in rats peculiar to red cells, or is it possible that you are damaging other kinds of cells, thereby exposing histocompatibility antigens? Damaged liver cells, for example, might have the same effect. Have you tried similar experiments using other cell types?

Jarra: Phenylhydrazine does have other effects besides causing anaemia and erythropoiesis, although, as Brown & Hills (1981) point out, it is difficult to envisage how these can contribute to the effects we have described, which appear to be associated with red cells. We haven't used other cell types.

Phillips: The mouse has histocompatibility (H-2) antigens on the surface of its red cells. I don't know about the rat. Man is slightly different; only the younger red cells are said to express HLA antigens. I am wondering if the protective effect is associated only with the destruction of red cells or whether, because of the unusual situation of having H-2 antigens on the red cells in mice, the protein may be related to histocompatibility antigens rather than, or in addition to, specific red cell antigens.

Brown: I can't answer that. We wanted to mimic the extensive red cell destruction of malaria. We can't exclude what you suggest. With *P. berghei* and August rats, one of the best ways to immunize older rats is to treat them with phenylhydrazine alone, leave them for a month and then challenge them. They are almost as immune as if we had given them lots of antigen.

Phillips: What is the state of the architecture of the spleen in these animals? Phenylhydrazine has the same effect as infection; you see grossly enlarged spleens.

Jarra: The spleen is slightly enlarged, but not on the scale that Dr Wyler showed for the infected spleens.

Wallach: Is there any binding of isoantibody to red cell precursors in the bone marrow?

Jarra: We haven't looked at this.

Sherman: The use of phenylhydrazine for inducing reticulocytosis has always bothered me. It gives lovely reticulocyte responses, but I wonder what would happen if you bled the animals. You wouldn't get nearly the same reticulocyte response, but it seems to be a more physiological way of creating reticulocytosis.

Jarra: This work actually began with experiments with Drs Trigg and McColm on *P. berghei* KSP11 cultivated *in vitro*. We were examining multiplication of the parasite in rat normocytes compared to reticulocytes, and Trigg & McColm (1976) showed that significant multiplication occurred only inside reticulocytes. We were aware of what you allude to, and we tried bleeding rats as an alternative to phenylhydrazine treatment. It didn't produce the same level of reticulocytes. I have since compared phenylhydrazine, bleeding, and the use of rabbit anti-erythrocyte serum in mice. Of these treatments, only phenylhydrazine, and to a lesser extent anti-erythrocyte serum, produced large numbers of reticulocytes. People claim to get 60 or 70% reticulocytes by bleeding, but we haven't achieved this.

Sherman: We were once interested in getting lots of juvenile red cells for amino acid incorporation studies. Before giving radioactive amino acids to the animals (ducklings) we wanted to see what effect reticulocytosis would have on subsequent infection with *P. lophurae*. We produced reticulocytosis using phenylhydrazine and waited for the red cells to mature. When we attempted to infect the animals with *P. lophurae*, although the erythrocytes were mature and looked normal to us, to *P. lophurae* they evidently looked different, since we obtained a poor infection; most of the ducklings didn't become infected. So I continue to wonder about the properties of red cells that are produced by phenylhydrazine treatment of the host.

Jarra: Certainly that doesn't seem to be true of *P. berghei*. Phenylhydrazine is used *because* it enhances infection of erythrocytes or reticulocytes to such a degree that we could produce by simple centrifugation, in a manner similar to that used for the preparation of the schizont-enriched layer in the *P. knowlesi* – rhesus monkey system, a very much enriched layer of parasitized cells.

Anders: Do you know anything about the target specificity of the cold agglutinins in your system, and is there any information from studies of these agglutinins in human populations in malarious areas that sheds light on their biological significance?

Jarra: We have no idea of the target for the cold agglutinins. We hope to study this using monoclonal antibodies. I don't know the relevance of these antibodies in experimental malaria infections, but Dr Facer could tell us if they are believed to be of any significance in man.

Facer: We found IgM anti-I and anti-i cold agglutinins in the Gambian children that we studied (Facer 1980, Facer & Sangster 1981). The titres were very low and they are probably not clinically significant because of this, and because of their low thermal range. They were unreactive at 37 °C. We have not yet looked for anti-Pr cold agglutinins.

Weatherall: To produce any agglutination or haemolysis *in vivo*, do these antibodies need a high thermal range and to be present at a high titre?

Facer: Yes; cold agglutinin titres and thermal amplitude in the presence of bovine albumin correlate better with haemolytic anaemia than reactions without albumin (Garratty et al 1977).

On the target antigen for cold agglutinins in mice, I do not have this information. I know that rabbit red cells are I positive, and the rat is i positive.

Jarra: There is an autoantibody found in some strains of mice which is believed to be directed against one of the I antigens.

Weatherall: When you talk about a positive Coombs' test in the mouse autoimmunity model, what was the Coombs' reagent, Dr Jarra?

Jarra: It was a polyspecific anti-globulin reagent provided by Dr Marshall-Clarke, raised against IgG.

REFERENCES

Brown KN, Hills LA 1981 Erythrocyte destruction and protective immunity to malaria: enhancement of the immune response by phenylhydrazine treatment. Tropenmed Parasitol 32:67-72

158 DISCUSSION

Carter R, Diggs CL 1977 Plasmodia of rodents. In: Kreier JP (ed) Parasitic protozoa. Academic Press, New York & London, vol 3:359-465

Fabia F, Gattegno L, Rousset J-J, Cornillot P 1979 *Plasmodium chabaudi*: modification des acides sialiques de surface des hématies au cours de l'infestation. Ann Parasitol 54:1-10

Facer CA 1980 Direct Coombs antiglobulin reactions in Gambian children with *Plasmodium falciparum* malaria. II. Specificity of erythrocyte-bound IgG. Clin Exp Immunol 39:279-288

Facer CA, Sangster J 1981 Chronic falciparum malaria and anti-I autoantibodies. Lancet 2: 1109-1110

Garratty G, Petz LD, Hoops JK 1977 The correlation of cold agglutinin titrations in saliva and albumin with haemolytic anaemia. Br J Haematol 35:587-595

Howard RJ, Smith PM, Mitchell GF 1982 Surface membrane proteins and glycoproteins of red blood cells from normal and anaemic mice. Comp Biochem Physiol 71B:713-721

Hunter KW, Finkelman FD, Strickland GT, Sayles PC, Scher I 1980 Murine malaria: an analysis of erythrocyte surface bound immunoglobulin by flow microfluorimetry. J Immunol 125:169-174

Jarra W, Brown KN 1980 Invasion and immunogenicity of *Plasmodium chabaudi* in mature and immature erythrocytes. Parasitology 82: xxiii

Lustig HJ, Nussenzweig V, Nussenzweig RS 1977 Erythrocyte membrane associated immunoglobulins during malaria infection of mice. J Immunol 119:210-216

Morell AG, Gregoriadis G, Scheinberg IH, Hickman J, Ashwell G 1971 The role of sialic acid in determining the survival of glycoproteins in the circulation. J Biol Chem 246:1461-1467

Poels LG, Van Niekerk CC, Franken MAM 1978 Plasmodial antigens exposed on the surface of infected reticulocytes: their role in induction of protective immunity in mice. Isr J Med Sci 14:575-581

Ronai Z, Avraham H, Sulitzenu D 1981 Autoantibodies to red blood cells in rats infected with *Plasmodium berghei*. J Parasitol 67:351-353

Trigg PI, McColm AA 1976 Cultivation of the erythrocytic stages of *Plasmodium berghei berghei*. Parasitology 73:xxxiii-xxxiv

Zuckerman A 1957 Blood loss and replacement in plasmodial infection. I. *Plasmodium berghei* in untreated rats of varying age and in adult rats with erythropoietic mechanisms manipulated before inoculation. J Infect Dis 100:172-206

Genetic variation in the host and adaptive phenomena in *Plasmodium falciparum* infection

L. LUZZATTO*†, O. SODEINDE**†, and G. MARTINI†

*Department of Haematology, Royal Postgraduate Medical School, Ducane Road, London W12 0HS, **Department of Paediatrics, College of Medicine, University of Ibadan, Ibadan, Nigeria, and †International Institute of Genetics and Biophysics, CNR, Napoli, Italy*

Abstract The *in vitro* culture of *Plasmodium falciparum*, after synchronization, lends itself well to an analysis of the asexual schizogonic cycle. We have found in this system that DNA synthesis and RNA synthesis are associated mainly with the trophozoite stage, with the latter peaking slightly ahead of the former. Distinctive patterns of protein synthesis are seen at serial times along the cycle, with a number of 'stage-specific' bands identifiable on SDS gels. The fate of the infection can be influenced by the genotype of the host cell. Thus, glucose-6-phosphate dehydrogenase (G6PD)-deficient erythrocytes are invaded normally, but maturation of intracellular parasites is delayed and impaired. However, the parasites that do develop will then have a normal behaviour in their next rounds in G6PD-deficient cells, suggesting that an adaptive change has taken place. These results fit well with the relative protection against *P. falciparum in vivo* of girls heterozygous for G6PD deficiency but not of hemizygous G6PD-deficient boys.

Among the many forms of symbiotic relationship between two organisms, intracellular parasitism exhibits extreme features of interaction and integration between parasite and host cell functions. In general, we find two genomes sharing the same *milieu*, and one exploiting to a greater or lesser extent the products, the energy supply, and even the macromolecule-synthetic machinery of the other. Often we tend to regard the parasite as the dependent, and to some extent the defective organism, and the host cell as the more competent partner in the symbiotic relationship. In this respect, the intraerythrocytic mammalian malaria parasite is a conspicuous exception (see Table 1). *Plasmodium* is the eukaryotic organism, fully competent for replication, protein synthesis and aerobic energy metabolism, inside a cell which has lost nucleus, ribosomes and mitochondria, and with them the

1983 Malaria and the red cell. Pitman, London (Ciba Foundation symposium 94) p 159-173

capacity to divide, to make protein, and most of its energy supply, except for glycolysis. Thus, while the erythrocyte certainly provides the malaria parasite with an extraordinarily rich nutrient environment, safely screened from immunological defences, we must certainly think of the *Plasmodium* as the more active component of the system. Indeed, the power of this active role is brought home to us only too forcefully when we consider how drastic a role *Plasmodium falciparum* has played in shaping human evolution. There is now overwhelming evidence that the three genetically determined pathological conditions that are most prevalent in the human species in absolute terms, namely sickle cell anaemia, the thalassaemia syndromes and glucose-6-phosphate dehydrogenase (G6PD) deficiency, are all related to selection by this parasite (reviewed by Luzzatto 1979, and see Friedman, this volume). On the other hand, as for any living organism, we can expect that a population of *Plasmodium* must be able not only to ensure its own propagation, but also to exhibit adaptive phenomena, in the way of either physiological changes in response to, or selection of, genetic variants by the environment—the environment being mainly the red cell itself. Although we have rather scanty knowledge of the physiology of the malaria parasite, and hardly any of its genetics and genetic variation, the revolutionary introduction by Trager & Jensen (1976) of the continuous culture of *P. falciparum* has given us recently an important tool that makes it possible, at least in principle, to investigate adaptive and selective phenomena.

We are reporting here some features of the intraerythrocytic cycle of *P. falciparum* as they are seen in cultures; and we shall discuss a specific case of host cell–parasite interaction in which adaptive changes in the parasite appear to take place.

The schizogonic cycle in culture

It is a well-known characteristic of the natural human infection with *P. falciparum* that, apart from the few, arresting images of gametocytes, only 'young' ring forms are seen in the peripheral blood. Evidently the more mature trophozoites and the schizonts tend to home very selectively to internal organs, such as the spleen and, when available, the placenta. By contrast, in a culture vessel in which the whole schizogonic cycle takes place, we have the privilege of observing the entire cycle. Another important consideration in comparing *in vivo* with *in vitro* parasites is the time course of schizogony. Classically, paroxysms of fever have been correlated with bursts of synchronous merozoite release. However, clinical experience with *P. falciparum*, especially in recurrent infections, has shown very variable temperature patterns, suggesting that synchrony has been disturbed and that

TABLE 1 Macromolecule synthesis in various parasite systems

Parasite					Host cell			
Taxonomic group	Organism	DNA content[a]	RNA	Protein synthesis	Type	DNA content[a]	RNA	Protein synthesis
Virus	*Vaccinia*	3.5×10^5	0	0	HeLa	6×10^9	+	+
Rickettsia	*Rickettsia rickettsii*		+	+	Lymphoid	6×10^9	+	+
Bacteria	*Mycobacterium leprae*	4×10^6	+	+	Macrophage	6×10^9	+	+
Protozoa	*Leishmania donovani*		+	+	Macrophage	6×10^9	+	+
Protozoa	*Plasmodium falciparum*		+	+	Erythrocyte	0	0	0

[a] Expressed in base pairs per cell.

the timing of schizogony is largely randomized. The same happens in culture after a few passages. However, the parasite population can become synchronized again, whether by accident or by manipulation. It is common experience that when a fresh culture is grown from an infected patient the existing

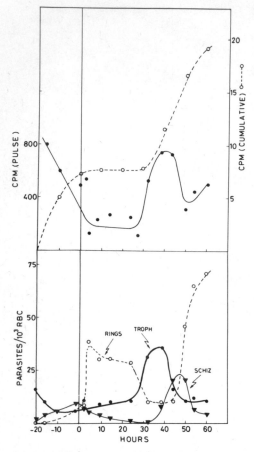

FIG. 1. DNA synthesis by *P. falciparum in vitro. Top:* radioactive hypoxanthine incorporation, in two-hour pulses, into DNAase-sensitive, trichloroacetic acid-insoluble material. *Bottom:* total and differential parasite counts in the course of the experiment. It is seen that DNA synthesis parallels closely the trophozoite stage.

rings give rise to a virtually pure population of schizonts within the first 48 hours (see Fig. 1). The same happens when parasitized cells stored frozen are grown up again after thawing: only rings survive the ordeal of hibernation, because mature forms are more susceptible to being damaged, whether by the procedure itself or through selective toxic effects of the 'cryoprotective' agents used. Alternatively, considerable enrichment of mature forms from an ordinary culture can be obtained by gelatine sedimentation (Pasvol et al 1978). In practice, we have found that if this technique is applied to a culture having a parasite rate of about 10%, we can obtain preparations with up to 70% of the red cells containing parasites, all of them mature (Table 2). If

TABLE 2 Preparation of synchronous cultures of malarial parasites

Experiment	Before physiogel[a]		After physiogel	
	Total parasites per 100 red cells	% mature	Total parasites per 100 red cells	% mature
1	3.5	31	40	78
2	9.4	38	30	98
3	10.2	45	61	100
4	8.2	51	70	100

[a] Physiogel: separation of parasites by a gelatine technique (see Pasvol et al 1978).

these are added as an inoculum to fresh unparasitized erythrocytes, a fairly synchronous course of infection is obtained.

Since there is hardly any information on the mode of DNA replication and nucleic acid synthesis in general in *P. falciparum*, we thought this would be a suitable system with which to attack the problem. A clear temporal pattern of DNA synthesis is seen during the schizogonic cycle (Fig. 1), with a sharp peak at the late trophozoite stage. Since synchronization of the culture is not perfect, the low rate of DNA synthesis between 15 and 25 hours can probably be attributed to contaminating trophozoites. If a correction for this is made, and the amount of DNA synthesis in the individual pulses is cumulated, one finds that in this particular experiment an approximately threefold increase in DNA takes place in one cycle. Also RNA synthesis is mostly associated with the trophozoite stage, peaking at about six hours before the schizont peak. RNA synthesis, as measured in these experiments, is completely absent during most of the ring form phase. Protein synthesis takes place at low level throughout the cycle, but again there is a steep rise associated with trophozoites. Indeed, there is an exponential increase in the rate of protein synthesis during this stage. A second peak in protein synthetic rate corresponds to the schizont peak, suggesting that different protein species are produced. This is born out by analysis on sodium dodecyl sulphate–polyacrylamide gels, which reveal a number of polypeptide bands apparently produced throughout the schizogonic cycle, and others that are stage-specific (O. Sodeinde & L. Luzzatto, in preparation). The data on stage-specific proteins extend the previously reported finding by Kilejian (1980) of a histidine-rich protein, and the pattern of macromolecule synthesis by *P. falciparum* agrees in general terms with previous observations on *P. knowlesi* (Cohen et al 1969, Gutteridge & Trigg 1978).

Glucose-6-phosphate dehydrogenase deficiency mosaics in vitro

Deficiency of erythrocyte glucose-6-phosphate dehydrogenase (G6PD) is an X-linked genetic trait with high frequencies in many human populations (Livingstone 1971, Luzzatto & Testa 1978). It was suggested over 20 years ago that the corresponding Gd^- gene was selected for over a number of generations by *P. falciparum* (sub-tertian) malaria (Allison 1960, Motulsky 1960), and since then much evidence has accumulated to support this concept (reviewed in Luzzatto 1979, Friedman 1980). The precise mechanism of protection, however, remained unclear. Early studies suggested a decreased rate of red cell invasion (Luzzatto et al 1976), while more recently it was shown that intracellular development of the parasite in G6PD(−) erythrocytes is impaired, especially if these are subjected to oxidative stress (Friedman 1979). An unexplained paradox has been that the Gd^{A-} gene in Nigeria seems to protect only Gd^+/Gd^- heterozygous females, who have in their blood a mixture of G6PD(+) and G6PD(−) cells (as a result of X-chromosome inactivation: Lyon 1972), but not hemizygous males, who have only G6PD(−) cells (Bienzle et al 1972). This has caused some controversy (Martin et al 1979, Luzzatto & Bienzle 1979, Bienzle et al 1979).

The mechanism of protection can now be tested *in vitro* by using again the synchronous culture system, in which mature parasites are inoculated in parallel in G6PD(+) and G6PD(−) recipient erythrocytes. It is clearly seen that the two types of cells are infected at about the same rate, but the growth curves diverge markedly by the second schizogonic cycle (Fig. 2, bottom and Table 3). In order to explain this divergence, we analysed the various forms of the parasites at successive times. In G6PD(+) cells, an orderly development of mature trophozoites (Fig. 2, middle) and of schizonts (Fig. 2, top) is seen, confirming that good synchronization had been achieved. In G6PD(−) cells, the development of mature trophozoites is retarded and the number of schizonts is markedly reduced. As a result, few merozoites are produced from these cells, and this explains the reduced slope of the growth curve in the second cycle of schizogony. Since the number of second-generation rings is even lower than would be expected from the number of first-generation schizonts, we infer that many of the schizonts either were not viable or produced a lower than average number of merozoites, or both. We find, then,

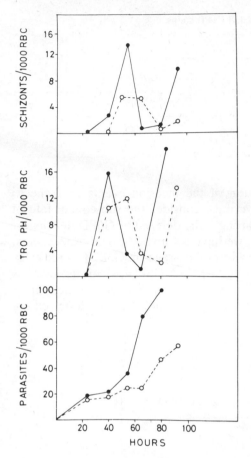

FIG. 2. Retarded development of *P. falciparum* in G6PD-deficient erythrocytes. ●——●, G6PD(+); ○---○, G6PD(−). The time course of total parasite rate (*bottom*) is virtually the same during the first cycle of infection, but grossly lowered in G6PD(−) cells during the second cycle. We presume this is due to retarded maturation to trophozoites (*middle*) and to schizonts (*top*), which may also release a decreased number of viable merozoites.

that G6PD(−) red cells can be invaded normally by *P. falciparum* but that only a fraction of these parasites are able to complete their asexual cycle.

These experiments show clearly that some maturation step along the schizogonic cycle is impaired in G6PD(−) red cells. However, there are two conceptual difficulties we must contend with. Firstly, it could be that the poor development of the parasite is due to some *in vitro* lesion of these cells, compared to normal cells. It might be, for instance, that after two days in the artificial culture conditions, G6PD(−) erythrocytes undergo metabolic changes that make them no longer competent to support the growth of *P.*

TABLE 3 In vitro infection by P. falciparum and G6PD status

Hours since inoculum	Parasites/1000 'recipient' red cells				
	G6PD(+)			G6PD(−)	
	Total	'Mature'		Total	'Mature'
48	50 ± 15	16 ± 6		25 ± 12	6 ± 3
72	88 ± 21	23 ± 8		36 ± 13	13 ± 5

falciparum. Secondly, since a fraction of the invasion events do come to fruition in the form of schizonts, we must consider the subsequent fate of those parasites which are 'leaking through' the defence of G6PD deficiency. In order to investigate these points, we have set up additional experiments. Firstly, if parasites are grown through several passages in G6PD(−) red cells, and their competence to infect G6PD(+) and G6PD(−) erythrocytes is tested, eventually no difference is observed (Fig. 3). Secondly, synchronous infection of G6PD-deficient red cells was again established and followed up,

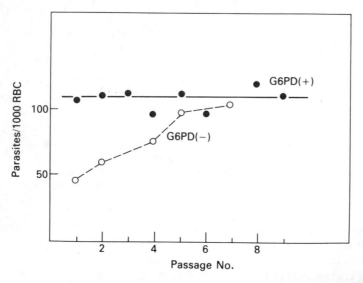

FIG. 3. Adaptive change in *P. falciparum.* Figures on the ordinate are parasite counts at 72 hours after each passage. Each passage consisted of a 1:4 dilution of a culture with fresh uninfected red cells, and this was done every four days. It is seen that the rate of multiplication is fairly steady in G6PD-normal red cells (filled circles). In G6PD-deficient red cells (open circles) the rate of multiplication is initially much lower (when parasites come from normal cells), but it tends gradually to the same steady-state level found in normal cells.

TABLE 4 Growth of P. falciparum in vitro depends on G6PD status of donor and recipient erythrocytes

Type of transfer	Efficiency of transfer		
	Rings/1000 red cells at 24 h	Schizonts/1000 red cells at 50 h	Total parasites/1000 red cells at 75 h
G6PD(+) → G6PD(+)	24	8.9	85
G6PD(+) → G6PD(−)	26	4.5	53
G6PD(−) → G6PD(−)	25	9.8	87

starting this time from parasites already matured (through several cycles) in the same cells. It now became clear (Table 4) that there was hardly any difference in the way *P. falciparum* developed: the parasite had apparently become adapted to this type of erythrocyte, which is fully competent under these circumstances to support the parasite cycle.

It has previously been pointed out that interruption of the malaria parasite cycle in human blood could take place through (a) failure of infection, (b) abortive infection or (c) suicidal infection (Luzzatto et al 1969). The experiments reported here show that in the transfer to G6PD(−) red cells, mechanism (b) does operate. Moreover, our findings may provide a specific explanation for the paradox mentioned earlier in this section. Indeed, in a *Gd⁺/Gd⁻* heterozygous female who has, on the average, 50% G6PD(+) and 50% G6PD(−) red cells, there is an even chance that a parasite emerging from a G6PD(+) cell will invade a cell of either type. From the results in Fig. 2 and Table 4, we infer that when a G6PD(−) cell is entered, the chance of successful development of the parasite is only about 1:2 to 1:4, compared to when a G6PD(+) cell is entered, thus limiting significantly the probability that high, life-threatening levels of parasitaemia are reached in these subjects (Bienzle et al 1972). It is important to point out that the experiments described here were done on red cells with the Mediterranean type of G6PD deficiency. However, we also did three experiments with G6PD(−) Mahidol erythrocytes (kindly supplied by Dr S. Fucharoen and Professor P. Wasi), and one with G6PD(−) A⁻ erythrocytes (kindly supplied by Dr P. McCurdy). All of these showed normal invasion but delayed and decreased maturation of *P. falciparum*, and this has been verified with several strains of the organism.

Biological changes in *Plasmodium* are not without precedent in the study of experimental malaria. The fact that the capacity to produce gametocytes is lost by *P. berghei* after a number of blood passages has been known for a long time (see Garnham 1966), and recently the time course of this phenomenon has been carefully investigated (Dore et al 1980) and shown to correlate with a decrease in repetitive DNA (Birago et al 1982). In our system the change taking place is more rapid and is probably more subtle: we do not yet know its nature. However, we can point out that the mechanism of malaria protection emerging from the combination of *in vivo* and *in vitro* findings is quite characteristic. While in sickle cell and in thalassaemia heterozygotes the erythrocyte population is homogeneous, and in some way or other less hospitable for the parasite, in G6PD deficiency heterozygotes it is the dual

TABLE 5 Potential biological advantages associated with X-inactivation-linked mosaicism

1. Selection AGAINST one of the two coexisting cell types:
   Elimination of cells with chromosomal abnormality
   Elimination of cells with disadvantageous allele
2. Selection FOR mosaicism:
   Within the whole organism: cells with either X chromosome active may be at an advantage in one or the other tissue
   Within one tissue or organ: coexistence of two cell types may itself be an advantage (e.g. malaria and the red cell)

population itself that is protective. Perhaps (see Table 5) the biological significance of the genetic mosaicism resulting from X-chromosome inactivation does not lie just in dosage compensation, but also in other selective advantage, such as is described here.

Acknowledgements

We thank Dr M. J. Friedman for many discussions and collaboration; Dr M. D'Urso for help with the cultures; and Mr A. De Falco for technical assistance. Dr W. Trager, Dr L. Perrin, Dr P. I. Trigg, Dr G. Butcher, Dr G. Mitchell and Dr F. A. Akinkugbe have kindly provided malaria-infected red cells. Financial support was received from the UNDP/WHO/World Bank Tropical Diseases Research Programme.

REFERENCES

Allison AC 1960 Glucose-6-phosphate dehydrogenase deficiency in red blood cells of East Africans. Nature (Lond) 186:531-532

Bienzle U, Ayeni O, Lucas AO, Luzzatto L 1972 Glucose-6-phosphate dehydrogenase and malaria: greater resistance of females heterozygous for enzyme deficiency and of males with non-deficient variant. Lancet 1:107-110

Bienzle U, Guggenmoos-Holzmann I, Luzzatto L 1979 Malaria and erythrocyte glucose-6-phosphate dehydrogenase in West Africa. Am J Trop Med Hyg 28:619-621

Birago C, Bucci A, Dore E, Frontali C, Zenobi P 1982 Gametogenesis is directly related to the amount of repetitive DNA in *Plasmodium berghei*. Parasitology, in press

Cohen S, Butcher GA, Crandall RB 1969 Action of malarial antibody *in vitro*. Nature (Lond) 223:368-371

Dore E, Birago C, Frontali C, Battaglia P 1980 Kinetic complexity and repetitivity of *Plasmodium berghei* DNA. Mol Biochem Parasitol 1:199-208

Friedman MJ 1979 Oxidant damage mediates variant red cell resistance to malaria. Nature (Lond) 280:245-247

Friedman MJ 1981 The biology of inherited resistance to malaria. In: Levandowsky M, Hutner SH (eds) Biochemistry and physiology of protozoa. Academic Press, New York, vol 4:463-493

Friedman MJ 1983 Expression of inherited resistance to malaria in culture. This volume, p 196-201

Garnham PCC 1966 Malaria parasites and other haemosporidia. Blackwell Scientific Publications, Oxford

Gutteridge WE, Trigg PI 1978 Periodicity of nuclear DNA synthesis in the intra-erythrocytic cycle of *Plasmodium knowlesi*. J Protozool 19:378-385

Kilejian A 1980 Stage-specific proteins and glycoproteins of *Plasmodium falciparum*: identification of antigens specific to schizonts and merozoites. Proc Natl Acad Sci USA 77:3695-3699

Livingstone FB 1971 Malaria and human polymorphisms. Annu Rev Genet 5:33-64

Luzzatto L 1979 Genetics of red cells and susceptibility to malaria. Blood 54:961-976

Luzzatto L, Testa U 1978 Human erythrocyte glucose-6-phosphate dehydrogenase: structure and function in normal and mutant subjects. Curr Top Hematol 1:1-70

Luzzatto L, Bienzle U 1979 The malaria/G6PD hypothesis. Lancet 1:1183-1184

Luzzatto L, Usanga EA, Reddy S 1969 Glucose-6-phosphate dehydrogenase deficient red cells: resistance to infection by malaria parasites. Science (Wash DC) 164:839-842

Luzzatto L, Okoye VCN, Williams AIO 1976 Fetal haemoglobin and malaria. Lancet 2:523-524

Lyon MF 1972 X chromosome inactivation and developmental patterns in mammals. Biol Rev Camb Philos Soc 47:1-35

Martin SK, Miller LH, Alling D et al 1979 Severe malaria and glucose-6-phosphate-dehydrogenase deficiency: a reappraisal of the malaria/G6PD hypothesis. Lancet 1:524-526

Motulsky AG 1960 Metabolic polymorphisms and the role of infectious diseases in human evolution. Hum Biol 32:28-62

Pasvol G, Wilson RJM, Smalley ME, Brown J 1978 Separation of viable schizont-infected red cells of *Plasmodium falciparum* from human blood. Ann Trop Med Parasitol 72:87-88

Trager W, Jensen JB 1976 Human malaria parasites in continuous culture. Science (Wash DC) 193:673-675

DISCUSSION

Howard: Is there any change in the ratio of erythrocytes of the G6PD-deficient phenotype in the female heterozygote made anaemic by means other than by malaria?

Luzzatto: If a G6PD-deficient heterozygotic female has a haemolytic episode triggered by drugs or by eating fava beans, the cells destroyed are (selectively) the G6PD-deficient cells (Panizon et al 1970). Thus, if we include in the definition of her phenotype the ratio of the two cell types, there will be a transient change in the phenotype, followed by regeneration of both cell populations, G6PD(+) and G6PD(−).

Howard: So in a malaria infection, the ratio of G6PD phenotypes might actually vary with time, depending on the history of the individual and the course of infection? The selective effect on parasite multiplication would then also vary.

Luzzatto: As I said, the phenotype could be defined quantitatively as the ratio of the two cell types. Normally, it is simply referred to as being 'intermediate' 'between normal and enzyme-deficient'. Because we know what range of phenotypes to expect in Gd^+/Gd^- heterozygotes, we feel quite confident that we are actually looking at this *genotype*.

Howard: Basically I am saying that the evidence for a selective effect of the G6PD phenotype on malaria parasites may be much more impressive if you measure their phenotype at, and during, infection, rather than in uninfected individuals.

Luzzatto: Yes.

Sherman: You say that there is no selection by the merozoite of the G6PD($+$) red cell and that there is an even chance of entry into positive and negative cells, which are distributed roughly 50/50. You also say that in the G6PD-deficient cells, a proportion of the parasites, from 1 in 2 to 1 in 4, will not develop. What is the mechanism of this abortion?

Luzzatto: I have a working hypothesis here, but without any proof yet. We know that parasites emerging from the G6PD($+$) cells are different from those emerging from the deficient cells, as judged by their capacity to infect further deficient cells (see Fig. 2).

Sherman: Do the parasites produce fewer merozoites in G6PD-deficient red cells?

Luzzatto: They produce the same numbers once they are adapted to the deficient cells. I don't know about the period before adaptation; they may produce fewer then. In other words, we don't know whether they abort before or after the schizont stage. We can only speculate on the difference in the parasites emerging from the two kinds of red cell. Does the parasite have its own G6PD, and what does it do with the host enzyme? Iain Wilson has produced some evidence in favour of a parasite-specific G6PD (Hempelmann & Wilson 1981). Perhaps this is insufficient for the needs of the parasite and it uses the host cell's G6PD if it is there. If it is not there, it has to turn on its own enzyme. There may be a lag in doing that, and many parasites die. But once the parasite grows in G6PD-deficient cells, the G6PD gene is derepressed and the host enzyme isn't required. That is entirely hypothetical!

Sherman: I know of no direct evidence, where the malaria parasite uses a host enzyme, or a situation where the host enzyme crosses the parasitophorous vacuole membrane and enters the parasite through its plasma membrane, or an enzyme of host origin can survive passage through the cytostome and the food vacuoles.

Wallach: The damage to the parasite might derive from some kind of oxidative stress, perhaps through the production of free radicals. In the normal red cell there is an oxygen free radical trap in the form of the enzyme superoxide dismutase which limits the level of free radical activity within the erythrocyte. The inhibition of red cell superoxide dismutase leads to the destruction of parasites. Superoxide dismutase is an adaptive enzyme, and one might investigate whether the parasite can turn this enzyme on and off. The enzyme hasn't yet been studied in protozoans at all.

Luzzatto: The problem to me is not so much why the parasite should do better in G6PD(+) cells than in G6PD(−) cells. The problem is that in fact only heterozygous mosaics, and not G6PD(−) hemizygotes, are protected. Any explanation of why parasites suffer in the G6PD(−) red cells is not sufficient. We must also explain how they eventually adapt to that same environment.

Pasvol: I am interested that you have been studying the Mediterranean type of G6PD deficiency. Dr Iain Wilson and I studied cells from G6PD(−) individuals in The Gambia. These included cells from African hemizygotes, homozygotes and female heterozygotes. We found no difference between normal and G6PD(−) cells in either invasion or the maturation of parasites (Pasvol & Wilson 1982). We were using 21% oxygen tensions in these studies, which is a relatively high oxygen stress. Dr Friedman also used the African type of G6PD(−) cells in his studies which showed damage to parasites (Friedman 1979), but there are differences in our culture systems. We used Medium 199, which has for example a higher concentration of reduced glutathione. This and the differences in oxygen tension might be factors accounting for the differences in our findings.

Turning to parasite rates, I find these difficult to interpret, particularly in the context of protection, which is often subtle. I wonder why you felt that the parasite rates in the two groups of young children were significantly different in Fig. 1 in Bienzle et al (1979)? Have you any comment on the problem of looking at parasite rates at an epidemiological level rather than, say, at parasite densities or mortality from the disease?

Luzzatto: There are others here more qualified to comment on that. I agree that if one finds no difference in the field in parasite rates, it may not mean anything. But if you *do* find differences, they are sure to mean something!

Wyler: In hypothesizing that the maintenance of the high incidence of G6PD deficiency depends on *P. falciparum* infection, aren't you implying that this depends on mortality rather than on parasitaemia? Have you investigated whether the frequency of potentially fatal complications such as pulmonary oedema or cerebral involvement differs in G6PD-deficient patients?

Luzzatto: This has never been looked at. An unpublished study by A. Adeniyi of the nephrotic syndrome in children has shown a paucity of G6PD heterozygotes. That is a complicated matter because it seems to be related to *P. malariae*, not to *P. falciparum* malaria.

Greenwood: One way of studying this problem is to look at the distribution of red cell haemoglobin abnormalities in a population in relation to age. If the abnormality has a harmful or a protective effect on mortality its distribution should change with age.

Luzzatto: In males, there was no difference between newborns and adults in the frequency of G6PD deficiency. But you need a relatively strong selection to detect such a difference. It has been found for haemoglobin AS heterozygotes, but here you have to balance, against the protective trait, a nearly fatal condition (homozygous sickle cell anaemia). With G6PD deficiency you need to balance relatively little pathology, so you need only a tiny advantage to get selection of heterozygotes.

Friedman: Except in the Mediterranean region, where G6PD-deficient individuals experience haemolytic episodes after eating fava beans.

Luzzatto: Probably even in the Mediterranean, because only about 20% of G6PD-deficient subjects develop favism, and they don't all die. But I agree that selection will be stronger than with the A^-(African) variant.

Howard: Can we obtain any information from the study of contemporary human populations and their distribution on the nature of the phenotype of the first humans? It would obviously be of interest for studies on innate resistance to malaria, as well as the genetics of immune responsiveness. The distribution of the Duffy-negative phenotype appears to confirm the hypothesis that as man migrated to areas away from the initial foci, where malaria was less prevalent, the reduced selection pressure allowed genetic drift to the Duffy-positive phenotype. Is there any area of the world in which there is no malaria but there is a high ratio of some of these polymorphisms that are related to resistance to malaria? The situation in China would be of interest, as I believe there is debate as to whether man evolved separately there or migrated there from an initial focus in Africa.

Luzzatto: I know of no areas without malaria and with a high frequency of these genes. There is, or has been, quite a lot of malaria in South China, and there is G6PD deficiency in the people there. The Canton variant is quite prominent: reported by Chan & Todd (1972).

Anders: In Papua New Guinea the number of G6PD variants is unusually high. I believe some of these are functionally silent G6PD variants, with no overt G6PD deficiency. What is the significance of this large number of variants, and what is the mechanism of selection for functionally silent variants?

Luzzatto: There are at least 25 polymorphic G6PD-deficient variants. This means there are many others that are deficient but not yet known to be polymorphic, and some that are polymorphic but not deficient. The total number has reached about 190. On the question of whether there could be selection of polymorphic variants that are not deficient in enzyme activity, but are detected by electrophoresis or other qualitative changes, there is little information (but see Modiano et al 1979). Why are there so many variants? Several people have tried to calculate whether it could be due simply to ascertainment bias: indeed, there has been very much work done on this enzyme, and if we looked hard enough at another gene maybe we would find as many variants. That is still a possibility. Others have suggested that the G6PD gene has a higher frequency of mutation, but that should be the last resort as an explanation.

REFERENCES

Bienzle W, Guggenmoos-Holzmann I, Luzzatto L 1979 Malaria and erythrocyte glucose 6-phosphate dehydrogenase variants in West Africa. Am J Trop Med Hyg 28:619-621

Chan TK, Todd D 1972 Characteristics and distribution of glucose 6-phosphate dehydrogenase-deficient variants in South China. Am J Hum Genet 24:475-484

Friedman MJ 1979 Oxidant damage mediates variant red cell resistance to malaria. Nature (Lond) 280:245-247

Hempelmann E, Wilson RJM 1981 Detection of glucose-6-phosphate dehydrogenase in malarial parasites. Mol Biochem Parasitol 2:197-204

Modiano G, Battistuzzi G, Esan GJF, Testa U, Luzzatto L 1979 Genetic heterogeneity of 'normal' human erythrocyte glucose-6-phosphate dehydrogenase: an isoelectrophoretic polymorphism. Proc Natl Acad Sci USA 76:852-856

Panizon F, Zacchello F, Sartori A, Addis S 1970 The ratio between normal and sensitive erythrocytes in heterozygous glucose-6-phosphate dehydrogenase deficient women. Acta Haematol 43:291-295

Pasvol G, Wilson RJM 1982 The interaction of malaria parasites with red blood cells. Br Med Bull 38:133-140

Glycophorins and red cell invasion by *Plasmodium falciparum*

GEOFFREY PASVOL and MICHELE JUNGERY

Tropical Medicine Unit, Nuffield Department of Clinical Medicine, John Radcliffe Hospital, Oxford, OX3 9DU, UK

Abstract The major red cell sialoglycoproteins, the glycophorins, play a central role in the invasion of human red cells by *Plasmodium falciparum*. En(a−) cells deficient in glycophorin A (α) and S − s − U − cells deficient in glycophorin B (δ) are relatively resistant to invasion, while trypsin treatment of S − s − U − cells, which removes most of the remaining sialoglycoprotein, renders these cells almost totally resistant to invasion. Parasites inside these glycophorin-deficient cells develop normally. Invasion of erythroid precursors *in vitro* by merozoites of *P. falciparum* parallels the appearance of glycophorins on the surface of these nucleated cells, even though parasites fail to develop inside them. However, another type of cell from an erythroleukaemic line (K562) which expresses glycophorins on its surface is resistant to invasion. Furthermore, the observed increased invasion of young cells as opposed to an older cell population is not related quantitatively to the presence of glycophorins on the cell surface. Thus, although the role of glycophorins is both specific and important in the invasion of cells by *P. falciparum*, it is clearly only part of a complex process.

Invasion of the red cell by the malarial parasite is now recognized as a highly specific, predictable and ordered process. This is quite unlike previously held concepts, where the parasite was thought to 'push its way' into red cells in an undefined and non-selective manner. Invasion involves a number of complex stages which include (a) recognition of the red cell by the invading merozoite, (b) attachment of the merozoite to the red cell, (c) orientation of the apical end of the merozoite to the red cell membrane, (d) formation of a junction between merozoite and red cell, (e) deformation of the red cell, followed by entry (f) of the merozoite into the parasitophorous vacuole caused by invagination of the red cell membrane. At an earlier Ciba Foundation symposium evidence for specific receptors involved in the attachment and entry of malarial parasites into red cells was presented (Howard & Miller 1981). The process of parasite invasion, as well as the involvement of factors

1983 Malaria and the red cell. Pitman, London (Ciba Foundation symposium 94) p 174-195

such as host specificity, red cell age and blood group antigens in invasion, was described. The relationship of the Duffy antigen to *Plasmodium knowlesi* and *P. vivax*, and the ability of the monosaccharide *N*-acetyl-D-glucosamine to block invasion by *P. falciparum*, were discussed. However, at that time none of the molecules on the merozoite or red cell which interacted during attachment or the following stages in invasion had been identified. Since then, the importance of one such group of molecules, namely the glycophorins, has been emphasized in the invasion of human red cells by *P. falciparum* (Miller et al 1977, Perkins 1981, Pasvol et al 1982a), and in this paper we shall discuss in greater detail evidence for the role played by these molecules in the interaction between the host red cell and the parasite.

The glycophorins

The human red cell membrane contains four distinct sialic acid-rich glycoproteins called the glycophorins (Fig. 1). These are individually known as α (glycophorin A), β and γ (glycophorin C) and δ (glycophorin B) (see Anstee 1981 for nomenclature). Each red cell possesses at least 1×10^6 molecules of α

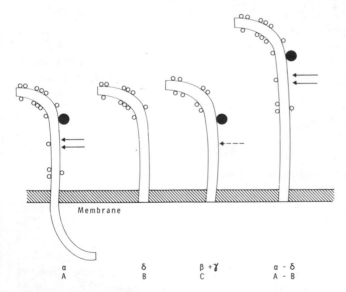

FIG. 1. A schematic representation of the major red cell sialoglycoproteins, glycophorins A, B and C (or α, β, γ and δ) (from Anstee 1981). The small circles represent *O*-glycosidically linked oligosaccharides; the large filled circles represent *N*-glycosidically linked oligosaccharides. The arrows indicate trypsin cleavage sites on intact cells. α—δ is a representation of the hybrid molecule obtained from an individual, A.G. (see text).

and 2.5×10^5 molecules of δ (Anstee et al 1982); the number of molecules of β and γ remains unknown. β and γ do however contribute about 10% of the sialic acid of the red cell surface, while the relative amounts for α and δ are 60% and 15% respectively. Despite being so highly represented on red cells, no function has been ascribed to these molecules and individuals with known deficiencies of these glycoproteins are haematologically quite normal.

The complete 131 amino acid sequence of the transmembrane α has been determined, but only partial sequence information is available for δ which shares the same 26 N-terminal residues with α. Alpha carries the M and N blood group antigens determined by the first five amino acids and oligosaccharides, whereas δ always carries a weak N antigen (N') and the S or s antigens, depending on the amino acid at position 29 from the amino end. The carbohydrate content of these molecules is largely in the form of sialic acid-rich tetrasaccharides which are O-glycosidically linked. There are 15 of these on α and 11 on δ. An N-glycosidically linked oligosaccharide, rich in N-acetylglucosamine and mannose, occurs at position 26 on α and also possibly on β and γ. There are also trypsin cleavage sites present on α (between residues 30 and 31, and 39 and 40), β and γ, but not on δ.

In investigations of the role played by these glycoproteins, naturally occurring cells deficient in α (En(a −) cells), deficient in δ (S − s − U − cells) and cells containing hybrid molecules of α and δ (AG cells) have proved to be extremely useful, particularly since these cells have been found to be functionally normal. We have also used cells from an erythroleukaemia line (K562), nucleated red cells from bone marrow aspirations, and cells of different metabolic age in attempting to clarify the role of the glycophorins in the invasion process.

En(a−) cells

Naturally occurring cells deficient in α have been described in fewer than 10 individuals worldwide. We have tested the rates of invasion by P. falciparum in cells from three such En(a−) individuals using standard micromethods of parasite culture (Pasvol et al 1980). Invasion of these cells was reduced to between 52 and 92% of the controls (Pasvol et al 1982a) (Table 1). Two of these samples had been tested earlier and inhibition of invasion using primate (Aotus monkey)-conditioned parasites was 39 and 47% respectively (Miller et al 1977). Both studies have emphasized the relative rather than absolute resistance of these cells to invasion. Once inside En(−) cells the parasites developed normally, indicating a specific effect on invasion.

The ability of sera from two En(a−) individuals to reduce invasion was also tested. We showed a significant reduction which correlated with the titre of

TABLE 1 Invasion of red cells deficient in glycophorins by P. falciparum

Cells	Samples tested	Sialic acid (% control)	Invasion (% control)
En (a−)	3	40	8–48
S − s − U −	4	85	28–53
S − s − U − + trypsin	4	24	7–33
α–δ hybrid	1	61	46
α–δ hybrid + trypsin	1	24	23
Wr[b]−	1	100	10
Tn	1	46	8

For a description of the cell types see text. Invasion rates in all controls exceeded five parasites per 100 red cells.

anti-En[a] antibody present, and this effect was removed by prior absorption of the sera with En(a+) cells (Pasvol et al 1982a). Antibodies against other commonly occurring antigens on the red cell surface, such as rhesus (C and c̄), Kidd (Jk[a]) and Duffy (Fy[a]), had no inhibitory effect on parasite invasion. However, since these anti-En[a] sera contain antibodies of numerous specificities directed against the trypsin-sensitive and insensitive portions of α and another red cell antigen, Wr[b] (which might exist on α; M. J. A. Tanner, personal communication 1982), none of these three determinants could be excluded as a specific receptor. In preliminary experiments using monoclonal antibodies we have shown marked inhibition of invasion with the antibody against the trypsin-sensitive portion of α and the Wr[b] antigen, but this inhibition occurred at titres which cause agglutination. A monoclonal antibody against band 3 (the main membrane anion transport protein) showed no inhibition.

Since the outer portion of α might be important in invasion we have tested invasion rates in MN, MM and NN cells but found no differences. This indicates that the merozoite is unable to distinguish between these two antigens. Finally, Perkins (1981) has purified α and shown that concentrations as low as 50 μg/ml are capable of 100% inhibition of invasion (Table 2). However, total sialoglycoprotein extract was required in significantly higher concentrations to bring about any inhibitory effect (Weiss et al 1981, M. Jungery, G. Pasvol, C. I. Newbold & D. J. Weatherall, unpublished work).

S − s − U − cells and cells bearing a hybrid α–δ molecule

S − s − U − cells are deficient in δ and the incidence of individuals with these cells reaches frequencies characteristic of a balanced polymorphism in

TABLE 2 Invasion of red cells by P. falciparum in the presence of various preparations of sialoglycoprotein extracts

Author	Preparation	Concentration (µg/ml)	% inhibition
Weiss et al 1981	Total sialoglycoproteins	500	28
		200	6
Perkins 1981	Aqueous phase (α)	200	100
		50	100
		10	21
	α (ex-rhesus monkey red cells)	200	100
		100	81
		50	49
M. Jungery, G. Pasvol, C. I. Newbold & D. J. Weatherall, unpublished results	Total sialoglyco-proteins	3800	100
		1900	60
		950	47
		475	10
		238	12

malarious areas in Africa. S − s − U − cells obtained from four different donors showed an invasion rate of between 28 and 53% of the control cells (Table 1). Moreover, treating these cells with trypsin, which removes α (and possibly also β and γ), further reduced the rate of invasion of S − s − U − cells, thus rendering them virtually resistant to invasion by P. falciparum (Pasvol et al 1982b).

Cells obtained from an individual (A.G.) with a hybrid glycophorin molecule consisting of the amino end of α and the carboxyl end of δ (denoted α–δ) showed relative (54%) resistance to parasite invasion which was increased even further (77%) on trypsin treatment (Table 1). (Such a hybrid molecule is both larger than α or δ alone and retains the trypsin-sensitive site of α; see Fig. 1.) Once again, as with En(a−) cells, the few parasites which penetrated these cells from A.G., deficient in sialoglycoprotein, whether untreated or trypsin-treated, developed normally.

Invasion of nucleated cells expressing glycophorin on their surface

Erythroid precursors

The appearance of α on the surface of erythroid precursors has been studied by Gahmberg et al (1978). By counting the number of staphylococci that bound to an anti-glycophorin A antibody, they demonstrated negligible

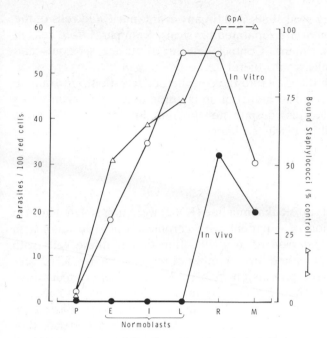

FIG. 2. The invasion of erythroid cells by *P. falciparum in vitro* (O——O) and *in vivo* (●——●) compared with the appearance of glycophorin A (GpA) on normal erythroid precursors. The amount of GpA was measured by the binding of staphylococci to an anti-glycophorin A antibody. The data for the appearance of GpA were adapted from Gahmberg et al (1978) (△ — △) and Lutz & Fehr (1979) (△ --- △). (The former did not distinguish between reticulocytes and mature erythrocytes.) P, pronormoblast; E, I, L, early, intermediate and late normoblasts, respectively; R, reticulocyte; M, mature erythrocyte.

amounts of glycophorin A on pronormoblasts, with increasing quantities on early, intermediate and late normoblasts and erythrocytes (Fig. 2). We have cultured schizonts of *P. falciparum* with the cells obtained from a bone marrow aspirate from an uninfected patient with erythroid hyperplasia and compared the rates of invasion of the various precursors *in vitro* with those seen in the marrow of a heavily infected patient. Parasites *in vitro* frequently invaded normoblasts, whereas pronormoblasts rarely contained parasites (Fig. 2). Maximal invasion was seen in late normoblasts and reticulocytes. This correlated well with the appearance of glycophorin on the surface of such cells and is in agreement with our previous findings on the increased invasion of metabolically young cells, both *in vitro* and in acutely ill patients (Pasvol et al 1980). Differential counts from the bone marrow of a heavily infected individual showed that *in vivo* none of the nucleated red cells were infected (Fig. 2). The absence of infected nucleated cells in bone marrow biopsies is well recognized (Smalley et al 1980) and, in any event, nucleated cells of the bone marrow compartment are separated physically from parasitized cells in the intravascular compartment. Contact between rupturing schizonts and uninfected nucleated cells would therefore be unlikely *in vivo* except when erythroid precursors are released into the peripheral circulation, for example under conditions of stress. The reduction in invasion in mature erythrocytes as compared to reticulocytes, despite no apparent loss of glycophorin as indicated on Fig. 2, will be discussed later.

K562 cells

Cells from the human erythroleukaemia line (K562) were first isolated in 1975 from the pleural effusion of a patient with chronic myeloid leukaemia in terminal blast crisis (Anderson et al 1979). Infection of these cells with malarial parasites was attempted for a number of reasons. Firstly, K562 cells are known to express glycophorins on their surface and can be maintained continuously in culture. They can also be induced by haemin (40 μM) to produce small quantities (10–15 pg) of haemoglobin. Moreover, Eisen et al (1977) have succeeded in infecting mouse erythroleukaemia (Friend) cells with *P. berghei* and *P. yoelii* and noted apparently normal morphological development of these parasites inside these cells.

We have attempted to infect uninduced and induced K562 cells with *P. falciparum* schizonts without success. No merozoites were seen bound to the K562 cell surface despite the presence of active schizogony. No invasion of the tumour line was seen. However, a 1% suspension of K562 cells bound only 5.2% of monoclonal antibody (R10) directed against α when compared to a similar suspension of red cells, indicating subtle differences in the α glycoprotein of red cells and that of the K562 line. At 48 hours after the start of the cultures, infected red cells with non-viable parasites (pyknic and hyperchromatic) were seen in close association with the K562 cells, suggesting toxicity.

Parasite invasion and the relationship to glycophorin in red cell ageing

We have previously speculated that the greater invasion of 'young' than 'old' red cells is related to one of three possible mechanisms, namely the increased number of receptor sites, increased metabolic activity, or the increased deformability displayed by relatively young cells (Pasvol et al 1980). We therefore tested the rates of invasion in red cells separated on the basis of age by centrifugation and correlated these with the binding of monoclonal antibodies directed against α (R10). Although there was clearly a greater rate of invasion in the relatively 'young' cells in the top fraction of the centrifuged red cells than in the old cells in the bottom fraction, the binding assay showed no significant difference in the binding of R10 to these cells (Table 3). Our

TABLE 3 The relationship of red cell age and the presence of glycophorins to the invasion of red cells by P. falciparum

Fraction	Reticulocytes (%)	Binding of anti-α (c.p.m. $\times 10^{-3}$)	Rings per 100 red cells
Whole blood	6.7	30.9	20.7
Top ('young')	24.6	31.3	30.1
Middle	4.7	31.2	15.3
Bottom ('old')	0.3	32.4	12.6
Top/bottom	82	1.0	2.4

The binding assay represents the mean of duplicate counts.

binding assay confirms the study by Lutz & Fehr (1979), who found the degree of surface iodination of glycophorins to be the same in young and old cells. These authors also showed that the total sialic acid content per glycophorin molecule is identical in young and old cells and that sialic acid loss could be accounted for by loss of intact glycophorin together with membrane. The density of sialylated glycophorin would therefore remain unchanged.

Since there is no evidence of loss of glycophorin during red cell ageing, the observed decrease in the invasion of old red cells cannot be attributed to decreased 'receptor' availability. Nor is there any evidence to suggest that the red cell remains anything other than a passive partner during invasion, which excludes decreased metabolic activity of old red cells as an explanation for their reduced invasion. The third possibility, decreased deformability of old cells, could therefore be of relevance. The decreased invasion of cells displaying decreased deformability, such as cells containing Hb S or Hb C, heat-treated cells, and ovalocytes, and the presence of anti-spectrin antibodies, would support this possibility (Pasvol & Wilson 1982).

Glycophorin as a specific receptor for P. falciparum

Quantitative aspects

From the evidence presented earlier it would seem that the predominant red cell sialoglycoproteins α and δ, and possibly β and γ, are in some way essential for the successful entry by merozoites of P. falciparum into red cells, and that this is a specific interaction. It might equally be argued that the relationship is a quantitative rather than qualitative one, so that the more glycoprotein is removed, the less invasion is seen. This in turn could be related to the negative charge of the cell surface provided by the sialic acid residues, so that the more glycophorin is removed the more resistant such cells become to invasion. However, since the merozoite is itself negatively charged, albeit less than the red cell (Miller et al 1973), removal of negative charge from the red cell would be expected to facilitate rather than reduce invasion. Moreover, such a non-specific mechanism might be expected to transcend the different species. It fails to do this in P. knowlesi, where neuraminidase, which strips the red cell of most of its sialic acid residues, leaves invasion unaffected. Although neuraminidase treatment of human red cells reduces invasion by P. falciparum, the reduction is less than that seen after trypsin treatment, which leaves many sialic acid residues intact (Miller et al 1977). However, Perkins (1981) has found that either trypsin or neuraminidase treatment of red cells can abolish invasion by P. falciparum merozoites.

We have also tested Wr[b]-negative cells, which retain the full complement of sialic acid residues and electrophoretic charge, in an invasion assay. On a single sample obtained from the only known donor, we found that these cells were extremely resistant to invasion (Table 1). Moreover, Tn cells, which are incompletely glycosylated, thus exposing Tn, a cryptantigen (Anstee 1981), and have about 46% of the normal amount of sialic acid, were particularly resistant to infection (Table 1). Taking all these results together, an effect of charge alone seems to be an unlikely basis for the role of glycophorins in the invasion of red cells by P. falciparum merozoites.

Another problem in our studies has been the relative rather than absolute resistance of many of these glycophorin-deficient red cells to invasion. This applies particularly to the trypsin-treated $S - s - U -$ cells, which are effectively lacking in glycophorin. A number of explanations are possible. Firstly, even trypsin-treated $S - s - U -$ cells retain a sizeable portion of α (± 33 amino acids and three 15-O-glycosidically linked oligosaccharides), which is below the trypsin cleavage site and external to the membrane surface. This remaining portion of the molecule might also possess specific receptor sites. Secondly, invasion might require only relatively few molecules of glycophorin, which are inevitably present even after trypsin treatment. Thirdly, alternative receptors for parasite invasion not located on glycophorins might exist. Finally, it is tempting to implicate glycophorins in the initial specific recognition of the red cell, facilitating the attachment and subsequent orientation of merozoites, rather than in junction formation or in interaction with the red cell cytoskeleton. The triggering of parasite entry could conceivably occur in the absence of glycophorin by random collision of the apical end of the merozoite with the cell, but only when the merozoite is orientated correctly. The testing of cells from patients homozygous for a deficiency in α and δ (Mk/Mk), of whom only two have been described (Tokunaga et al 1979), would be particularly relevant to answering some of these questions.

Qualitative aspects

The involvement of glycoproteins such as the glycophorins in the attachment of the malarial parasite to red cells points to the possibility of the binding involving a lectin–ligand type of interaction. Carbohydrate-binding proteins, similar in their properties to the well-known plant lectins, are well documented for the attachment of microorganisms to epithelial cells. Among the protozoa in particular, such an interaction is not without precedent. *Acanthamoeba castellani*, for example, has been shown to agglutinate horse blood cells, a reaction which can be inhibited by mannose, fructose and α-methyl-D-mannoside (Brown et al 1975). Kobiler & Mirelman (1980) found that the trimer and tetramer, but not the monomer, of N-acetyl-D-glucosamine inhibited the agglutination of human red cells by extracts of *Entamoeba histolytica*.

Recently, the specific inhibition of invasion by *P. falciparum* of human red cells by N-acetylglucosamine has been reported (Weiss et al 1981). They found significant invasion inhibition by this sugar at concentrations of 100, 50 and 25 mM and demonstrated that these concentrations did not prevent the intracellular development of the parasite. Independently, we have found similar effects of N-acetylglucosamine on invasion at concentrations of the order of 10 mM and have also detected some invasion inhibition by relatively high concentrations of the related sugars N-acetylgalactosamine (75 mM) and N-acetylneuraminic acid (25 mM) (Fig. 3). Invasion was unaffected by other sugars such as D-glucose, D-galactose, fucose or mannose.

It is important in experiments of this kind to exclude the possibility that these sugars prevent the development of the parasite. No toxicity of N-acetylgalactosamine or N-acetylneuraminic acid was detected in our system, even at high concentrations. However, N-acetylglucosamine did retard parasite development at high concentrations (>20 mM). Toxicity was assessed in two ways. In the first, ring forms of the parasite were cultured to the schizont stage in media containing the sugars, and maturation was assessed. In the second, parasites were grown to the schizont stage in sugar concentrations of up to 20 mM, then washed free of the sugar and placed back into culture. There was no reduction in the subsequent rate of invasion, even

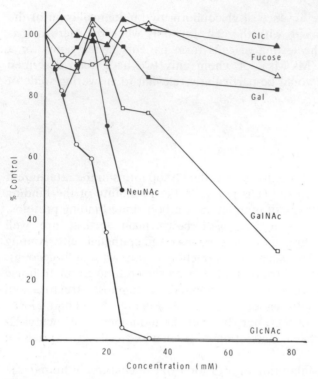

FIG. 3. Invasion of red cells by *P. falciparum* in the presence of various sugars, as a percentage of control. Glc, glucose; Gal, galactose; GalNAc, *N*-acetyl-D-galactosamine; NeuNac, *N*-acetyl-neuraminic acid; GlcNac, *N*-acetyl-D-glucosamine.

though maturation had occurred in the presence of the sugar. This suggests that these sugars do inhibit the invasion process itself, rather than acting via a deleterious effect on maturation.

These results point to the specificity of the interaction between the merozoites of *P. falciparum* and red cells and support the possibility of a lectin–ligand type of interaction. *N*-Acetylglucosamine, *N*-acetylgalactosamine and *N*-acetylneuraminic acid, which we have shown to inhibit invasion, are structurally similar when in the pyranose configuration. However, each sugar might not represent a 'perfect fit' and might therefore result only in a relative inhibition of invasion. It could be hypothesized that the merozoite recognizes clusters of *O*-linked oligosaccharides present on glycophorin (be it α, β, γ or δ) through a receptor on the parasite surface. This model would resemble that of Baenziger & Fiete (1980), where a mammalian lectin on rat hepatocytes must recognize specific *O*-linked oligosaccharides for the glycoprotein to be endocytosed. Thus certain homologous portions present on the various glycophorins might be involved which provide specific attachment sites prior to parasite entry. Events subsequent to attachment may in turn require further specific interactions between host cell and parasite.

Conclusions

We have identified a group of well-characterized molecules, located on red cell membranes, that are important in the invasion of human red cells by the malarial parasite *P. falciparum*. The exact role of these sialoglycoproteins in the invasion process remains unknown, but the initial binding of merozoites to red cells might be consistent with a model in which the parasite specifically recognizes and then binds to a portion of the glycoprotein or clusters of oligosaccharides on glycophorin, such as sialic acid, which conform to a particular spatial arrangement. Once merozoites have attached to red cells and orientation of the apical end has occurred, further conformational alterations might take place which trigger the process of red cell deformation and parasite entry.

Acknowledgements

We should like to thank Drs D. J. Anstee and M. J. A. Tanner for the supply of many of the cells, antisera and monoclonal antibodies used in these studies. We are also grateful to Dr H. Zeitlin for the K562 cells, Dr S. Abdalla for the bone marrow aspirates, and Mrs T. Patel for her technical assistance.

REFERENCES

Anderson LC, Nilsson K, Gahmberg CG 1979 K562—A human erythroleukemic cell line. Int J Cancer 23:143-147

Anstee DJ 1981 The blood group MN Ss-active sialoglycoproteins. Semin Hematol 18:13-31

Anstee DJ, Mawby WJ, Tanner MJA 1982 Structural variation in human erythrocyte sialoglycoproteins. In: Martonosi AN (ed) Membranes and transport. Plenum Publishing Corporation, New York, vol 2:427-433

Baenziger JU, Fiete D 1980 Galactose and *N*-acetylgalactosamine-specific endocytosis of glycopeptides by isolated rat hepatocytes. Cell 22:611-620

Brown RC, Bass H, Coombs JP 1975 Carbohydrate binding proteins involved in phagocytosis by *Acanthamoeba*. Nature (Lond) 254:434-435

Eisen H, Furusawa M, Tanabe K, Takada S, Ostertag W 1977 Interactions of rodent malarial parasites with Friend erythroleukemia cells *in vitro*. Bull WHO 55:367-372

Gahmberg CG, Jokine M, Andersson LF 1978 Expression of the major sialoglycoprotein (glycophorin) on erythroid cells in human bone marrow. Blood 52:379-387

Howard RJ, Miller LH 1981 Invasion of erythrocytes by malaria merozoites: evidence for specific receptors involved in attachment and entry. In: Adhesion and microorganism pathogenicity. Pitman Medical, London (Ciba Found Symp 80) p 202-219

Kobiler D, Mirelman D 1980 Lectin activity in *Entamoeba histolytica* trophozoites. Infect Immun 29:221-225

Lutz HU, Fehr J 1979 Total sialic acid content of glycophorins during senescence of human red blood cells. J Biol Chem 254:11177-11180

Miller LH, Powers KG, Finerty J, Vanderberg JP 1973 Difference in surface change between host cells and malarial parasites. J Parasitol 59:925-927

Miller LH, Haynes JD, McAuliffe FM, Shiroishi T, Durocher JR, McGinniss MH 1977 Evidence for differences in erythrocyte surface receptors for the malarial parasites, *Plasmodium falciparum* and *Plasmodium knowlesi*. J Exp Med 146:277-281

Pasvol G, Wilson RJM 1982 The interaction of malaria parasites with red blood cells. Br Med Bull 38:133-140

Pasvol G, Weatherall DJ, Wilson RJM 1980 The increased susceptibility of young red cells to invasion by the malarial parasite *Plasmodium falciparum*. Br J Haematol 45:285-295

Pasvol G, Wainscoat JS, Weatherall DJ 1982a Erythrocytes deficient in glycophorin resist invasion by the malarial parasite *Plasmodium falciparum*. Nature (Lond) 297:64-66

Pasvol G, Jungery M, Weatherall DJ, Parsons SF, Anstee DJ, Tanner MJA 1982b Glycophorin as a possible receptor for *Plasmodium falciparum*. Lancet 2:947-950

Perkins M 1981 Inhibitory effects of erythrocyte membrane proteins on the in vitro invasion of the human malarial parasite (*Plasmodium falciparum*) into its host cell. J Cell Biol 90:563-567

Smalley ME, Abdalla S, Brown J 1980 The distribution of *Plasmodium falciparum* in the peripheral blood and bone marrow of Gambian children. Trans R Soc Trop Med Hyg 75:103-105

Tokunaga E, Sasakawa S, Tamaka K, Kawamata H, Giles CM, Ikin EW, Poole J, Anstee DJ, Mawby W, Tanner MJA 1979 Two apparently healthy Japanese individuals of type M^kM^k have erythrocytes which lack both the blood group MN and Ss-active sialoglycoproteins. J Immunogenet (Oxf) 6:383-390

Weiss MM, Oppenheim JD, Vanderberg JP 1981 *Plasmodium falciparum:* assay *in vitro* for inhibitors of merozoite penetration of erythrocytes. Exp Parasitol 51:400-407

DISCUSSION

Wallach: You say there is no effect of charge on invasion, Dr Pasvol, but have you measured the charge on the red cell? Have you used gangliosides as inhibitors of invasion?

Pasvol: We haven't measured the surface charge, or tested the effects of gangliosides.

Cabantchik: We used a mixture of gangliosides from sheep brain and showed that they had no effect on invasion (W.V. Breuer et al, unpublished).

Friedman: We have unpublished results which add to what Dr Pasvol has said and are complementary to his data, if not to his conclusions! In one experiment we treat red cells with neuraminidase for various times and look at the rate of invasion by *P. falciparum* merozoites. We see a steady decrease in the extent of invasion with an increasing amount of sialic acid removed. So there is a correlation between sialic acid on the cell and invasion, as you showed.

In another experiment we also used neuraminidase-treated red cells but we varied the serum component of the medium, to investigate a serum factor that interacts with enzyme-treated cells. With control cells in baboon serum, we saw invasion of about 10% of the cells. In neuraminidase-treated cells there were about 0.2% rings. If human serum is added to the system, with enzyme-treated cells, invasion rises to about 4%. So something in human serum restores invasion levels in neuraminidase-treated cells. This factor is orosomucoid (α_1-acid glycoprotein). You can get the same effect with the purified glycoprotein.

When we treat red cells with trypsin we find two different effects. With low concentrations (0.15 mg/ml) invasion is rare, only about 0.8%. Invasion levels can be restored to 4% by adding the glycoprotein. With high trypsin concentrations (1 mg/ml) invasion is again low (0.2%) and cannot be restored with the glycoprotein. We examined the surface charge of the neuraminidase-treated cells and trypsin-treated cells in the presence of the glycoprotein (M.J. Friedman & T. Tenforde, unpublished work). Neuraminidase treatment decreases the charge by 85%; when the glycoprotein is added the charge increases by about 15%. After trypsin the charge is not reduced so much, presumably because sialoglycolipid is still on the surface. Both trypsin treatments (0.15 and 1 mg/ml) decreased the surface charge by about 50%, so higher trypsin levels do not remove any more glycoprotein. When we add the α_1-acid glycoprotein the charge increases by about the same amount in both cases, so the glycoprotein is binding to the cell after both trypsin treatments. This all suggests that you can remove a negative charge with either trypsin or neuraminidase and restore the potentiality for invasion with a completely different protein that binds to the surface and provides negative charge. In treating with 1 mg/ml trypsin, we may be taking off something else as well, as yet unidentified.

Wallach: Can you restore susceptibility to invasion with gangliosides?

Friedman: I haven't done any experiments with gangliosides.

Pasvol: Charge as related to sialic acid content has been measured in the deficient cells but I still don't think that it alone can be involved. Monsigny et al (1980) showed that a specific interaction, negative charge, and an avidity effect were important in the binding of wheat germ agglutinin (WGA) to glycoconjugates containing N-acetylneuraminic acid. Charge alone cannot be responsible, since when polyanionic substances such as hyaluronic acid, heparan and keratan sulphate are added they do not block the binding of WGA to glycoconjugates (Bhavanandan & Katlic 1979). Perhaps the binding of WGA to glycoconjugates resembles the binding of the merozoite to red cells. Results obtained by Breuer et al (1982) would support this notion.

Tanner: It seems clear from Dr Pasvol's results that as well as sialic acid other factors, such as the Wr[b] antigen, are involved in the invasion process. The Wr[b]-

negative cells that are not invaded have an entirely normal sialic acid content and sialoglycoprotein staining pattern on SDS gels. We know that the Wr^b antigen is on the α sialoglycoprotein, from immunoprecipitation experiments (K. Ridgewell, D.J. Anstee & M.J.A. Tanner, unpublished work), and we think that the Wr^b-negative variant has some sort of mutation which does not affect the sialic acid of α but is elsewhere in the molecule. The reactivity of the Wr^b-negative cells with anti-α sialoglycoprotein monoclonal antibodies is also normal (Anstee & Edwards 1982).

Pasvol: We have shown that Wr^b-negative cells are resistant to invasion (Table 1) (Pasvol et al 1982). This was confirmed with anti-Wr^b monoclonal antibodies obtained from three separate fusions (Anstee & Edwards 1982). Such

TABLE 1 (Pasvol) Invasion of Wr^b-negative cells by P. falciparum

Expt no.	Parasites per 100 cells		
	Control	Test	Test/control (%)
1	7.0	0.7	10
2	7.6	0.7	9
3	8.4	0.8	10
			Mean: 10

antibodies block invasion into Wr^b-positive cells (Table 2). We think that this determinant is located on α close to the membrane. Since Wr^b-negative cells are not carbohydrate-deficient we hypothesize that a second specific step occurs after the merozoite has recognized and attached to the red cell. This second step could have something to do with orientation, junction formation, red cell deformation and so on, and in this context the Wr^b determinant could act as a trigger.

Friedman: I would argue only that charge is important to bring the cells together, and that a second interaction is then necessary. In fact, polyanions do block invasion.

Pasvol: But it's a charge *difference*, so how would that help? Since merozoites are thought to carry a negative charge (Miller et al 1973) and neuraminidase decreased that charge in your experiments, that would allow approximation of negatively charged cells rather than repulsion. Stripping off negative charge should theoretically bring parasite and red cell together.

Cabantchik: We have to define our terms. Are we talking about charge density, or about a charge involved in binding? Dr Pasvol is presumably referring to charge density, which is a very general physico-chemical term, as

TABLE 2 (Pasvol) Invasion by *P. falciparum* of Wr^b-positive cells in presence of anti-Wr^b monoclonal antibodies

Source of antibody	Haemagglutinating titre (reciprocal)	Final dilution (reciprocal)	Parasites per 100 cells[a]		
			Control	Test	Test/control (%)
Ascites R7	25 000	200	16.0	0.1	1
Supernatant BRIC[b] 13	64	2	16.0	4.4	27
Supernatant BRIC 15	64	2	16.0	6.8	43

[a]These results are the means of two experiments.
[b]Bristol Immunochemistry.

compared to an affinity for a particular ligand which happens to carry a negative charge. I think one can eliminate charge density as a factor in invasion. However, a charged group may be necessary in order for merozoite–cell interaction to occur at a specific membrane site. So Dr Pasvol cannot eliminate the need for a discrete negative charge at a specific site on the relevant receptor molecule.

Pasvol: The model of WGA goes further than that. Bhavanandan & Katlic (1979) looked at the density of charge on the glycoconjugates and found them to be important in the binding of the lectin to the receptor. But that may be different from the binding of parasite to red cell.

Cabantchik: Yes, this is a different matter. As to the second point, I want to make a cautionary comment, particularly regarding enzyme treatment and its effect on invasion. The important parameter to assess is what is left in the red cell membrane after enzymic treatment and not only what has been excised. This is particularly important for comparing results obtained with different enzyme treatments. For example, one may specify how much sialic acid and/or how much membrane protein is left, and on which membrane components they are located.

Pasvol: For that reason, it seems so advantageous to look at these well-characterized, naturally occurring red cell variants, where you don't have to involve these often confusing procedures, such as enzymic treatment.

Cabantchik: However, there is also the effect of chymotrypsin, which can remove up to 30% of the sialic acid from the erythrocyte membrane, changing the charge density considerably but hardly affecting invasion. This reinforces the previous comment that reduction in charge density has no effect on parasite invasion.

Friedman: In that experiment it matters greatly what else is in the system. All these experiments are done in the presence of human serum and therefore of α_1-acid glycoprotein. The ability of this glycoprotein to restore invasion in a cell that has no glycophorin A on it indicates that it can provide a missing interaction.

Wallach: Do you completely restore invasion with this glycoprotein?

Friedman: Not completely; at high concentrations, α_1-acid glycoprotein inhibits invasion, as do other polyanions. The concentrations at which it inhibits are found during infection.

Pasvol: If you do invasion assays with oligosaccharide-deficient Tn cells in the presence of human serum, you don't reinstate invasion, so this would not support your argument.

Friedman: That is an important point. So these Tn cells, and also the cells treated with 1 mg/ml trypsin, lack something else.

Holder: Dr Jungery, when you inhibit invasion with monosaccharides, do you see a synergistic effect when you use a combination of sugars?

Jungery: We have not yet tested the effect of combinations of monosaccharides on invasion.

Sherman: We saw the beautiful electron micrographs of Dr Aikawa earlier in the symposium. 'Invasion' covers a multitude of sins, so to speak. There is an attachment phase; then the formation of a dense layer of the red cell membrane (junction formation); and then endocytosis of the merozoite. In the term 'invasion' you are measuring the end result of all these processes. I visualize the rhoptry as a kind of toothpaste tube with its end closed; adjacent to the rhoptry tip is the merozoite ligand, specific for a complementary site on the red cell surface (Fig. 1). The red cell has a kind of molecular 'needle' on its surface

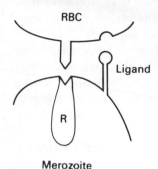

FIG. 1 (Sherman). Possible invasion mechanism of the merozoite. RBC, host red blood cell. R, rhoptry.

which fits into the closed end of the rhoptry. The binding of the merozoite ligand to the red cell surface receptor constitutes the attachment phase. Then, as the red cell membrane is brought into close apposition to the tip of the rhoptry, the 'needle' on the red cell surface punctures it. There follows discharge of the material from the rhoptry and invagination of the red cell membrane. There must be at least two steps, but perhaps there are three steps, or more, involved. Invasion is the end result of all these steps, and we must be able to separate out these events.

Aikawa: We have shown that trypsin treatment of Duffy-negative human erythrocytes allowed their invasion by the merozoites. Could you speculate, Dr Pasvol, on how trypsin acts on the membrane of the Duffy-negative erythrocyte to permit its invasion by the merozoite?

Pasvol: One can hypothesize that the initial attachment of the merozoite, which can be lateral or apical, might be the first step required to allow the parasite now to make contact with something physically closer to the red cell membrane. If you treat with trypsin a Duffy-negative red cell you might expose a cryptantigen, which acts as a trigger for parasite entry. The Duffy antigen *per se* has not been shown to be essential for invasion. It might be something close to it.

Howard: We have results (Howard et al 1982) on the trypsin treatment of S+s+U+ and S−s−U− red cells which agree with yours, Dr Pasvol. However, we interpret them a little differently. Trypsin-treated S+s+U+ cells lack the portion of glycophorin A which bears the MN blood group determinants but possess glycophorin B, whereas trypsin-treated S−s−U− cells lack the MN-bearing portion of both glycophorin A and glycophorin B. Since the treated S−s−U− cells showed an even greater loss of susceptibility to invasion than the treated S+s+U+ cells, we conclude that glycophorin B might have a role in merozoite recognition, although it appears less important than glycophorin A. Does your study show directly that glycophorin A is the receptor, or do your results admit the possibility that glycophorin B is also involved?

Pasvol: Since there is a reasonable amount of homology between α and δ one can argue that they present a similar conformation to the parasite. α may merely be a 'better' receptor because there is more of it; there are at least a million copies of α but only a quarter of that number of δ on each red cell. There is also no reason why there should not be any cooperation between the two.

Howard: I point this out because it might be wrong to chase the Wr antigen as the exclusive requirement for attachment and invasion.

Tanner: Trypsin-treated red cells are still Wr^b positive. They still have the Wr^b antigen.

Howard: Where is the Wr^b antigen located?

Tanner: We think it probably lies between residue 57 and the membrane, because erythrocyte variants such as MiV contain (α–δ) hybrid sialoglycoproteins which lack the Wr^b antigen. A characteristic of all En(a−) cells is that they are all Wr^b negative.

Howard: Dr Pasvol, we have shown the same results as you with K562 cells. They were not invaded by *P. falciparum*, even when they were induced for haemoglobin synthesis. *P. knowlesi* was also unable to invade these cells.

Pasvol: The K562 cell and the Friend cell are very different. Some people would say that the glycophorin on K562 is not the same as on red cells. Also, binding of our anti-α monoclonal antibody to K562 cells showed under 10%, relative to the binding of this monoclonal to normal red cells.

Howard: Dr Facer, do you know whether the distribution of sialic acid on different glycoproteins is the same in Wr^b-negative and positive phenotypes?

Facer: No, I do not have that information.

Howard: That being so, one cannot conclude from the fact that the *content* of sialic acid in Wr^b-negative is identical to the normal phenotype, that sialic acid does not bear a relationship to invasion. Could the Wr^b-negative phenotype be refractory to invasion because of a different sialic acid *distribution*? In the

En(a−) phenotype, some oligosaccharides are differently distributed on membrane proteins, by comparison with normal cells.

Facer: We have also been investigating En(a−) and S−s−U− cells and found a similar reduction in invasion (unpublished results). K562 cells, normal and haemin-induced, were not invaded. We were unable to induce our line of K562 with sodium butyrate.

Pasvol: There is evidence that induction of K562 cells leads to no increase in the expression of α on the surface of these cells (Tonkonow et al 1982).

Facer: Kidson investigated invasion of *P. falciparum in vitro* into ovalocytes from Melanesians and found them resistant to invasion (Kidson et al 1981). Ovalocytic cells from homozygotes show a widespread but selective depression in blood group antigens and are not agglutinated by anti-Wr^b serum (Booth et al 1977). However, they believe that the resistance of ovalocytes is probably the result of an altered and rigid cytoskeleton which may physically prevent penetration by the merozoite. We have examined the susceptibility of red cells from a patient with hereditary elliptocytosis to invasion. Elliptocytes have a different cytoskeletal defect to that found in ovalocytes (the heat sensitivity of spectrin is different). These cells were not resistant. It would be interesting to obtain red cells from a case of the rare condition, hereditary pyropoikilocytosis, and to examine their susceptibility to invasion.

Anders: May I amplify Dr Facer's comments on the ovalocytic cell? Serjeantson et al (1977) first described the apparent resistance of Papua New Guineans with ovalocytic erythrocytes to the three malaria parasites, *P. falciparum*, *P. vivax* and *P. malariae*. A feature of the ovalocytic cells was the reduced expression of a number of blood group antigens (Booth et al 1977). Dr Kidson's group at the Queensland Institute of Medical Research, Brisbane has been attempting to define the abnormality in the ovalocytic cell. Such cells are relatively resistant to invasion by *P. falciparum in vitro* although the degree of resistance varies with different ovalocytic individuals, suggesting heterogeneity within the group (Kidson et al 1981). The abnormality has not been identified. Electrophoretic analysis of membrane proteins has not shown differences between ovalocytes and normocytes, and, although ovalocytic cells were shown to deform at slightly higher temperatures than normal cells, the temperature at which isolated spectrin denatures is no different from that found for normal red cell spectrin.

Weatherall: What is the frequency of the defect in that population?

Anders: It is more than 20% in some areas of Papua New Guinea.

Luzzatto: I have never seen any genetics on this condition. Has anything been done?

Anders: Three families have been studied in Australia where there is a Melanesian mother with the ovalocytic phenotype and a normocytic Caucasian father. These studies (Castelino et al 1981) have demonstrated the dominant inheritance of ovalocytosis. In one family the four children were all ovalocytic and had red cells resistant to invasion by *P. falciparum*. In another, all children were normal. In the third family, two of three children studied were ovalocytic.

Luzzatto: If the incidence is 20%, and if the gene is dominant, homozygotes should be found. One wonders about their phenotype. I think this must be different from elliptocytosis in its textbook form. Several people, including myself, have observed beautiful infection by *P. falciparum* in elliptocytic cells.

Anders: Competitive invasion studies were done by Kidson et al (1981). The ovalocytic cells did not compete with normal cells, indicating that merozoites did not bind irreversibly to the ovalocytic cells.

Pasvol: It would be interesting to know the sialic acid content of the ovalocytic cells. This is the first instance where we can really say that the parasite 'prefers' normal cells to ovalocytes; that is, that the merozoite might detach from ovalocytes and then invade normal cells. This is an important point because it gives the merozoite an active role, rather than the particular host cell type showing an increased or decreased susceptibility to invasion.

Holder: If there is a defective cytoskeletal system in these ovalocytes and this prevents their invasion by the parasite, one should look at the functional characteristics of the ovalocytic cell; for example, the relationship between its energy state and the degree of cytoskeletal phosphorylation. Perhaps there is a particular defective protein kinase in these cells.

Anders: Kidson's group is now looking for more subtle abnormalities such as defective phosphorylation.

Cabantchik: One of the problems we find with the present *in vitro* assays of *P. falciparum* invasion into human erythrocytes is that they do not allow us to separate the initial attachment step from the subsequent penetration into the cell. Among other things, these assays may give erroneous values for inhibitory doses of agents which interfere with attachment via competition with putative merozoite receptors. For glycophorin, the inhibitory doses required are unusually high, in comparison with the amounts present in the native system. Moreover, the present assays do not allow us to draw definite conclusions about the presence or absence of receptors for merozoites in variant red blood cell types, particularly when the basis of the assay is inhibition of invasion into invasion-competent cells. The main problem with the assays is that they measure the appearance of rings approximately 12 hours after schizonts have been added to uninfected cells. By analogy with enzymic reactions, merozoite invasion is an irreversible reaction which is preceded by a reversible receptor-mediated binding step. Therefore, any competition between free ligands and cell receptors for merozoite binding sites should be looked for at the initial stages of the reaction or, better, as a function of time. To my knowledge, most of the published studies have not dealt with this problem. The only work that comes close to measuring a kinetically meaningful inhibitory dose of glycophorin is that of Perkins (1981). However, as I understand it, that work is open to criticism because of the poor invasion capacity of the isolated merozoites.

REFERENCES

Anstee DJ, Edwards PAW 1982 Monoclonal antibodies to human erythrocytes. Eur J Immunol 12:228-232

Bhavanandan VP, Katlic AW 1979 The interaction of wheat germ agglutinin with sialoglycoproteins; the role of sialic acid. J Biol Chem 254:4000-4008

Booth PB, Serjeantson S, Woodfield DG, Amato D 1977 Selective depression of blood group antigens associated with hereditary ovalocytosis among Melanesians. Vox Sang 32:99-110

Breuer WV, Ginsburg H, Cabantchik ZI 1982 Red cell membrane components involved in *P. falciparum* invasion into human erythrocytes. J. Cell Biochem, in press

Castelino D, Saul A, Myler P, Kidson C, Thomas H, Cooke R 1981 Ovalocytosis in Papua New Guinea—dominantly inherited resistance to malaria. Southeast Asian J Trop Med Public Health 12:549-555

Howard RJ, Haynes JD, McGinnis MH, Miller LH 1982 Studies on the role of red blood cell glycoproteins as receptors for invasion by *Plasmodium falciparum* merozoites. Mol Biochem Parasitol, in press

Kidson C, Lamont G, Saul A, Nurse GT 1981 Ovalocytic erythrocytes from Melanesians are resistant to invasion by malaria parasites in culture. Proc Natl Acad Sci USA 78:5829-5832

Miller LH, Powers KG, Finerty J, Vanderberg JP 1973 Difference in surface charge between host cells and malarial parasites. J Parasitol 59:925-927

Monsigny M, Roche A-C, Sene C, Maget-Dana R, Delmotte F 1980 Sugar–lectin interactions: how does wheat-germ agglutinin bind sialoglycoconjugates? Eur J Biochem 104:147-153

Pasvol G, Jungery M, Weatherall DJ, Parsons SF, Anstee DJ, Tanner MJA 1982 Glycophorin as a possible receptor for *Plasmodium falciparum*. Lancet 2:947-950

Perkins M 1981 Inhibitory effects of erythrocyte membrane proteins in the in vitro invasion of the human malarial parasite (*Plasmodium falciparum*) into its host cell. J Cell Biol 90:563-567

Serjeantson S, Bryson K, Amato D, Babona D 1977 Malaria and hereditary ovalocytosis. Hum Genet 37:161-167

Tonkonow BL, Hoffman R, Burger D, Elder JT, Mazur EM, Murnane MJ, Benz EJ Jr 1982 Differing responses of globin and glycophorin gene expression to hemin in the human leukemia cell line K562. Blood 59:738-746

Expression of inherited resistance to malaria in culture

MILTON J. FRIEDMAN

Department of Medicine, Division of Experimental Hematology, and Howard Hughes Medical Institute, University of California, San Francisco, CA 94143, USA

Abstract Inherited resistance to *Plasmodium falciparum* malaria is primarily determined by genes affecting red blood cell function, but the expression of resistance genes is influenced by non-erythrocytic factors. Some of these factors were studied in cultures of the malaria parasite in genetically variant red cells, and it was found that both oxygen tension and medium components could modify resistance-gene expression.

Falciparum malaria is the result of an interaction between one of the simplest eukaryotic organisms and one of the most complex. In the last few years we have been able to isolate the simple component, *Plasmodium falciparum*, from its complex host and to define the conditions under which it grows and multiplies. The *in vitro* culture of the malaria parasite has been especially useful in studying its interactions with the human red blood cell. We can study how the parasite recognizes, invades, catabolizes, alters and finally destroys its host cell—all in the absence of other cells, tissues, and organs. In doing so, we are also able to define many of the factors that determine virulence of infection and death.

Some of the factors that determine virulence are genetically controlled characters of the host cell itself. We assume that by culturing *P. falciparum* in abnormal red blood cells, we are looking at the effects of single alterations of human genes on host susceptibility or resistance to infection. Unfortunately, by isolating the parasite and red cell from uncontrollable and possibly interfering *in vivo* factors, we also isolate them from the milieu in which genetic variations arise, are expressed, and are selected for or against. The expression of resistance *in vitro* may require aspects of that milieu.

The nature of this problem is well exemplified by the relationship between *P. falciparum* and sickle cell haemoglobin (Hb S). The first attempts to grow

1983 Malaria and the red cell. Pitman, London (Ciba Foundation symposium 94) p 196-205

P. falciparum in Hb S-containing red cells *in vitro* showed that haemoglobin type made no difference in parasite development (Raper 1959), though by then it was known that individuals with sickle cell trait were resistant to falciparum malaria (Allison 1957). Luzzatto et al (1970) later found that parasitized deoxygenated sickle trait red cells sickled more rapidly than unparasitized cells. They suggested that the parasitized cells sickle in circulation and are destroyed by phagocytic cells of the spleen and that the sickle cell gene acts beneficially only in concert with splenic function. This mechanism could not be demonstrated fully *in vitro*, but the investigators attempted to mimic events as they might occur *in vivo*. Our more recent studies have focused on this experimental paradigm. We have studied how specific conditions of *in vitro* culture influence the expression of resistance in variant red cells, and we have attempted to relate these conditions to possible *in vivo* events.

Oxygen tension, for example, has a profound effect on parasites in Hb S-containing red cells. Lowered oxygen concentration (1–5%) inhibits growth in sickle cells, but has little effect on parasites in normal cells (Friedman 1978, Pasvol et al 1978). Low oxygen tension and the decreased pH of the infected red cell together cause the Hb S-containing host cell to sickle. The host cell plasma membrane then becomes leaky to potassium cations, and the parasite dies (Friedman et al 1979). We believe that low *in vitro* oxygen tension represents the environment that the falciparum parasite encounters when trophozoite-infected cells adhere to the venous endothelium in the later stages of the erythrocytic developmental cycle. Again, *in vitro* data suggest a mechanism in which the expression of resistance depends on an event that cannot be seen *in vitro*, the sequestration of infected cells in the venous environment. The sickle cell example demonstrates that both chemical and cellular environments *in vivo* may modify parasite growth in variant red cells.

P. falciparum growth is also inhibited in other variant red cells under special conditions. Thalassaemic, glucose-6-phosphate dehydrogenase (G6PD)-deficient, and fetal red cells are all sensitive to oxidant stress, and parasite growth is inhibited in these cells when reduced glutathione, a component of RPMI 1640 medium, is left out of the culture (Friedman 1979). Reduced glutathione normally protects parasite cultures against oxidant damage. Without it, the oxidant stress of the culture is great enough for infected sensitive cells to be damaged just as they might be damaged *in vivo*. Although it is difficult to assess the extent of oxidant stress during actual infection, several factors which vary *in vivo* can be studied in culture.

One substance that contributes to oxidant stress is oxygen, and parasite multiplication in sensitive cells is inhibited at higher oxygen levels (25–30%). Rodent malaria parasites produce hydrogen peroxide (Etkin & Eaton 1975), and we therefore tested the possibility that the oxygen levels of *P. falciparum* cultures affected the rate of H_2O_2 production by these parasites. The evolution of H_2O_2 can be measured by adding aminotriazole to infected red cells and determining the rate of catalase inactivation. Aminotriazole forms a reversible complex with red cell catalase but, in the presence of H_2O_2, this complex becomes irreversible and inactive (Margoliash et al 1960). As shown in Fig. 1, catalase activity decreases after aminotriazole is added to infected

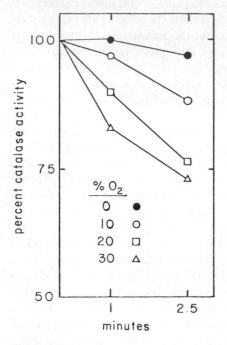

FIG. 1. Effect of varying oxygen levels on H_2O_2 production as measured by catalase inhibition. A 1% (v/v) suspension of parasitized cells (32%) was equilibrated with 3% CO_2/N_2 in an Instrumentation Laboratory tonometer at 32 °C. Five seconds before 0 time, oxygen was introduced to the level indicated, and at 0 time, aminotriazole was added to 50 mM. At 1.0 and 2.5 minutes, aliquots were removed and spun in a Beckman microfuge for 10 seconds and the supernatant was replaced with 0.1 ml 0.04% saponin in Tris-buffered saline. The free parasites were spun out and the catalase and Hb concentrations were determined in the lysate. Catalase was measured by the rate of decrease of absorbance (between 30 and 60 seconds after enzyme addition) at 240 nm of a 0.05% solution of H_2O_2 in 50 mM Tris-HCl, pH 7.2. There was no decrease in catalase activity in uninfected cells.

red cells equilibrated with different oxygen tensions. The faster decrease at higher oxygen levels indicates a greater production of H_2O_2. We can expect, therefore, that the level of H_2O_2 production and the subsequent parasite inhibition in oxidant-sensitive red cells *in vivo* will vary according to local oxygen tension and that cells sequestered in low oxygen environments will be less susceptible to inhibition than those in circulation. *Plasmodium* species that are not sequestered, such as *vivax* or *malariae*, may be especially sensitive to oxidant-mediated resistance.

Other modifiers of inhibition in oxidant-sensitive red cells are redox catalysts, such as riboflavin or menadione (Friedman 1979). These compounds may either enhance H_2O_2 production (menadione) or react with H_2O_2 to produce free radicals (riboflavin). In either case, the rate of parasite multiplication decreases. The significance of these results *in vitro* lies in the possibility that certain foods contain similar substances and that regular ingestion of such foods enhances the protective advantage of red cell oxidant sensitivity in malarial regions.

One such food is the fava bean. Ingestion of this bean causes oxidant-mediated haemolytic anaemia in some individuals with G6PD deficiency, and so it is likely that a component or metabolite of fava beans would enhance oxidant-mediated resistance. In collaboration with Gian-Franco Gaetanni and Lucio Luzzatto, I tried to test this possibility. Although this study remains incomplete, I will describe its design and initial results so that others may be inspired to explore this area further. We fed a meal of fava beans to seven normal individuals and collected serum samples after 3, 6 and 20 hours. These sera were added at a final concentration of 33% to cultures of *P. falciparum* in normal, G6PD-deficient, or β-thalassaemia trait red cells. After two days, parasites were counted in each culture, and we found that some sera collected after fava ingestion were inhibitory to parasites in variant cells but not to those in normal cells (Fig. 2). Not all individuals produced inhibitory sera, but those sera that were inhibitory acted in both G6PD-deficient and thalassaemia trait cultures. There is individual variation in the ability to produce inhibitory serum (just as there is variation in the response of G6PD-deficient individuals to fava beans), but the finding that some sera were inhibitory supports the hypothesis that diet influences variant gene expression of resistance.

The last topic I would like to discuss is the fate of the oxidatively damaged, infected red cell. If the damage is sufficient, the cell membrane will leak potassium and the parasite will die, but it is possible that an earlier fate intervenes. Knyszynski et al (1979) have reported on the increased phagocytosis of thalassaemic red cells by mouse macrophages *in vitro*. Their studies suggest that surface alterations on these cells result in increased recognition and uptake by unstimulated phagocytes. The effects of parasitization on oxidant-sensitive cells may also lead to enhanced phagocytosis. I mention this possibility because normally we do not include phagocytes in *in vitro* culture. By ignoring the role of phagocytes in recognizing abnormal cells, we may be missing a significant mechanism by which genes for thalassaemia and G6PD deficiency could confer selective advantage. These genes may enhance the

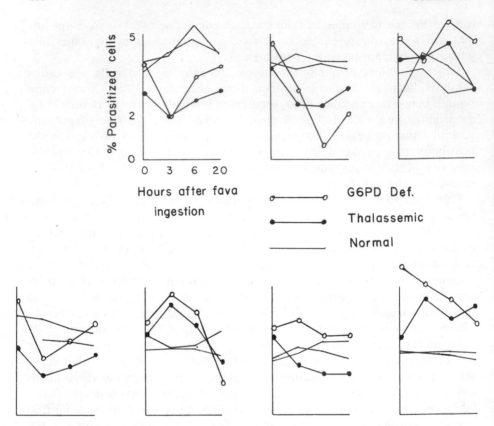

FIG. 2. Percentage of parasitized cells grown in variant red cell cultures with sera collected after fava bean ingestion. Serum donors were fed a meal of fava beans and sera were collected at 0, 3, 6 and 20 hours after ingestion. Sera were added to a final concentration of 33% to *P. falciparum* cultures started two days earlier in either normal, G6PD-deficient (Gd^{Med}), or β-thalassaemia trait red cells. After two more days (in 18% O_2), slides were made and the number of parasites per 1000 red cells was determined. (M. J. Friedman, G.-F. Gaetanni & L. Luzzatto, unpublished results.)

recognizable difference between uninfected and infected cells by amplifying the effect of parasitization on the red cell surface. Parasitized cells would then be more efficiently removed from circulation and the parasite load better controlled. The selective advantage of genes causing red cell oxidant sensitivity is not only determined by the parasite–red cell interaction as represented by *in vitro* culture. Local oxygen tensions, foods, and phagocytes may all interact to form the milieu in which these genes evolve.

The laboratory is a controlled environment. We make our measurements on simple systems wherever possible, and in doing so we may 'control out' significant events. This is a danger we are all aware of. I have attempted here to suggest some aspects of inherited resistance to malaria that are not represented in standard *in vitro* cultures. Our increasing ability to consider the factors of cellular interactions, nutrition and varying physiological conditions will accompany our increasing understanding of the ways in which red cell variation influences resistance to falciparum malaria.

REFERENCES

Allison AC 1957 Malaria in carriers of the sickle-cell trait and in newborn children. Exp Parasitol 6:418-447
Etkin NL, Eaton JW 1975 Malaria-induced erythrocyte oxidant sensitivity. In: Brewer J (ed) Erythrocyte structure and function. Liss, New York, p 219-232
Friedman MJ 1978 Erythrocytic mechanism of sickle cell resistance to malaria. Proc Natl Acad Sci USA 75:1994-1997
Friedman MJ 1979 Oxidant damage mediates variant red cell resistance to malaria. Nature (Lond) 280:245-247
Friedman MJ, Roth EF, Nagel RL, Trager W 1979 *Plasmodium falciparum*: physiological interactions with the human sickle cell. Exp Parasitol 47:73-80
Knyszynski A, Danon D, Kahane I, Rachmilewitz EA 1979 Phagocytosis of nucleated and mature β-thalassaemic red blood cells by mouse macrophages in vitro. Br J Haematol 43:251-255
Luzzatto L, Nwachuku Jarrett ES, Reddy S 1970 Increased sickling of parasitized erythrocytes as mechanism of resistance against malaria in the sickle-cell trait. Lancet 1:319-322
Margoliash E, Novogrodsky A, Schejter A 1960 Irreversible reaction of 3-amino-1,2,4-triazole and related inhibitors with the protein of catalase. Biochem J 74:339-348
Pasvol G, Weatherall DJ, Wilson RJM 1978 Cellular mechanism for the protective effect of haemoglobin S against *P. falciparum* malaria. Nature (Lond) 274:701-703
Raper AB 1959 Further observations on sickling and malaria. Trans R Soc Trop Med Hyg 53:110-117

DISCUSSION

Howard: Your study of the effects of sera from people who have eaten fava beans was obviously difficult to do. There are two technical factors that you may or may not have controlled for. You didn't show results for the same group of subjects, or another group, who had eaten something other than fava beans. Secondly, there appeared to be a large variation in the effect of a particular serum on the three cell types at time zero, *before* bean consumption. The serum from individual number 7, for example, in Fig. 2 showed a 100% difference in effects on parasitization of G6PD-negative or thalassaemic cells. In contrast, serum from individual number 1 at time zero has an equal effect on parasitization of normal and G6PD-deficient cells. This situation, *before* the experiment, makes it extremely difficult to look at the kinetics of serum effects *after* ingestion of fava beans.

Friedman: I agree that other controls are necessary, such as different foods. I wanted to present this preliminary result as a way for us to start thinking about these interactions, and how we might answer the problems raised. The interactions are there, and if we never try to study them because of experimental difficulties, there will always be questions.

Sherman: What is the evidence that malaria parasites produce peroxide in red cells?

Friedman: The best evidence is from the inhibition of catalase by aminotriazole, which complexes irreversibly with catalase only in the presence of peroxide (Fig. 1). This inhibition is not found when aminotriazole is added to uninfected cells.

Sherman: There are many things that don't occur in uninfected red cells! I suggest that what is happening is that the peroxide is acting on the outside of the red cell, to affect those cells which are already labile, and therefore the parasite is affected indirectly. You showed that if you used menadione or riboflavin, or you increased the oxygen concentration, you de-stabilized a red cell with a parasite in it. However, you are looking only at the infected cells. Perhaps lysis of other red cells occurs, but you are not paying attention to those. I know of no direct evidence for the production of hydrogen peroxide by malaria parasites. Eugene Roth looked for changes in the malonyldialdehyde content of membranes of *P. falciparum*-infected red cells and found no change (unpublished results).

Wallach: Do you see lipid peroxidation?

Friedman: The evidence for membrane damage in infected thalassaemic cells is indirect. The inhibition of parasite growth in these cells is prevented by vitamin E or by incubation in medium containing high potassium concentrations (0.1 M) (Friedman 1979). Vitamin E is a membrane antioxidant and the high potassium medium maintains potassium levels within a leaky red cell. These two observations suggest that a potassium leak is the direct cause of inhibition and that this leak is caused by oxidant damage.

Cabantchik: You don't have to assume that leakiness to cations is necessarily the result of membrane damage. Any mechanism leading to higher intracellular calcium concentration, and/or to pH reduction, will induce potassium leakage. Such a mechanism has been recently demonstrated to operate in various abnormal red blood cells (Bookchin & Lew 1981).

Wallach: A drop in ATP would lead to all these effects.

Weatherall: You have shown membrane-bound haemoglobin in these haemoglobin mutants.Were the studies done on homozygotes or heterozygotes?

Friedman: I was studying whether the polymorphic haemoglobins S, C, E, O_{Arab} and D_{Punjab} bound to the red cell membrane with higher affinity than normal and whether this property could confer resistance to malaria by causing increased oxidant damage to the membrane during infection (Friedman 1981). To measure binding affinity, we used lysates from heterozygotes containing both normal and abnormal haemoglobin. The relative binding affinity was calculated from the ratio of the two haemoglobins on the membrane, compared to the ratio of the two haemoglobins in the lysate. In all cases there was a greater proportion of abnormal haemoglobin on the membrane than in the soluble fraction. Eisinger et al (1982) have now described a method to measure the amount of haemoglobin bound to the red cell membrane, in the intact cell. That has not yet been applied to the abnormal haemoglobins.

Wallach: This has now been done in the sickle cell. Dr Helen M. Ranney has shown intensified binding of sickle cell haemoglobin (unpublished results).

Sherman: I wonder very much whether the abundance of malarial pigment in infected red cells might influence measures of catalase activity. One tends to use standard assays on infected red cells. Sam Granick once suggested the mode of evolution of catalase: iron itself had slight catalase-like activity, but when the iron was put into a porphyrin, it had a little more activity. And if you linked the iron-porphyrin to a protein, as in catalase, the breakdown of peroxide was enhanced. Remember that an infected cell has something that is absent from an uninfected cell, namely the iron-containing malarial pigment, or haemozoin. That might influence the measurements. Since one uses a standard assay, it is assumed that one is measuring the expected reaction. Perhaps another kind of control is needed in experiments with these infected red cells? This is why I asked you about the direct measurement of hydrogen peroxide. There may be hydrogen peroxide in infected red cells, but I don't know of any direct estimate of it. It remains possible that when one adds substances such as riboflavin or menadione one is influencing the red cell, which in turn affects the parasite. The mechanism is operating from outside in, rather than the proposed model, which is an action from the inside out. The end result, however, might be the same.

Friedman: It is precisely because of the presence of catalytic factors in red cells that hydrogen peroxide cannot be measured directly. Hydrogen peroxide is detected by the catalase inhibition assay in infected cells. The site and mode of its production are unknown.

Jarra: In relation to membrane-bound haemoglobin, do sickle cells or other abnormal red cells contain Heinz bodies?

Weatherall: Sickle cells don't. Only thalassaemic cells or cells from patients with unstable haemoglobins do, and usually only after splenectomy.

Luzzatto: And also G6PD-deficient cells, which under stress induced by a variety of haemolytic agents develop Heinz bodies, massively.

Jarra: And is it correct that these bodies are sometimes associated with the red cell membrane?

Weatherall: Yes. In phenylhydrazine-induced Heinz body anaemia and in haemoglobin H disease they are. This is not the case in β-thalassaemia (Polliack et al 1974).

Wallach: A technical point on your culture conditions, Dr Friedman. Is there any way of controlling the reducing levels inside the cultured cells?

Friedman: One method that I have used to counteract the deleterious effects of, say, G6PD deficiency is to add the reducing agent, dithiothreitol, to cultures. This maintains normal levels of growth of *P. falciparum* in oxidant-sensitive variant cell cultures.

Howard: The level of glutathione in sheep red blood cells is controlled by a single pair of autosomal alleles giving rise to two types: (1) 'high glutathione' sheep (approx. 90 mg glutathione/100 ml red cells) and (2) 'low glutathione' sheep (approx. 30 mg glutathione/100 ml red cells) (Agar 1975). Although sheep are not susceptible to malaria they do become infected by other haemosporidia—*Babesia,* for example. In your studies on the effect of intracellular redox potential on the growth of intraerythrocytic parasites, Dr Friedman, you might be interested to compare the growth of parasites in sheep red cells of high or low glutathione type.

Brown: As a general point on how parasites get into red cells, it seems unlikely that a red cell can have a true receptor for a merozoite. A receptor, as I understand it, is something that initiates a transmembrane signal which then produces a regulatory response in the cell. As I see the situation, a merozoite receptor interacts with a ligand on a red cell. If it does so sideways-on, a merozoite transmembrane signal will do nothing because the right organelles are not located beneath that part of the merozoite membrane. If it approaches head-on, where the rhoptries are, the merozoite receptor for the erythrocyte ligand will initiate a rhoptry or microneme response. Thus the actual attachment site on the red cell might be quite simple, and all the response is in the merozoite, and it is not necessarily a reversible reaction. In inhibition studies, by adding the right sugar for example, you may irreversibly set a merozoite off on the cell entry response.

Fitch: So the receptor is on the parasite, not on the red cell?

Brown: Absolutely.

Howard: May I bring in the old experiments by McGhee (1953) on the invasion of mixtures of chicken and duck erythrocytes? He showed that *P. lophurae* merozoites invaded more duck erythrocytes than chick erythrocytes when exposed to both, even though chick erythrocytes were in excess. This introduced the concept that multiple collisions of a merozoite may occur before invasion and that the frequency of invasion could depend on subtle properties of the erythrocyte receptors, other than their mere presence or absence.

REFERENCES

Agar NS 1975 Glutathione polymorphism in sheep red blood cells. Int J Biochem 6:843-852

Bookchin RM, Lew VL 1981 Effect of a 'sickling pulse' on calcium and potassium transport in sickle cell trait red cells. J Physiol (Lond) 312:265-280

Eisinger J, Flores J, Salhany JM 1982 Association of cytosol hemoglobin with the membrane in intact erythrocytes. Proc Natl Acad Sci USA 79:408-412

Friedman MJ 1979 Oxidant damage mediates variant red cell resistance to malaria. Nature (Lond) 280:245-247

Friedman MJ 1981 Hemoglobin and the red cell membrane: increased binding of polymorphic hemoglobins and measurement of free radicals in the membrane. In: Brewer GJ (ed) The red cell. Alan R. Liss. New York (Fifth Ann Arbor Conference) p 519-531

McGhee RB 1953 The infection by *Plasmodium lophurae* of duck erythrocytes in the chicken embryo. J Exp Med 97:773-782

Polliack A, Yataganas X, Rachmilewitz E A 1974 Ultrastructure of the inclusion bodies and nuclear abnormalities in β-thalassemic erythroblasts. Ann N Y Acad Sci 232:261-282

bolism and surface transport of parasitized erythrocytes in malaria

IRWIN W. SHERMAN

Department of Biology, University of California, Riverside, CA 92521, USA

Abstract Plasmodium requires a living cell for growth and reproduction. Intraerythrocytically the parasite stores no reserve carbohydrate, relying entirely on host-supplied glucose and certain amino acids (glutamic acid) for its energy. Plasmodia are microaerophiles degrading glucose primarily to lactate rather than to CO_2. The limited amounts of oxygen utilized may serve for biosynthetic purposes (e.g. pyrimidine biosynthesis) rather than being involved in an energy-yielding electron transport chain. Evidence for a parasite pentose pathway is weak since glucose-6-phosphate dehydrogenase has rarely been found; paradoxically, activity for 6-phosphogluconate dehydrogenase, the next enzyme in the pathway, is consistently identified. The parasites synthesize pyrimidines *de novo*, but being incapable of *de novo* purine biosynthesis they require preformed purines. Exogenously supplied purine, notably hypoxanthine derived from catabolism of erythrocytic ATP, is taken up and incorporated whereas pyrimidines are not. The capacity for *de novo* amino acid biosynthesis is limited and presumably haemoglobin supplies most of the amino acids required by the parasite. Degradation of haemoglobin, involving parasite proteases, notably a cathepsin D-like enzyme, leaves a characteristic golden-brown residue, haemozoin. Haemozoin consists of dimers of ferriprotoporphyrin IX, methaemoglobin and plasmodial proteins. For some species, isoleucine and methionine must be supplied exogenously for good plasmodial growth. Infected erythrocytes characteristically show altered permeability properties, changes which in large part contribute to parasite growth while at the same time impairing red cell function.

'Science', George Gaylord Simpson wrote, 'is a study of errors slowly corrected'. Having spent the better part of 25 years studying the metabolism of a variety of malaria parasites I find that Simpson's description applies not only to science in general, but particularly to the biochemistry of *Plasmodium*. In this review I shall sketch some of what we think we know about metabolism and transport in the infected red cell as well as in parasites removed from the red cell. But, in highlighting the biochemistry of malarial

1983 Malaria and the red cell. Pitman, London (Ciba Foundation symposium 94) p 206-221

parasites, I shall focus attention on areas where there is reason to be sceptical, and suggest critical kinds of investigations that might further our understanding of intracellular parasitism as practised by *Plasmodium*.

Prologue

All too rarely has it been appreciated that metabolic studies of parasitized erythrocytes, as well as those of free parasites, are fraught with difficulties. Recognition of these pitfalls—I shall call them 'The Perils of *Plasmodium*'—is a prerequisite for interpreting the literature. Some of these 'perils' are:

1. Parasites may reside in red cells of differing ages, and therefore the metabolic capacities of infected cells can vary widely.

2. During their intraerythrocytic existence parasites undergo differentiation; consequently the metabolism of the parasitized cell may reflect stage specificity.

3. Varying parasitaemias may influence metabolic parameters.

4. Parasitized erythrocytes may be contaminated by cellular elements such as leucocytes or platelets as well as microbes, and these may affect the measurements made on the infected cell, directly or indirectly.

5. High parasitaemias, obtained by manipulation of *in vitro* culture conditions, may provoke red cell alterations that are not inherent metabolic characteristics of an individual infected cell.

6. Virulent strains may so affect host metabolism that the changes observed in infected red cells are more a consequence of deranged host physiology than changes provoked by the parasite *per se*.

7. The highly active metabolism of the infected red cell may require that measurements be made on a time scale different from that used for uninfected erythrocytes.

8. The fragile nature of the infected red cells and free parasites, with attendant *in vitro* lysis, leads to cytosolic components being released into the medium which may affect the metabolism of infected cells and/or create artifacts.

9. *In vitro* conditions optimal for normal erythrocytes may be unsuitable for infected ones.

10. Standard methodologies (e.g. enzyme assays) may not be directly applicable because of unique attributes of the plasmodium.

11. Misinterpretations of biochemical data may result from a lack of understanding of parasite biology.

12. Reagent contaminants may markedly affect findings.

Glucose metabolism and transport

Erythrocytic stages of malaria store no reserve carbohydrate; therefore parasites must be supplied with a directly utilizable energy source. Glucose is that source. Glucose is readily metabolized by the infected red cell. The exact amount of sugar consumed depends on the stage of the parasite, the degree of parasitaemia and the species. In the primate and rodent malarias the principal end-product of glucose catabolism is lactate, but in the bird malarias both CO_2 and lactate are formed. The consumption of glucose by free parasites is equal to or exceeds that of infected cells, but the end-products are reported to be formate and acetate, as well as lactate (reviewed by Sherman 1979, 1983). In my view the production of volatile acids by free parasites is more likely to be a consequence of damage incurred in removing parasites from host cells than a true reflection of their metabolism.

The enzymes of glycolysis have been identified, more or less, in all plasmodia studied; however, since all the enzymes have not been described in a single species it is more an act of faith than accurate documentation that leads us to conclude that glucose is degraded to lactic acid via the Embden–Meyerhof pathway. And, although there is suggestive evidence for a citric acid cycle in avian malarial parasites, the only enzymes identified have been isocitrate and succinate dehydrogenases. Malate dehydrogenase, which appears to be cytosolic, is found in both the avian and mammalian parasites (Sherman 1979).

Avian and mammalian erythrocytes also metabolize glucose via the hexose monophosphate shunt (HMS), but overall shunt activity tends to be low. Similarly, the activity of the parasitized red cell is also low. In *Plasmodium knowlesi*-infected erythrocytes the mean percentage of glucose metabolized via the shunt was reported to be 4%, whereas in the normal cell the value was 10% (Barnes & Polet 1969). Similar trends were obtained by E. F. Roth (unpublished) for *P. falciparum*-infected erythrocytes.

The only enzyme of the HMS consistently identified in malarial parasites is 6-phosphogluconate dehydrogenase, and only rarely is evidence found for activity of glucose-6-phosphate dehydrogenase (G6PD). Recently, Hemplemann & Wilson (1981) identified G6PD activity in *P. knowlesi* merozoites and *P. falciparum* schizonts by electrophoretic separation and histochemical visualization. Unfortunately, no other stages in the developmental cycle were studied. No activity was found for *P. chabaudi*-infected cells, however. Additionally, in *P. vinckei*- and *P. lophurae*-infected erythrocytes the activity of G6PD decreased during intraerythrocytic growth, suggesting that the activity being measured was of host cell origin, and that enzyme was being destroyed during parasite development. Why, we might ask, has it been so difficult to find G6PD in parasites? Is it because the enzyme is so labile, or are very special conditions required for assay, or is it that the enzyme just doesn't exist in all species of *Plasmodium*?

The HMS is a major mechanism for production of NADPH, which is specifically utilized in the biosynthesis of long-chain fatty acids and sterols, in the reduction of dihydrofolate to tetrahydrofolate, in hydroxylation reactions involved in the production of unsaturated fatty acids, and in pentose formation. If indeed G6PD is absent from plasmodia, then how is the substrate, 6-phosphogluconic acid, formed and what role can be served by the sole presence of 6-phosphogluconate dehydrogenase? And, how does the parasite obtain NADPH and pentoses? Possibly, NADPH is formed by cytosolic glutamic dehydrogenase, which is universally found in *Plasmodium* (and not in red cells), and pentoses might be formed by the action of purine nucleoside phosphorylases. The latter mechanism for pentose formation, incidentally, has never been shown.

In what manner does the parasite obtain the glucose needed for growth and reproduction? Glucose enters the red cell by facilitated diffusion, and in the human red cell the D-glucose transport protein is associated with band 4.5. In avian erythrocytes the rate of sugar uptake can be increased by anoxia (presumably due to an acceleration of a carrier-mediated process). When studies were done with *P. lophurae*-infected duckling red cells, the transport constant (K_t) for D-glucose was similar for normal and infected red cells, and the K_t was unchanged whether parasites were schizonts or trophozoites. In contrast the V_{max} was significantly higher ($\sim 9\times$) in infected red cells, but was independent of the stage of parasite development. Increased sugar entry, by simple diffusion, was shown by using the non-metabolizable 3-*O*-methylglucose (Sherman & Tanigoshi 1974a). Neame & Homewood (1974) reported that the diffusional entry of L-glucose was increased for *P. berghei*-infected mouse erythrocytes, but neither normal nor uninfected red cells from an infected host took up L-glucose. In the latter case, *N*-ethylmalcimide and D-glucose were without effect on L-glucose entry. It may be that with *P. lophurae*- and *P. berghei*-infected erythrocytes, alterations in the cholesterol content of the erythrocyte membrane, and the consequent change in its fluidity, contribute to the increased entry of glucose by passive diffusion. In the case of *P. lophurae*-infected cells, anoxia may alter the V_{max} without affecting the K_t, as was reported by Wood & Morgan (1969) for avian erythrocytes. Unfortunately, the studies with *P. lophurae*-infected red cells were done over protracted periods of time (30 min) and there was no measure of substrate modification. Studies of the effects of cytochalasin B and trypsin on membrane transport of glucose by infected cells would be of considerable interest. Perhaps future investigations, carefully conducted, will provide alternative explanations for the observed properties of infected red cells toward glucose.

Oxygen utilization and the electron transport system

Malaria-infected red cells showed enhanced O_2 uptake with glucose by comparison with uninfected red cells (reviewed by Sherman 1983). Some of this increased respiratory activity may be due to stimulation of host cell metabolism, but the favourable effects of low oxygen levels ($<5\%$) on the *in vitro* growth of infected cells suggest that the parasites are microaerophilic (Scheibel et al 1979b).

Save for the presence of cytochrome oxidase, no cytochromes have been isolated from plasmodia. So what is the functional significance of O_2 utilization and the presence of cytochrome oxidase? It has been suggested that the cytochrome oxidase does not function as a component of an aerobic energy-generating system, but instead is involved in the *de novo* synthesis of pyrimidines. In the proposed scheme, dihydroorotate dehydrogenase catalyses the conversion of dihydroorotate to orotate and the electrons from this reaction are passed first to ubiquinone, then to cytochrome and then to oxygen (Gutteridge et al 1979). Dihydroorotate dehydrogenase has been found in extracts of *P. gallinaceum*, *P. berghei* and *P. knowlesi* and such activity was inhibited by cyanide. Scheibel et al (1979a) reported that Antabuse (tetraethylthiuram disulphide), as well as low concentrations of KCN (5 μM), inhibited the *in vitro* growth of *P. falciparum*; this suggests that metalloprotein oxygenases other than cytochrome oxidase could be involved in O_2 utilization. It is not known for any of these systems whether the electrons are passed directly to O_2 with the formation of water, or where such systems are localized.

The notion that *Plasmodium* uses O_2 for the biosynthesis of nucleic acids is particularly intriguing in light of work carried out 40 years ago by Velick (1942), where a marked increase in O_2 consumption by *P. cathemerium*-infected cells was shown to occur at the time of schizogony.

Amino acid transport and protein synthesis

Malarial parasites spend most of their time suspended in a viscous (30%) solution of haemoglobin. Haemoglobin is ingested via the cytostome, which buds off food vacuoles at its base. Within the food vacuoles haemoglobin is digested and malarial pigment (haemozoin) is deposited (Aikawa & Seed 1980). The electron microscopic appearance of haemozoin is quite variable among the malarias studied. Mammalian plasmodia have a crystalline-appearing haemozoin that is distributed uniformly in the cytoplasm within small food vacuoles, whereas in avian species the food vacuoles are fewer and larger, and the abundant malarial pigment appears rather amorphous. The chemical nature of haemozoin remains controversial, and it probably differs from one species to another. The method of isolating haemozoin, by breakage of free parasites followed by differential centrifugation and chemical extraction, rather than by direct separation of intact food vacuoles from the remainder of the plasmodial organelles, may result in adventitious binding of haemozoin to other cellular constituents. Thus, what is finally recovered as haemozoin may be rather far removed from what it was inside the food vacuole. Aware of these limitations, we nevertheless did undertake a characterization of the haemozoin from *P. lophurae*. It consisted of insoluble monomers and dimers of ferriprotoporphyrin IX, insoluble methaemoglobin and proteins of plasmodial origin (Yamada & Sherman 1979). Unfortunately, no other haemozoin has been analysed in a similar way, so that direct comparisons cannot be made. And for all haemozoins the functional significance, if any, remains speculative. But, as you will hear subsequently from Dr Fitch, it has been suggested that the chloroquine receptor is ferriprotoporphyrin IX prior to its sequestration as haemozoin.

Malarial parasites fabricate limited amounts and kinds of amino acids (glutamic acid, aspartic acid and alanine) via CO_2 fixation; subsequent incorporation into plasmodial proteins is exceedingly low. However, the parasites do have access to the free amino acid pools of the red cell and the plasma. Indeed, infected erythrocytes avidly take up and incorporate exogenously supplied amino acids, especially methionine, isoleucine and leucine (see Sherman 1977).

Mature mammalian erythrocytes possess specific, but not concentrative amino acid transport systems, mostly of the facilitated-diffusion type of mechanism. Despite 30 or more years of study, the data on transport remain rather fragmentary. With the possible exception of glycine and alanine, sodium ion dependence of transport has not been observed. Although it was earlier claimed that human red cells had both a low capacity, high affinity transport system and a high capacity, non-saturable route of entry, recent evidence suggests that the low affinity system may be an artifact that resulted from the use of stored erythrocytes (Young & Ellory 1977). Reticulocytes on the other hand do show differences in amino acid transport systems from mature erythrocytes, but definition of the route of entry has proved to be difficult because of rapid transport, overlapping systems and a high degree of metabolic alteration.

No detailed studies of the mechanism of uptake (or transport) by mammalian malaria parasites have been reported on, but the study by McCormick (1970) purportedly showed the accumulation of isoleucine, methionine, leucine, cystine and histidine. However, in this study there were no indications whether substrate modification had occurred. In studies with *P. lophurae*-infected duckling erythrocytes (Sherman & Tanigoshi 1974b) evidence was given for increased entry by simple diffusion (alanine, leucine, histidine, methionine and cysteine) as well as a reduced affinity for the carrier (glycine, serine, threonine, lysine and arginine).

The changes in amino acid transport by the parasitized red cells could be due to alterations in the carrier itself; to a modification of the lipid milieu; and to a depletion of intracellular ATP. In no case have compartments been defined, and no information exists on sodium ion dependence. Moreover, it is simply not known whether the alterations in amino acid transport occur in all red cells of an infected host, whether the changes are restricted solely to infected cells, or whether the changes are stage-related.

In 1962 Moulder suggested, primarily on the basis of the observation that highly polar molecules such as ATP and coenzyme A were beneficial to the extracellular growth of *P. lophurae*, that the parasites had lost many of the active transport systems which serve to regulate the passage of molecules across its surface, and was freely permeable to all sorts of molecules which were now obtained from the host cell. Such a notion seems quite attractive. Indeed, we spent several years chasing after the transport systems of free parasites, and claimed that the parasites were, as Moulder put it, 'leaky'. However, in recent years we have come to recognize distinct flaws both in the hypothesis and in the manner whereby the supporting data were obtained.

Many laboratories have worked with parasites removed from the host cell by a wide variety of methods. Although some workers questioned the purity of such preparations, little attention was given to the integrity of the plasmodia. Recently we had the occasion to evaluate the metabolic capabilities of parasites obtained by what some have come to believe is the most gentle procedure for removing parasites—haemolytic antiserum plus complement. When such preparations were evaluated for integrity by measuring leakage of cytosolic enzymes (lactate dehydrogenase and adenosine deaminase) into the medium, as well as the ability of the plasmodia to maintain a constant volume, we were astounded by the lability of the plasmodia (Yamada & Sherman 1981). No method of preparation used by us, or for that matter any environmental condition we tested, provided parasites that maintained their integrity for the time required for transport studies. Moreover, it remains to be ascertained whether all or only a fraction of the parasites are damaged during isolation, or if the leaky state of plasmodia exists *in situ*. My own feeling is that the parasites are damaged by the isolation methods currently in vogue, and that the leaky condition does not exist intraerythrocytically. Indeed, if parasites were really nothing more than 'living sieves', how could they maintain their integrity for days during intracellular growth and reproduction?

Haemoglobin is digested in the food vacuoles by the concerted action of an acidic endopeptidase (cathepsin D) and aminopeptidases (Sherman & Tanigoshi 1981). The amino acids, derived both from proteolysis of haemoglobin and from the free pool of the plasma, are fabricated into plasmodial proteins by what appear to be typical eukaryotic mechanisms. That is, protein synthesis is sensitive to cycloheximide and puromycin, but not to chloramphenicol or streptomycin. Plasmodial ribosomes are entirely a product of the parasite itself and are not, as was once claimed, a hybrid of host and plasmodial subparticles (reviewed by Sherman 1983). Indeed, studies of plasmodial ribosomes may be one of the best examples of how biochemical confusion may result from ignorance of the biology of *Plasmodium*.

In an early study the delay in the labelling of the plasmodial 60S subparticle with ^{32}P, and the recovery of radioactivity in its 40S subparticle, were interpreted as giving evidence for the large ribosomal RNA being derived from host ribosomes (Tokuyasu et al 1969). For some unexplained reason there was little concern with the dilemma: how do host ribosomes placed in food vacuoles where digestion takes place provide intact, large subparticle RNA that can be combined with plasmodial 40S RNA to yield a functional 80S ribosome? And, in mature red cells that lack ribosomes, where do the plasmodia get their 60S ribosomal RNA? The answer, provided by several subsequent studies, was that nuclease activity degraded the plasmodial 60S particle, and it was for this reason that radioactivity was not recovered—an example of Simpson's errors being slowly corrected.

There is only one report of the cell-free translation of plasmodial mRNA (Eggit et al 1978). Nothing is known about plasmodial initiation factors or other components necessary for the fabrication of parasite proteins. And of all of the proteins made by plasmodia only one, the histidine-rich protein (HRP) of *P. lophurae*, has been characterized as to molecular weight, amino acid composition and cellular location (Kilejian 1974). Unequivocal evidence for the presence of HRP in other species is still lacking, and its function remains unexplained.

It has been reported that a malarial parasite may destroy up to 75% of the intracellular haemoglobin. Some may dispute this value and surely there is need of verification. But even more critical is the need to know exactly how much the haemoglobin and plasma amino acids each contribute to the total amount of amino acids required by the intracellular parasite.

Nucleic acid metabolism and purine transport

Malarial parasites synthesize pyrimidines *de novo*, and all or many of the half-dozen enzymes involved in the complete sequence have been identified in several species (reviewed by Sherman 1983). Thymidine kinase appears to be absent from malarial parasites; consequently, all attempts to label plasmodial DNA with tritiated thymidine have failed. The folate enzymes associated with the *de novo* pyrimidine pathway have been found in extracts of malarial parasites, and together form a thymidylate synthesis cycle.

The situation with purines, however, is entirely different from that of pyrimidines: all species of *Plasmodium* are unable to synthesize purine *de novo*, and instead the parasites rely on the salvage of preformed purines. It has been suggested (Yamada & Sherman 1981) that during parasitization, despite significant changes in the absolute levels of ATP, ADP and AMP, the adenylate energy charge (AEC) ratio is maintained precisely at 0.93. Regulation of the AEC of the infected cell depends on the activities of adenylate deaminase and kinase, which serve to reduce the AMP level and raise the ATP/ADP ratio. Concomitantly, there is increased production of hypoxanthine. This purine, which cannot be used by the red cell for nucleotide synthesis, is taken up by the parasite and fabricated into plasmodial nucleic acids. In effect, the plasmodium takes advantage of the normal process of purine turnover in the erythrocyte, accelerates its pace, utilizes its end-product, hypoxanthine, and avoids direct competition for adenosine, a purine essential to red cell survival.

Some years ago we studied the uptake of purines by the *P. lophurae*-infected red cell and suggested that purines competed for shared transport sites. However, the periods of incubation were long (5 min) and metabolic conversions had obviously occurred. Recently, we used a rapid sampling technique to study hypoxanthine transport in *P. falciparum*-infected cells, and found no change in K_t. Presumably the red cell carrier was unaltered by the presence of the parasite. Attempts to do similar studies with adenosine failed because of its rapid conversion to inosine. Clearly, this is an area in need of further work.

Although earlier we claimed that free parasites had a single transport locus for hypoxanthine, inosine and adenosine and recently Hansen et al (1980) found dramatic changes in the K_t and V_{max} for free parasites, such contentions are highly suspect because of the leaky nature of the parasites. Similarly, Manandhar & Van Dyke's conclusion (1975) that adenosine is not directly transported, but is deaminated and deribosylated on or just outside the free parasite membrane, and the resultant hypoxanthine is transported, is unwarranted for the reasons given above. The rapid metabolic conversion of added substrate in the medium and the instability of free plasmodia makes it impossible to do meaningful transport studies with free parasites.

Lipid metabolism and transport

Malarial parasites contain no lipid reserves, so all their lipids are membrane-associated. Despite the limited number of studies of lipids of infected erythrocytes a constant feature is that such cells are lipid-rich by comparison with the normal erythrocyte. This is not surprising when one considers that after parasite invasion and growth the cytosol of the red cell is occupied by an abundance of membranous organelles—the plasmodium. Characteristic of infected red cells is an increased ratio of phospholipid to cholesterol, and elevated amounts of saturated fatty acids, notably palmitic (16:0) and oleic (18:1). The enhanced amounts of 18:1 in the erythrocyte are not solely due to the lipids of the parasite, but are associated with the red cell membrane itself. This, coupled with reports of the loss of cholesterol from the parasitized red cell and increased fluidity of the outer membrane of red cells parasitized with *P. berghei* (Howard & Sawyer 1980), suggests that there is a parasite-induced remodelling of the erythrocyte membrane. Such modifications in the composition of the host cell interface undoubtedly contribute to the increased permeability and osmotic fragility that are characteristic of the parasitized red cell.

The reported compositional analyses of parasite membrane lipids must be taken with some degree of scepticism since the isolated 'free' parasites are frequently associated with host membranes. Nevertheless it does appear to be true that the membranes of the parasite are richer in unesterified fatty acids, triacylglycerols, 1,2-diacylglycerols, diacylphosphatidylethanolamine and phosphatidylinositol than are the membranes of the red cell; on the other hand, the plasmodial membranes contain less cholesterol, phosphatidylserine and sphingomyelin.

The rapid and extensive incorporation of fatty acids and cholesterol by free parasites (*P. knowlesi*) and infected red cells, together with the lack of evidence for *de novo* fatty acid synthesis, suggest that the parasites depend on the host for fatty acids and cholesterol. *Plasmodium* is able to maintain a lipid composition distinct from that of the normal host cell by limited activity of desaturases and chain-elongation enzymes as well as by exchange with the blood plasma and erythrocytic fatty acids, phospholipids, and cholesterol. The mechanism whereby such exchanges are accomplished has not been described.

Sodium transport

Cationic imbalance, especially an increased level of intracellular sodium, is characteristic of parasitized red cells. Dunn (1969) found with *P. knowlesi*-infected erythrocytes that the sodium content increased disproportionately to the parasitaemia, and that this abnormality persisted for several days after drug therapy had eradicated the infection. In addition he found that both unparasitized as well as parasitized erythrocytes were abnormal in their capacity to extrude sodium. He postulated that the elevated sodium levels were a consequence of a circulating toxin that diminished the efflux of sodium while promoting its influx. However, cross-incubation experiments with malarious plasma failed to produce sodium transport changes identical to those observed in infected monkeys. Since *P. knowlesi* infections are rather severe in the rhesus monkey, and the disruption of the cation gradient was found to develop gradually, it seems more plausible to ascribe such changes to a modification in the sodium pump itself or to a changed lipid milieu rather than to a circulating toxin. Unfortunately, no further studies on cation alterations in malaria have appeared in the literature since that time.

Acknowledgements

The research in my laboratory has been supported by the National Institute of Allergy and Infectious Diseases, NIH (AI–05226) and the World Health Organization Special Programme for Research and Training in Tropical Diseases.

REFERENCES

Aikawa M, Seed TM 1980 Morphology of plasmodia. In: JP Kreier (ed) Malaria. Academic Press, New York, vol 1:285-345

Barnes MG, Polet H 1969 The influence of methylene blue on the pentose phosphate pathway in erythrocytes of monkeys infected with *Plasmodium knowlesi*. J Lab Clin Med 74:1-11

Dunn MJ 1969 Alterations of red blood cell sodium transport during malarial infection. J Clin Invest 48:674-684

Eggit MJ, Tappenden L, Brown KN 1978 Synthesis of *Plasmodium knowlesi* polypeptides in a cell-free system. Bull WHO 57 (Suppl):109-114

Gutteridge WE, Dave D, Richards WHG 1979 Conversion of dihydroorotate to orotate in parasitic protozoa. Biochim Biophys Acta 582:390-401

Hansen BD, Sleeman HK, Pappas PW 1980 Purine base and nucleoside uptake in *Plasmodium berghei* and host erythrocytes. J Parasitol 66:205-212

Hemplemann E, Wilson RJM 1981 Detection of glucose-6-phosphate dehydrogenase in malarial parasites. Mol Biochem Parasitol 2:197-204

Howard RJ, Sawyer WH 1980 Changes in the membrane microviscosity of mouse red blood cells infected with *Plasmodium berghei* detected using N-(9-anthroyloxy) fatty acid fluorescent probes. Parasitology 80:331-342

Kilejian A 1974 A unique histidine-rich polypeptide from the malarial parasite, *Plasmodium lophurae*. J Biol Chem 249:4650-4655

Manandhar MSP, Van Dyke K 1975 Detailed purine salvage metabolism in and outside the free malarial parasite. Exp Parasitol 37:138-146

McCormick GJ 1970 Amino acid transport and incorporation in red blood cells of normal and *Plasmodium knowlesi*-infected rhesus monkeys. Exp Parasitol 27:143-149

Moulder J 1962 The biochemistry of intracellular parasitism. University of Chicago Press, Chicago, p 13-42

Neame KD, Homewood CA 1974 Alterations in the permeability of mouse erythrocytes infected with the malaria parasite *Plasmodium berghei*. Int J Parasitol 5:537-540

Scheibel W, Adler A, Trager W 1979a Tetraethylthiuram disulfide (Antabuse) inhibits the human malaria parasite *Plasmodium falciparum*. Proc Natl Acad Sci USA 76:5303-5307

Scheibel LW, Ashton SH, Trager W 1979b *Plasmodium falciparum*: microaerophilic requirements in human red blood cells. Exp Parasitol 47:410-418

Sherman IW 1977 Transport of amino acids and nucleic acid precursors in malarial parasites. Bull WHO 55:211-225

Sherman IW 1979 Biochemistry of *Plasmodium* (malarial parasites). Microbiol Rev 43:453-494

Sherman IW 1983 Metabolism. In: Peters W, Richards WHG (eds) Antimalarial drugs. Springer-Verlag, Heidelberg (Handbook of Experimental Pharmacology vol 68), in press

Sherman IW, Tanigoshi L 1974a Glucose transport in the malarial (*Plasmodium lophurae*) infected erythrocyte. J Protozool 21:603-607

Sherman IW, Tanigoshi L 1974b Incorporation of ^{14}C-amino acids by malarial plasmodia (*Plasmodium lophurae*). VI. Changes in the kinetic constants of amino acid transport during infection. Exp Parasitol 35:369-373

Sherman I, Tanigoshi L 1981 The proteases of *Plasmodium*: a cathepsin D-like enzyme from *Plasmodium lophurae*. In: Slutzky GM (ed) Biochemistry of parasites. Pergamon Press, Oxford and New York, p 137-149

Tokuyasu K, Ilan J, Ilan J 1969 Biogenesis of ribosomes in *Plasmodium berghei*. Mil Med 134:1032-1038

Velick SF 1942 The respiratory metabolism of the malaria parasite, *P. cathemerium*, during its developmental cycle. Am J Hyg 35:152-161

Wood RE, Morgan HE 1969 Regulation of sugar transport in avian erythrocytes. J Biol Chem 244:1451-1460

Yamada KA, Sherman IW 1979 *Plasmodium lophurae*: composition and properties of hemozoin, the malarial pigment. Exp Parasitol 48:61-74

Yamada K, Sherman IW 1981 Purine metabolism by the avian malarial parasite *Plasmodium lophurae*. Mol Biochem Parasitol 3:253-264

Young JD, Ellory JC 1977 Red cell amino acid transport. In: Ellory JC, Lew VL (eds) Membrane transport in red cells. Academic Press, London, p 301-325

DISCUSSION

Holder: Is there any indication of an association of the glycolytic enzymes, by analogy with the glycosome found in trypanosomes?

Sherman: No; there seems to be no sign of a glycosome in malaria parasites.

Wallach: What medium caused the parasites to collapse?

Sherman: We tried RPMI 1640 with Hepes, glucose-saline and ordinary saline. The best medium for maintaining the parasites was 30% red cell extract. We can't do many studies in that, unless we can get rid of some of the enzymes which catalyse conversion of substrates.

Wallach: So an isoionic, isotonic medium did not work?

Sherman: No. We tried to make up something similar in amino acid composition to the normal red blood cell, but this doesn't help. I think G.G. Simpson is absolutely right: 'Science is a study of errors slowly corrected'!

Wilson: To some extent I share your scepticism about the evidence for the existence of G6PD in malaria parasites. We didn't use any special techniques to isolate the enzyme, but others using our method have also found what may be a high molecular weight form of the enzyme. Our procedure was simply to separate an extract of concentrated frozen and thawed parasites or infected red cells by polyacrylamide gel electrophoresis and stain the gel for enzymic activity (Hemplemann & Wilson 1981). The uninfected red cell has a large amount of G6PD activity. Parasitized cells have an additional, less intense band of slower electrophoretic mobility. We have not excluded the possibility that this is a modified form of the host cell enzyme but it doesn't look like a degraded form because of its large size. Clearly, more work has to be done on it.

Sherman: You found G6PD in merozoites (*P. knowlesi*); have you looked at it through development? The question is whether it is made at only one point in the life cycle, or continuously.

Wilson: We looked at schizonts as well as merozoites but not at earlier forms. It was very apparent that the slow-moving band was the main source of G6PD in extracts of merozoites of *P. knowlesi* freed from host cells, unlike in schizonts where the red cell band predominated.

Sherman: Were controls run? There are problems with contamination of reagents—for example, of glucose 6-phosphate by 6-phosphogluconate. Is the pattern of 6-phosphogluconate dehydrogenase of the same high molecular weight as G6PD?

Wilson: We looked at that, and the electrophoretic mobility of the 6-phosphogluconate dehydrogenase activity is distinctly different.

Sherman: It makes sense for the parasites to have G6PD, because they always have this other enzyme.

Friedman: Not only are there different developmental stages to consider, but also exo-erythrocytic parasites, and the mosquito stages. G6PD activity has been reported in exo-erythrocytic parasites (Howells & Bafort 1970). It is possible that this enzyme is expressed only in non-red cell stages. It may be repressed in the red cell forms to prevent the diversion of glucose 6-phosphate from the glycolytic cycle when it is not needed.

Luzzatto: Dr Wilson, why do you say that the activity is of high molecular weight? These were not SDS gels, but ordinary acrylamide gels. So you don't know whether that is a charge difference or a molecular weight difference. That is important, because the G6PD activity attributed to the parasite could be a modification of a host enzyme. I hope we shall repeat this work in collaboration with you, after having grown the parasites in G6PD-deficient cells: this would eliminate any such ambiguity.

Wallach: Can any of these enzymes move back and forth between the cytoplasm of the red cell and of the parasite? Could the parasite use the host enzyme in this way?

Sherman: I don't know. Enzymes ordinarily do not cross the barrier of the parasitophorous vacuolar membrane or plasma membranes.

Friedman: Does cytochemical staining show enzyme only in the red cell cytoplasm or in the food vacuoles of the parasite, but not in the parasite cytoplasm?

Sherman: I don't think we know. This whole speculation on transfer of enzymes and substrates is not well-documented. Further, it would be difficult to investigate this phenomenon.

Wallach: If there is a transfer between the two, this would have implications for G6PD deficiency. You mentioned the effect of Antabuse, inhibiting growth of *P. falciparum*. Can you say more on that?

Sherman: Scheibel et al (1979) suggested that there might be metalloprotein oxygenases in the parasite, other than cytochrome oxidase. These oxygenases, if identified, might be involved in the utilization of the small amounts of oxygen that seem to be essential for the growth of *P. falciparum*.

Wallach: The enzyme that is most sensitive to inhibition by Antabuse is superoxide dismutase. The parasite presumably doesn't have that enzyme, though the red cell does. Could this effect be operating at the cellular level, through the dissipation of superoxide?

Sherman: I don't know. There are many protozoans where oxygenases have been looked for and are now being found. In *Entamoeba histolytica*, for example, there is a non-cytochrome oxidation-reduction system (Lo & Reeves 1979). Scheibel et al (1979) did Dr Friedman's type of experiment, of ingesting Antabuse, preparing their own serum and growing parasites in serum containing Antabuse. There was some inhibition of growth, but one is limited by using only 10% serum in the culture medium.

Cabantchik: Do you attach any physiological significance to the fact that infected cells seem to show very high permeability to so many kinds of compounds? Is this increased permeability the traumatic result of the parasite growing and expanding and stretching the red membrane, or is there an 'intentional' insertion of new proteins into the red cell membrane for the purpose of growing and acquiring compounds which otherwise permeate very slowly? For instance, amino acid transport in red cells is usually very slow.

Sherman: Many of these mechanisms might operate. In *P. lophurae* the red cell doesn't enlarge, but when one is using red cells from a heavily infected animal, one with an altered physiology, there could well be an alteration in the lipid composition of the red cell membrane. This has been shown for some species of *Plasmodium* (Beach et al 1977). Such a change may alter the transport functions of some of the erythrocyte membrane proteins. I know of no evidence for the insertion of a new transport protein in the red cell membrane, but perhaps it hasn't been looked for. When we studied the transport of hypoxanthine in *P. falciparum*-infected cells, using the silicone oil centrifugation technique, and with a 10% parasitaemia, we found no difference between normal and infected red cells (Ting & Sherman 1981). It is important that transport studies be carried out within five seconds or so, and this rapid sampling technique makes that possible. Centrifugation through the oil layer quickly separates the cells from the medium without a change in substrate. If there is a change in the substrate, then you are not looking at its transport. Once you get into the minute range, and if you don't determine the products inside those cells, claims about transport cannot be made. Glucose, for example, would be difficult to measure without a rapid sampling technique.

Cabantchik: Yes. If I may add something on some non-physiological experiments that we did, we were intrigued by your results and therefore decided to study two questions: whether there is a permselectivity change in the host cell membrane and, if so, at which developmental stage it occurs and what is its nature. Our studies relied on a battery of modern techniques for measuring transport. We found that at the trophozoite stage the permselectivity properties of the red blood cell membrane changed dramatically (Kutmer et al 1982). Compounds which were otherwise impermeant, could easily gain access to the host red cell cytoplasm. Some of these were very bulky, hydrophilic compounds of up to 500 M_r. Glucose and various hexitols penetrated apparently through the same pathway; however, seven-carbon saccharides and disaccharides were excluded. Despite the fact that various organic acids could penetrate rapidly through a similar pathway, we observed that these infected cells retained their osmotic barrier, inasmuch as incubation with isotonic sorbitol selectively haemolysed these cells and released the compounds which penetrated inside. We interpreted that not as a general permeabilization of the host cell membrane, but as a modification of a more discrete nature, such as the appearance of new membrane pores. They need not be associated with the insertion of parasite proteins into the host cell membrane. They could arise also from changes in lipid organization, induced by modification of cytoskeletal elements or changes in lipid composition.

Sherman: I would agree that the changes induced by the parasite become more apparent as the parasite gets larger, and that there must be selectivity, otherwise the red cell could not maintain its integrity. It is important that the erythrocyte be maintained as an intact cell until schizogony is complete. We measured the adenylate energy charge (AEC) during one growth cycle of *P. lophurae*. The AEC did not change until late in schizogony; then it dropped very dramatically to 0.6, the value for a non-viable cell. That makes great sense, because if the fall in ATP concentration were sufficient to lower the AEC earlier, the cell would be inviable and the parasite would perish. It is beautifully coordinated. Although there is a decline in total ATP at early stages of parasite development, there are compensatory mechanisms, namely a switching to the formation of hypoxanthine, so the relative amounts of nucleotides are maintained; therefore, the AEC is also maintained. So I agree with the idea of selectivity, although we ourselves found no evidence of it.

Cabantchik: We have evidence that the host cell membrane selectivity towards cations relative to anions is largely retained, and this is all that is needed in order to preserve the membrane potential and the osmotic properties (Kutner et al 1982). However, I wonder whether the discrete changes in the permselectivity properties of infected cells can now be used to design drugs which will selectively affect infected cells. This would provide a new and rational approach to malaria chemotherapy.

REFERENCES

Beach D, Sherman IW, Holz GG 1977 Lipids of *Plasmodium lophurae*, and of erythrocytes and plasmas of normal and *P. lophurae*-infected pekin ducklings. J Parasitol 63:62-75

Hemplemann E, Wilson RJM 1981 Detection of glucose-6-phosphate dehydrogenase in malarial parasites. Mol Biochem Parasitol 2:197-204

Howells R E, Bafort J M 1970 Histochemical observations on the pre-erythrocytic schizont of *Plasmodium berghei*. Ann Soc Bel Med Trop 50:587-594

Kutner S, Baruch D, Ginsburg H, Cabantchik ZI 1982 Alterations in membrane permeability of malaria-infected human erythrocytes are related to the growth stage of the parasite. Biochim Biophys Acta 687:113-117

Lo HS, Reeves RE 1979 *Entamoeba histolytica*: flavins in axenic organisms. Exp Parasitol 47: 180-184

Scheibel W, Adler A, Trager W 1979 Tetraethylthiuram disulfide (Antabuse) inhibits the human malaria parasite *Plasmodium falciparum*. Proc Natl Acad Sci USA 76:5303-5307

Ting AW, Sherman IW 1981 Hypoxanthine transport in normal and malaria-infected erythrocytes. Int J Parasitol 13:955-958

Mode of action of antimalarial drugs

COY D. FITCH

Department of Internal Medicine, Saint Louis University School of Medicine, 1402 South Grand Boulevard, Saint Louis, MO 63104, USA

Abstract Chloroquine, quinine, quinacrine and related drugs are effective antimalarial agents only against parasites that degrade haemoglobin. This fact prompted an examination of the role of ferriprotoporphyrin IX (FP), a product of haemoglobin degradation, in the mode of action of chloroquine. FP was identified as a high affinity drug receptor of malaria parasites by showing that it has the appropriate affinity for chloroquine, with a dissociation constant on the order of 10^{-8} M, and specificity for amodiaquine, quinacrine, quinine and mefloquine. Moreover, FP and its complex with chloroquine impair the ability of cell membranes to maintain cation gradients, and they lyse normal erythrocytes, *Plasmodium berghei* and *P. falciparum*. The amount of FP required for lysis is less than 0.1% of the haem in erythrocytic haemoglobin. Recently, evidence has been obtained that FP in the parasite forms transient, non-toxic complexes with cytoplasmic haem binders and that FP in this form can interact with chloroquine. Thus, chloroquine and related drugs may act as antimalarial agents by shunting FP away from natural haem binders and into toxic drug–FP complexes. In addition FP released from haemoglobin, either spontaneously or by oxidant drugs, may contribute to haemolysis and protection against malaria in patients with Heinz body haemolytic anaemias.

At least since 1894 (Marchiafava & Bignami) there has been a hypothesis that malaria parasites are susceptible to treatment with quinine only when they degrade haemoglobin and produce malaria pigment. This hypothesis can be extended to include quinacrine, chloroquine and related drugs. In its favour, susceptible malaria parasites invariably produce pigment, and parasites that fail to produce pigment are invariably resistant to quinine, quinacrine and chloroquine (Peters 1970). Moreover, when chloroquine-resistant, non-pigmented parasites revert to pigment production, they simultaneously revert to chloroquine susceptibility (Peters 1970). The hypothesis does not predict that all parasites that degrade haemoglobin will be susceptible to quinine, quinacrine and chloroquine. On the contrary, chloroquine-resistant strains of *Plasmodium falciparum* are known to produce malaria pigment (Schmidt

1983 Malaria and the red cell. Pitman, London (Ciba Foundation symposium 94) p 222-232

1978). Apparently, the generation of haemoglobin degradation products by the parasite is necessary but not sufficient to ensure drug susceptibility.

In the past three years, evidence has been developed which indicates that ferriprotoporphyrin IX (FP) is the chloroquine receptor of malaria parasites and that FP and its complex with chloroquine are toxic for cellular membranes, including those of malaria parasites and erythrocytes. This evidence is the basis for modern hypotheses designed to explain the mode of action of chloroquine, the mechanism of chloroquine resistance in malaria, the protective effect against malaria of glucose-6-phosphate dehydrogenase deficiency and certain abnormalities of haemoglobin structure, and the mechanism underlying Heinz body haemolytic anaemias.

Identification of FP as a chloroquine receptor

By 1967, sufficient information had accumulated to permit Macomber et al to propose that FP might serve as a receptor for chloroquine in malaria parasites. The basis for their hypothesis may be summarized as follows. The relationships between haemoglobin degradation, pigment production, and drug susceptibility were receiving considerable attention (Peters 1970); it was well known that FP binds nitrogenous bases, including chloroquine (Cohen et al 1964, Schueler & Cantrell 1964); a molecular explanation was needed for the new observation that erythrocytes infected with chloroquine-susceptible malaria parasites accumulate exceptionally large quantities of chloroquine (Macomber et al 1966); and the ability of chloroquine and related drugs to induce pigment clumping (Bock 1939) had just been rediscovered (Warhurst & Hockley 1967, Macomber et al 1967). Unfortunately, Macomber et al (1967) failed to demonstrate chloroquine binding to malaria pigment, in which FP is sequestered (Yamada & Sherman 1979), and the hypothesis received little further consideration for more than a decade.

Additional support for the hypothesis became available in 1980 when comparisons of affinities and specificities revealed a close correspondence between FP in aqueous solution and the chloroquine receptor of malaria parasites (Chou et al 1980). The dissociation constant (K_d) was estimated to be 10^{-8} M for the chloroquine–receptor complex in infected erythrocytes (Fitch 1969) and 3.5×10^{-9} M for the chloroquine–FP complex. When the K_d of chloroquine–FP was estimated in the presence of biological membranes a value of 2.3×10^{-7} M was obtained. Clearly, FP has an affinity for chloroquine in the range expected from studies of the chloroquine receptor. One molecule of chloroquine can bind 2.3 molecules of FP (Chou et al 1980). With regard to specificity, amodiaquine and quinacrine are more potent competitive inhibitors of chloroquine binding to FP than are quinine and mefloquine.

The inhibitor dissociation constants are on the order of 10^{-7} M for amodiaquine and quinacrine, 10^{-6} M for quinine and 10^{-5} M for mefloquine. These values agree reasonably well with values obtained from studies of the chloroquine receptor in infected erythrocytes (Fitch 1972). Together with information previously available, the new data led us to conclude that FP is the high affinity chloroquine receptor of malaria parasites (Chou et al 1980).

From this conclusion we predicted that exogenous FP added to cell-free preparations of malaria parasites should become sequestered in a form inaccessible to chloroquine binding. This prediction proved to be correct (Fitch & Chevli 1981). First, we confirmed the observation of Macomber et al (1967) that the chloroquine receptor is ordinarily undetectable in cell-free preparations of malaria parasites, regardless of the amount of FP sequestered in pigment. Then we discovered that the receptor could be trapped transiently in an accessible form as a drug complex by preincubation with chloroquine, followed by disruption of the parasites in the cold. These cell-free preparations now contained large quantities of the receptor; but, when they were incubated at room temperature or 37 °C, the receptor rapidly became sequestered in a form that was unavailable for chloroquine binding (Fitch & Chevli 1981). The transient existence of the receptor in an accessible form explains why high affinity binding of chloroquine to malaria pigment was not detected by Macomber et al in 1967. To demonstrate that exogenous FP is likewise rapidly sequestered, we added a chloroquine–FP complex to cell-free preparations of malaria parasites. As predicted, authentic FP became sequestered in a form inaccessible to chloroquine, with a time course similar to that of the endogenous receptor (Fitch & Chevli 1981). This similarity of behaviour in cell-free preparations strengthens the conclusion that FP is the chloroquine receptor.

Toxicity of FP and the chloroquine–FP complex

With convincing evidence in hand that FP is the high affinity chloroquine receptor of malaria parasites, we asked next whether or not FP might mediate the chemotherapeutic action of chloroquine and related drugs. By this time, Meshnick et al (1977) had demonstrated that FP lyses the protozoan parasite, *Trypanosoma brucei*. We soon found that FP in a concentration of 10 μM or less lyses normal erythrocytes (Chou & Fitch 1980, 1981), chloroquine-susceptible and chloroquine-resistant *P. berghei* (Orjih et al 1981), and chloroquine-susceptible and chloroquine-resistant *P. falciparum* (Fitch et al 1982). Mixing chloroquine with the FP to form a complex enhanced the toxicity of FP for erythrocytes (Chou & Fitch 1980) and reduced somewhat the toxicity of FP for malaria parasites (Orjih et al 1981, Fitch et al 1982). The amount of FP required for lysis represents less than 0.1% of the haem present in haemoglobin in the erythrocyte. The amount of chloroquine–FP complex required for lysis is less than the amount of chloroquine–receptor complex which accumulates when erythrocytes infected with malaria parasites are exposed to chloroquine *in vitro* (Fitch 1969, 1970). Lysis was demonstrated by showing that the turbidity of suspensions of the cells decreases and that the cells swell and release their intracellular contents (Orjih et al 1981). In the case of *P. falciparum*, lysis was confirmed by electron microscopy, which revealed loss of internal detail, swelling and, ultimately, rupture (Fitch et al 1982). Chloroquine alone did not cause lysis of erythrocytes or malaria parasites in these experiments.

The mechanism of cell lysis by FP and the chloroquine–FP complex has been studied using normal erythrocytes as an experimental model (Chou & Fitch 1980, 1981). The earliest abnormality was an impaired ability to maintain cation gradients. Thus, 90% of the intracellular potassium was lost within 30 minutes of exposing erythrocytes to 5 μM-FP. In association with potassium loss, the erythrocytes swelled, became spherocytic, and developed exquisite susceptibility to hypotonic lysis (Chou & Fitch 1981). FP-induced haemolysis was not inhibited by incubation in the dark or by various free radical scavengers and was not associated with the production of malonyldialdehyde from membrane lipids. Cysteine, dithiothreitol and mercaptoethanol protected erythrocytes from FP, but the reason for the protection remains to be elucidated (Chou & Fitch 1981), as does the molecular basis of the impairment by FP of the ability to maintain cation gradients.

Returning to the effect of FP and the chloroquine–FP complex on malaria parasites, two related questions come to mind. How can the parasite survive when it degrades large quantities of haemoglobin and releases FP? And why would it be necessary to form a chloroquine–FP complex to kill malaria parasites? Answers to these questions are provided by some recent experiments (Banyal & Fitch 1982) in which albumin and parasite cell sap preparations were found to neutralize the toxicity of FP. One mg per ml of albumin or 0.56 mg per ml of cell sap protein completely eliminated the toxicity of 40 μM-FP for isolated *P. berghei* parasites. Cell sap from normal erythrocytes provided much less protection. Neither of the cell sap preparations nor albumin eliminated the toxicity of the chloroquine–FP complex for malaria parasites. These results are interpreted as evidence that malaria parasites possess soluble haem binders which can form non-toxic complexes with FP as it is released by haemoglobin degradation. Furthermore, we suggest that complexes of FP with soluble intracellular haem binders represent the transiently accessible form of FP that can be demonstrated in cell-free preparations of malaria parasites (Fitch & Chevli 1981).

Mode of action of chloroquine as an antimalarial drug (hypothesis)

From the foregoing observations we propose that chloroquine acts by diverting FP from non-toxic complexes with soluble, intracellular haem binders into a toxic chloroquine–FP complex (Banyal & Fitch 1982). We would suggest that this toxic complex impairs the ability of the parasite, the host erythrocyte, or both to maintain cation gradients and that the parasites die either because of the ionic changes or because of outright lysis. This hypothesis synthesizes all available information about the chloroquine susceptibility of malaria parasites, including the requirement for haemoglobin degradation, and it explains the selectivity of chloroquine as an antimalarial drug.

Mechanisms of chloroquine resistance (hypotheses)

For non-pigmented malaria parasites that do not degrade haemoglobin, the explanation for chloroquine resistance is straightforward. In the absence of haemoglobin degradation, no FP would be available to form a toxic complex, the parasite would not bind [14C]chloroquine with high affinity (Fitch 1969), and it would be expected to be as resistant as the host to chloroquine. A different hypothesis must be proposed for chloroquine resistance in *P. falciparum*, for this parasite is pigmented (Schmidt 1978). It is well established, however, that the FP produced by chloroquine-resistant *P. falciparum* is unavailable to bind chloroquine with high affinity (Fitch 1970, 1973). Consequently, to explain chloroquine resistance, it is necessary to account for the unavailability of FP. There could be an increase in the amount or affinity of intracellular haem binders, for example. Alternatively, the process of FP sequestration into pigment might be accelerated in chloroquine-resistant *P. falciparum*. These hypotheses merit further study.

Possible role of FP in Heinz body haemolytic anaemias

Abnormal haemoglobin molecules that have increased susceptibility to oxidation release FP and are precipitated as haem-depleted Heinz bodies (Jacob & Winterhalter 1970). Even normal haemoglobin can be induced to release FP by oxidation (Bunn & Jandl 1968). Since FP is such a lytic substance and since erythrocyte cell sap has a relatively limited capacity to neutralize the toxicity of FP (see Banyal & Fitch 1982), the hypothesis should be considered that FP plays an important role in erythrocyte lysis in Heinz body haemolytic anaemias (Chou & Fitch 1981). In support of the hypothesis, oxidant drugs (primaquine, for example), which cause haemolytic anaemia in patients with glucose-6-phosphate dehydrogenase deficiency, also cause potassium loss when incubated with erythrocytes *in vitro* (Weed 1961).

Finally, the hypothesis should be considered that FP plays an important role in the protection against malaria afforded by thalassaemia, glucose-6-phosphate dehydrogenase deficiency, and perhaps other Heinz body haemolytic anaemias (Luzzatto et al 1983). A central role for FP would explain why erythrocytes from patients with thalassaemia or glucose-6-phosphate dehydrogenase deficiency provide an exceptionally hostile environment for malaria parasites when they are exposed to high oxygen tension or oxidant drugs (Friedman 1979). It would also explain why extra potassium in the culture medium protects *P. falciparum* against oxidant stress (Friedman 1979), since the extra potassium would prevent the FP-induced loss of intracellular potassium.

Acknowledgements

This work was supported in part by a contract from the US Army Medical Research and Development Command and by a grant from the United Nations Development Programme/World Bank/World Health Organization Special Programme for Research and Training in Tropical Diseases.

REFERENCES

Banyal HS, Fitch CD 1982 Ferriprotoporphyrin IX binding substances and the mode of action of chloroquine against malaria. Life Sci 31:1141-1144

Bock E 1939 Über morphologische Veränderungen menschlicher malaria Parasiten durch Atebrineinwirbeung. Arch Schiffs Tropenhyg 43:209-214

Bunn HF, Jandl JH 1968 Exchange of heme among hemoglobins and between hemoglobin and albumin. J Biol Chem 243:465-475

Chou AC, Fitch CD 1980 Hemolysis of mouse erythrocytes by ferriprotoporphyrin IX and chloroquine. Chemotherapeutic implications. J Clin Invest 66:856-858

Chou AC, Fitch CD 1981 Mechanism of hemolysis induced by ferriprotoporphyrin IX. J Clin Invest 68:672-677

Chou AC, Chevli R, Fitch CD 1980 Ferriprotoporphyrin IX fulfills the criteria for identification as the chloroquine receptor of malaria parasites. Biochemistry 19:1543-1549

Cohen SN, Phifer KO, Yielding KL 1964 Complex formation between chloroquine and ferrihemic acid *in vitro* and its effect on the antimalarial action of chloroquine. Nature (Lond) 202:805-806

Fitch CD 1969 Chloroquine resistance in malaria: a deficiency of chloroquine binding. Proc Natl Acad Sci USA 64:1181-1187

Fitch CD 1970 *Plasmodium falciparum* in owl monkeys: drug resistance and chloroquine binding capacity. Science (Wash DC) 169:289-290

Fitch CD 1972 Chloroquine resistance in malaria: drug binding and cross resistance patterns. Proc Helminthol Soc Wash 39(suppl):265-271

Fitch CD 1973 Chloroquine-resistant *Plasmodium falciparum*: difference in handling of ^{14}C-amodiaquine and ^{14}C-chloroquine. Antimicrob Agents Chemother 3:545-548

Fitch CD, Chevli R 1981 Sequestration of the chloroquine receptor in cell-free preparations of erythrocytes infected with *Plasmodium berghei*. Antimicrob Agents Chemother 19:589-592

Fitch CD, Chevli R, Banyal HS, Phillips G, Pfaller MA, Krogstad DJ 1982 Lysis of *Plasmodium falciparum* by ferriprotoporphyrin IX and a chloroquine–ferriprotoporphyrin IX complex. Antimicrob Agents Chemother 21:819-822

Friedman MJ 1979 Oxidant damage mediates variant red cell resistance to malaria. Nature (Lond) 280:245-247

Jacob HS, Winterhalter KH 1970 The role of hemoglobin heme loss in Heinz body formation: studies with a partially heme-deficient hemoglobin and with genetically unstable hemoglobins. J Clin Invest 49:2008-2016

Luzzatto L, Sodeinde O, Martini G 1983 Genetic variation in the host and adaptive phenomena in *P. falciparum* infection. This volume, p 159-169

Macomber PB, O'Brien RL, Hahn FE 1966 Chloroquine: physiological basis of drug resistance in *Plasmodium berghei*. Science (Wash DC) 152:1374-1375

Macomber PB, Sprinz H, Tousimis AJ 1967 Morphological effects of chloroquine on *Plasmodium berghei* in mice. Nature (Lond) 214:937-939

Marchiafava E, Bignami A 1894 On summer–autumn malaria fevers. The New Sydenham Society, London (translated by Thompson JH)

Meshnick SR, Chang K-P, Cerami A 1977 Heme lysis of the bloodstream forms of *Trypanosoma brucei*. Biochem Pharmacol 26:1923-1928

Orjih AU, Banyal HS, Chevli R, Fitch CD 1981 Hemin lyses malaria parasites. Science (Wash DC) 214:667-669

Peters W 1970 Chemotherapy and drug resistance in malaria. Academic Press, London

Schmidt LH 1978 *Plasmodium falciparum* and *Plasmodium vivax* infections in the owl monkey (*Aotus trivirgatus*). I. The courses of untreated infections. Am J Trop Med Hyg 27:671-702

Schueler FW, Cantrell WF 1964 Antagonism of the antimalarial action of chloroquine by ferrihemate and an hypothesis for the mechanism of chloroquine resistance. J Pharmacol Exp Ther 143:278-281

Warhurst DC, Hockley DJ 1967 Mode of action of chloroquine on *Plasmodium berghei* and *P. cynomolgi*. Nature (Lond) 214:935-936

Weed RI 1961 Effects of primaquine on the red blood cell membrane. II. K[+] permeability in glucose-6-phosphate dehydrogenase deficient erythrocytes. J Clin Invest 40:140-143

Yamada KA, Sherman IW 1979 *Plasmodium lophurae*: composition and properties of hemozoin, the malarial pigment. Exp Parasitol 48:61-74

DISCUSSION

Wallach: Does methaemoglobin itself bind chloroquine?

Fitch: Methaemoglobin does not bind chloroquine with high affinity.

Wallach: Do you need the iron for binding?

Fitch: We haven't determined whether or not protoporphyrin IX binds chloroquine.

Wallach: Are the propionyl residues of haemoglobin necessary?

Fitch: We have not evaluated the effect of modifying the porphyrin molecule.

Wallach: Are oxyhaem or carbonmonoxyhaem inactive in chloroquine binding?

Fitch: Cyanide eliminates the toxicity of FP for erythrocytes, and, presumably, carbon monoxide would have a similar effect. We have not measured the effect of cyanide or carbon monoxide on chloroquine binding to FP.

Wallach: Would a protohaem work?

Fitch: We have tried only ferrihaem (ferriprotoporphyrin IX).

Wallach: Have you substituted another metal? For example, by testing chlorophyll (Mg instead of Fe)?

Fitch: No, but such studies would be of interest from the point of view of establishing the role of iron in chloroquine binding.

Tanner: I gather that FP affects both the outside and the inside of the red cell membrane. Is there any 'sidedness' in the membrane effects?

Fitch: We do not yet have a satisfactory way of placing FP inside the cell, so all our results were obtained with FP acting from the outside.

Tanner: Are there any effects of FP on Na^+, K^+-ATPase pumping activity?

Fitch: Chou and I (unpublished) found no effect of FP on Na^+, K^+-ATPase. Moreover, the potassium loss and swelling of erythrocytes exposed to FP precede any decrease in the concentrations of ATP or of reduced glutathione (Chou & Fitch 1981).

McGregor: Dr Fitch, you say you believe that FP has a receptor for chloroquine and that when the two substances bind a compound is formed which is lethal for the parasite. You have also found that other drugs, including quinine and mefloquine, also bind to FP, indicating that they may kill parasites by the same mechanism as chloroquine. If this is so, why then are quinine and mefloquine successful in treating chloroquine-resistant malaria? Do your findings indicate that it is only a matter of time before mefloquine-resistant parasites become common?

Fitch: Rodent malaria parasites that lack pigment show a high degree of cross-resistance against quinine, quinacrine, and even mefloquine compared to chloroquine-resistant *P. falciparum*, which is pigmented and therefore produces FP. I think the differences in effectiveness between quinine, mefloquine and chloroquine in the treatment of chloroquine-resistant *P. falciparum* malaria may be due to differences in accessibility to FP. Even amodiaquine may be more effective than chloroquine against certain strains of chloroquine-resistant *P. falciparum*, presumably because the ortho-cresol ring in its side-chain gives it more hydrophobicity and perhaps enables it to come closer to partially sequestered FP.

McGregor: Nonetheless, the fact that all these drugs cross-bind with the receptor is disquieting, from the point of view of looking for effective drugs against chloroquine-resistant parasites.

Fitch: Yes, and this fact causes me to predict that only minor adaptations of chloroquine-resistant *P. falciparum* may result in cross-resistance to other drugs in this class.

Anders: I am intrigued by the different mechanisms of chloroquine resistance in *P. falciparum* and *P. berghei*. Were the experiments with the haem binder done with both parasites? Are there equivalent or different affinities in the two systems?

Fitch: Nearly all the work with the haem binder has been done with *P. berghei*. We are just beginning to work with *P. falciparum*.

Luzzatto: Were the haemolysis experiments done in the light or in the dark?

Fitch: Since protoporphyrin is not lytic in the dark, we evaluated the effect of light on haemolysis by FP. FP is as toxic in the dark as in light.

Pasvol: Did you look at the total content of haemoglobin remaining in red cells containing chloroquine-resistant, mature *P. berghei* parasites? Was it left unchanged?

Fitch: No, we have not measured haemoglobin content.

Pasvol: When we talk about the protection afforded by various abnormal haemoglobins in malaria, it is probably the *functional* consequences of a given type of haemoglobin being present in the cell which leads to parasite damage, rather than structural aspects. The role of these abnormal haemoglobins could be clarified using chloroquine-resistant strains of parasite, which possibly utilize minimal amounts of intracellular haemoglobin. Are there strains of *P. falciparum* which produce no FP at all?

Fitch: Such a strain of *P. falciparum* has not yet been found.

Pasvol: We teach our students that chloroquine acts in malaria by intercalating between DNA base pairs and that it inhibits DNA polymerase in the parasite. Do you feel now that this has very little role to play in its therapeutic effect?

Fitch: I do not think intercalation with DNA has a role in the mode of action of chloroquine as an antimalarial drug. For intercalation, 10^{-5}M or more chloroquine is needed, whereas 10^{-9} to 10^{-8}M concentrations are sufficient for antimalarial effects.

Pasvol: Is the pharmacology of chloroquine compatible with the clinical observations that if you treat people with malaria you must wait 36–48 hours for an effect on the parasite? Secondly, one sees a clinical improvement quickly with the use of chloroquine. This has often been related to the anti-inflammatory effect of chloroquine. Can you relate this to your findings?

Fitch: As a biochemist, I add concentrations and adjust conditions to produce an effect in an hour or two. Very small concentrations of the chloroquine–FP complex might be toxic enough to kill the parasites during the course of

36–48 hours. Possibly, the anti-inflammatory effect of chloroquine may explain its immediate effect. Alternatively, very small concentrations of the chloroquine–FP complex might cause the parasite to cease production of a toxic substance long before the parasite dies.

Sherman: You mentioned that *P. berghei,* if it is unpigmented, is chloroquine-resistant. I gather that Paul Thompson had a *P. berghei* strain that was pigmented and resistant?

Fitch: Yes. I understand that he had a strain of *P. berghei* that behaved similarly to *P. yoelii.* When exposed to chloroquine it was not pigmented; but, when not exposed to chloroquine, it was pigmented.

Sherman: This is unlike *P. falciparum,* where chloroquine need not be present for stable drug resistance. A technical detail, and one that may be important: you talked about FP IX binding to chloroquine, but in fact what you are using for chloroquine binding is haematin. In the FP IX that we referred to (Yamada & Sherman 1979) in our paper on malarial pigment the exact chemical composition wasn't known, so we used a neutral term for the pigment monomers and polymers. There may be a difference between haematin and FP IX found in parasites. The other aspect is that *in vivo*, the action of chloroquine–FP may be quite different from what you show. Chloroquine must enter the cytostome, pass through the parasitophorous vacuole membrane, enter the cytoplasm of the parasite, and get into the food vacuole—because that is probably the only place where haem is liberated from haemoglobin. Then the chloroquine complex presumably would act on the food vacuole membrane, then perhaps on the parasite cytoplasm, and then on the red cell membrane. This is the reverse order of what you have demonstrated for the action of FP–chloroquine on membranes.

Fitch: I chose 'ferriprotoporphyrin' as a generic term because chloroquine binds either to haemin or to haematin. I'm not sure at which membrane the toxicity occurs. Every biological membrane that has been tested so far has been susceptible to FP toxicity. It might be sufficient only to damage the food vacuole with the chloroquine–FP complex to kill the parasite.

Sherman: Your haem-binding protein would, I assume, be in the food vacuole.

Aikawa: We have investigated the localization of chloroquine in the parasite by using electron microscope autoradiography (Aikawa 1972). ^{3}H-labelled chloroquine was concentrated exclusively within the food vacuoles. Several hours after the injection of chloroquine, the food vacuoles become enlarged and eventually the parasite's morphology disintegrates.

Fitch: On the point about chloroquine having to traverse several membranes, we find that chloroquine equilibrates across the erythrocyte membrane very rapidly. Presumably, it would behave similarly with regard to other membranes.

REFERENCES

Aikawa M 1972 High-resolution autoradiography of malarial parasites treated with 3H-chloroquine. Am J Pathol 67:277-284

Chou AC, Fitch CD 1981 Mechanism of hemolysis induced by ferriprotoporphyrin IX. J Clin Invest 68:672-677

Yamada KA, Sherman IW 1979 *Plasmodium lophurae*: composition and properties of hemozoin, the malarial pigment. Exp Parasitol 48:61-74

General discussion

Summary of symposium

Howard: I have been asked to attempt a summary of this symposium. Clearly, it can be only an incomplete statement of what seemed to me to be some of the major points of discussion. The symposium began with the topic of the *invasion of the red cell* by the malarial merozoite. Dr Aikawa presented electron micrographs that define the merozoite–red cell interaction as a *multistep process*, beginning with attachment of the merozoite via any part of its surface, followed by reorientation and apical attachment. This step is believed to be a critical interaction, involving the release of merozoite material from the rhoptry organelles at the apical complex into the red cell membrane. Freeze–fracture electron microscopy has been used by Dr Aikawa to study the distribution of intramembranous particles in the red cell membrane during invasion, showing clearly that the nature of the red cell membrane area invaginated by the merozoite is altered, by comparison with adjacent areas.

The experiments described by Dr Pasvol and Dr Friedman, and those published elsewhere by Dr Miller, made use of enzyme pre-treatments of red cells and of red cells of different serological phenotypes to show that the multistep process of invasion involves *specific interactions* at several levels. We can infer that there are specific molecules, or parts of molecules, on both the red cell and the merozoite required for invasion. Red cell glycoproteins are being examined in several laboratories, including those of Drs Tanner, Pasvol, Friedman and Miller, for a potential role as red cell receptors recognized by *P. falciparum* merozoites. The possibility was discussed that there might be molecular events during invasion that are specific for interaction of merozoites of particular malaria species with the red cell, while other molecular events might be shared by several malaria species. With the expanding interest in merozoite invasion as a step in the asexual parasites' life cycle that might be interrupted immunologically, we can predict that in the next few years some of the specific events during invasion will be described at a molecular level. The use of anti-malaria parasite monoclonal antibodies promises to be important in this direction, although this work was not discussed at this symposium.

A question which links our thinking on merozoite invasion and on changes in

1983 Malaria and the red cell. Pitman, London (Ciba Foundation symposium 94) p 233-245

the erythrocyte membrane of infected cells is whether there are new components inserted into the erythrocyte membrane during invasion that remain
there after parasite entry. Merozoite-derived proteins or lipids that remain on
the erythrocyte surface after invasion might constitute antigenic targets for
immunity on early ring-stage parasites. If invasion involves enzymic modification of erythrocyte membrane components, these altered components might
also constitute new target antigens. The use of monoclonal antibodies might
again prove useful for answering these questions. Dr Luzzatto described the
variety of red cell phenotypes that determine *innate resistance* (and degrees of
resistance) to the intraerythrocytic survival of malaria parasites. Other red cell
phenotypes determine the efficiency of merozoite attachment and invasion.
The elucidation of the molecular basis for differences in red cell phenotype
defined serologically, morphologically or enzymically will continue to provide
us with new experimental tools for investigating factors that determine parasite
survival. It was also pointed out that although many abnormal red cell phenotypes or relatively rare polymorphisms result from changing an allele at a single
locus, this may have multiple effects on the red cell phenotype. Alterations in
alleles at enzyme loci such as glucose-6-phosphate dehydrogenase, or at loci for
structural proteins such as spectrin, can be expected to alter many red cell
properties.

    Another complicating phenomenon with genetic abnormalities is evident
from the biochemical studies on membrane protein glycosylation accompanying the En(a−) phenotype. This phenotype is characterized by lack of the
MN-bearing sialoglycoprotein (glycophorin A). En(a−) red cells are also
characterized by increased galactose and *N*-acetylglucosamine on band 3 (Tanner et al 1976), suggesting that some of the enzymes which normally glycosylate
glycophorin A act on band 3 when the sialoglycoprotein is lacking. In this case a
change at a particular membrane protein locus results in an altered phenotype
for another membrane protein. These results indicate that we must be cautious
before ascribing the altered properties of red cells of rare or abnormal phenotype with respect to malaria invasiveness or intraerythrocytic growth to a
phenotypic change of a single component directly encoded in the altered
genotype.

    If we next consider the *intraerythrocytic stage*, including parasite maturation
from ring stage, to trophozoite, to schizont, we can consider changes in the
membrane properties of infected cells. Two types of *morphological changes in
the outer membrane* of infected cells have been described by electron microscopy.

    Vivax-and ovale-type malarias cause small invaginations of this membrane
(caveolae) that contain electron-dense material at the base of the caveolae.
Many small vesicles are seen connected to the caveolae, each vesicle delimited
by a unit membrane. This alteration in the membrane is called a *caveola–vesicle*

complex. Caveolae without the associated vesicles are seen with falciparum- and malariae-type parasites and *P. knowlesi*, as well as with the vivax- and ovale-type malarias. The numbers of caveolae or caveola–vesicle complexes increase as the intraerythrocytic parasite matures. Dr Bannister showed us that caveolae are seen even with immature ring stages of *P. knowlesi*. The function of this particular membrane change is unknown, some workers favouring the view that caveola–vesicle complexes are endocytic, others suggesting that they are exocytic. These complexes contain parasite antigens accessible to external antibody (Aikawa et al 1975). The molecular nature of the new antigens in the caveola is unknown, nor do we know whether antibody to these antigens kills the intracellular parasite.

The second type of morphological change in the outer membrane of infected erythrocytes are the *knob excrescences* of falciparum- and malariae-type parasites (occasionally also with ovale-type parasites). The molecular nature of these knobs and their function is currently the focus of work in several laboratories. Although the molecular nature of the membrane components making up the knobs is unknown, a variety of studies published before this symposium lead us to infer that several components must be present. Falciparum-type parasites are sequestered on the venous endothelium of the heart and other organs with the knobs on the infected erythrocyte's membrane providing the focal points of attachment to endothelial cells (Luse & Miller 1971). We conclude that some component of the knob mediates binding to endothelial cells. Support for this hypothesis comes from the observation that IgG in homologous immune sera inhibits or reverses the binding of *P. falciparum*-infected cells to cultured endothelial cells *in vitro* (I.J. Udeinya & L.H. Miller, unpublished results).

Knobs must contain other components, however, besides those required for endothelial attachment. In *P. malariae* and *P. brasilianum* infections knobs are seen on erythrocytes infected by asexual parasites or gametocytes, and yet these cells do not sequester. A minimal hypothesis would hold that knobs in these parasites contain structural components only, which may be similar to components of knobs in falciparum-type infections required similarly to produce the knob structure. Alternatively, the knobs of malariae- and ovale-type parasites (the latter seen only occasionally) may contain, in addition to structural components, other molecules with functions as yet unknown that are specific to these parasites or shared also by falciparum-type parasites. It is possible that knobs serve as localized regions of the infected erythrocyte's membrane where membrane permeability is altered by the insertion of parasite transport proteins to allow parasite uptake or excretion of metabolites. The predicted multicomponent nature of knobs in different malaria species (i.e. structural, endothelial-binding and other functional components) should be elucidated as monoclonal antibodies become available.

Two aspects of the expression of knobs on *P. falciparum*-infected cells were dealt with in some detail. Dr Wyler and Dr Barnwell stressed that the capacity of this parasite to produce knobs, and thereby to sequester to venous endothelium, enabled the parasite to evade *passage through the spleen*. Mature parasitized cells would clearly be most susceptible to non-specific 'pitting' of the parasitic inclusion on passage through the narrow fenestrations in the spleen. Furthermore, a variety of other splenic immune responses, both specific and non-specific, are probably also avoided by parasite sequestration. One immune response that the parasite would not be expected to avoid by its capacity to sequester would be humoral antibody. The capacity of homologous antibody to block the attachment of *P. falciparum*-infected cells to endothelium *in vitro* was mentioned above. We can now examine by the *in vitro* attachment assay (Udeinya et al 1981) whether sera from immune individuals block the attachment of infected cells to endothelium, while sera from infected non-immunes may not block attachment.

The second aspect of knob expression concerns the evidence for the *lability of different knob components* in the membrane on *in vitro* or *in vivo* passage. It had already been shown that prolonged *in vitro* culture of *P. falciparum* led to the loss of knobs from the surface of infected cells (Langreth et al 1979). Dr Barnwell presented new results on the lability of binding components in the knob structure. Parasites which bound via knobs to endothelial cells *in vitro* and which sequestered *in vivo* were passaged in splenectomized monkeys. After only one or two passages, parasites were recovered which still expressed knobs on the surface of the infected cell (seen by electron microscopic analysis) but failed to bind to endothelial cells *in vitro* and did not sequester *in vivo*. This not only provides additional evidence for the separate existence of structural and endothelial-binding components in the knobs of *P. falciparum*, but emphasizes the need for careful monitoring of the phenotype of malaria parasites passaged *in vitro* or *in vivo*. Changes in the molecular nature of the knobs are inferred from this study, but there was no evidence of morphological alterations.

The role of the spleen in the expression of *P. falciparum* knob components, also indicated by these studies, is a surprising one, and one for which as yet we have no idea of the mechanisms involved. The involvement of the host spleen in the expression of parasite antigens in the membrane of infected erythrocytes was also highlighted by Dr Barnwell's results with *P. knowlesi*. The SICA variant antigen on *P. knowlesi* schizont-infected cells is not expressed after passaging this parasite in splenectomized rhesus monkeys. SICA antigen expression *per se* appears to require some splenic factors. It is now apparent, from results presented here, that the ability of *P. knowlesi* to alter its antigenic phenotype from the expression of one variant antigen to the expression of another also depends on the host's spleen. The dependence of the malaria parasite on its host appears, therefore, to extend beyond a requirement for metabolites and the osmotic, temperature and ionic conditions of the vascular milieu, to a requirement for splenic factors which allow the parasite to modulate its expression of antigens on infected cells.

A question that has long intrigued malariologists is the mechanism for the *transport of new antigens to the surface* of parasitized erythrocytes. The antigens are presumed to originate from the intracellular parasite. Clefts bounded by unit membrane have been observed by electron microscopy in the erythrocyte cytoplasm, between parasite and erythrocyte outer membrane, in all malaria species. These clefts may be involved in antigen transport. At this symposium Dr Bannister and Dr Aikawa showed us vesicles blebbing out from the parasitophorous vacuole membrane. These electron micrographs support the contention that antigens are transported to the cell surface in membrane-bound form via vesicles and clefts. The next step will be to use the traditional methods of subcellular fractionation and membrane characterization, together with monoclonal antibodies to parasite antigens shown to be on the erythrocyte surface, in an effort to characterize the route of antigen transport and to see whether antigens are modified structurally along this route. If the erythrocyte surface antigens are always membrane-bound, it has been predicted that they will also be expressed on the plasma membrane of the intraerythrocytic parasite (Howard 1982). It will also be interesting to characterize the molecular basis for the failure of *P. knowlesi* parasites to express SICA antigen or the loss of endothelial-binding capacity of *P. falciparum* parasites after passage in splenectomized animals. These altered phenotypes may result from an interruption of the normal process of antigen transport from the intracellular parasite to the erythrocyte surface.

New antigens in the surface membrane of infected erythrocytes could arise by insertion of parasite-derived proteins, glycoproteins or glycolipids. Alternatively, host membrane components could be altered in structure or arrangement, for example by limited proteolysis or by forming new protein–protein complexes, to create new antigenic determinants specific for the surface of infected cells. Dr Jarra presented evidence from immunoelectron microscopy that *altered host antigens* exist on the surface of erythrocytes infected by murine plasmodia. It was suggested that the nature of such altered autoantigens and their degree of association with malarial antigens might affect the induction of immune responses directed against the surface of infected cells. Again we can predict that our understanding of the role of these altered host antigens in anti-malarial immunity will become clearer when monoclonal antibodies are available.

Other changes in the membrane of malaria-infected erythrocytes have been described, in addition to the morphological and antigenic alterations mentioned here. The uptake of glucose, certain amino acids and purines, and the release of lactate from infected cells, have been shown earlier to be greatly enhanced in infected erythrocytes by comparison with uninfected erythrocytes. There appear to be *specific permeability and selectivity alterations* in the barrier properties of the membrane of infected erythrocytes. It is not known whether these changes reflect the insertion of specific parasite transport components into the membrane, alterations in endogenous membrane transport components, or changes in the barrier properties through changes in membrane lipid composition. Dr Cabantchik described results from his laboratory which indicate a selective increased permeability of the membrane of infected cells to anionic compounds. This change did not appear to be due to a change in band 3, the endogenous erythrocyte anion transporter. Dr Wallach described a marked increase in calcium level within infected erythrocytes, due primarily to uptake by the intracellular parasite. It is not yet known whether the membrane barrier which maintains a high internal calcium level is only the parasite plasmalemma, or whether the parasitophorous vacuole and erythrocyte membranes are also involved in calcium uptake. It was suggested that regulation of calcium levels, both free and bound, within the parasite will be involved in many metabolic processes, perhaps including parasite invasion of erythrocytes.

We did not discuss the evidence for *alterations in lipid composition* of the erythrocyte membrane in malaria. Alterations in lipid composition have been calculated from total lipid analyses of infected cells, attempting to take the parasite's own lipid composition into account. Furthermore, the fluidity of the lipid phase of the outer membrane of infected cells is markedly increased (Howard & Sawyer 1980), and there are dramatic changes in the transbilayer phospholipid asymmetry in the host cell membrane of *Plasmodium knowlesi*-infected cells (Gupta & Mishra 1981). The effects of these changes in lipid composition and distribution on the activity of enzymes in the erythrocyte membrane of infected cells remain to be assessed.

It is apparent from all these studies on new morphological structures, new antigens, altered host antigens and altered lipid components of the infected red cell's membrane that a number of *antigenic targets* must exist on the red cell surface for potential parasiticidal immune responses. At this stage we are working towards a molecular description of these biochemical and antigenic changes. As these antigens are identified and as monoclonal antibody reagents are developed to them, we shall be able to investigate the induction of specific immune responses to these antigens and the quantitative importance for protective immunity of immune responses directed against the merozoite surface, as compared to those directed against surface antigens of infected cells.

Finally, some technical considerations. A recurring point in discussion has been the problem of how to prove that a particular antigen is actually on the surface of infected erythrocytes. Dr Sherman summarized some of the reasons for this problem: malaria-infected cells are notoriously fragile and may rupture during radiolabelling; they may be more permeable to radiolabelling probes than uninfected erythrocytes; traditional methods of subcellular fractionation, used to define the location of new radiolabelled antigens, are hampered by lack of defined markers for the different membranes involved. (Although markers for erythrocyte and parasite membranes exist, there is as yet none for the parasitophorous vacuole membrane.) Experiments in my laboratory and in Dr Brown's laboratory have shown that by adding antibody to preparations of schizont-infected erythrocytes, washing to remove unbound antibody and then extracting antigen–antibody complexes in non-ionic detergent, one can identify a very small subset of total malarial antigens of these cells. These antigens appear to be restricted to the cell surface. However, even if only a very small proportion of the cells lyse during incubation with antibody, internal antigens will be identified. The problem of lysis of infected cells also plagues attempts to demonstrate that an antigen is on the surface by showing that the appropriate antibody specificity is removed by adsorption with intact cells.

In our own attempts to prove the surface location of particular malarial antigens of interest, we are trying to produce monoclonal antibodies for immunoelectron microscopy with intact cells, broken cells and membranes. This approach may eventually tell us not only whether a particular antigen is actually on the surface membrane, but whether it is also present on clefts or vesicles presumed to be *en route* from the parasite to the erythrocyte surface.

Antigenic changes in parasitized erythrocytes

Anders: Is one looking at antigens that are parasite-derived, or modified host components? The usual method of establishing antigens as parasite-derived is by using biosynthetically labelled parasites and conventional immunoprecipitations and gel analysis, but this is not unequivocal evidence because of the problem of co-precipitation. This is a particular problem with membrane components. Most people solubilize membranes with non-ionic detergents which do not disrupt all the protein–protein interactions.

Wallach: Several laboratories have done cell-free translation of messenger RNA from malaria parasites, and have isolated peptide components which could be specifically immunoprecipitated.

Sherman: But you don't know where those peptides are localized in the parasite.

Wallach: We do! The precipitating antibody can be specifically absorbed out by intact infected cells, so the antigens are localized at the cell surface.

Sherman: But suppose it is a host red cell modified protein? The assumption is that a protein is from the red cell because it is absorbed out by intact cells.

However, if it is modified red cell protein, it would not be absorbed out by red cells. The conclusion that proteins are of parasite origin may not be true, if one uses absorption with normal red cells to discriminate among proteins. Also, as Dr Howard said, there is no good marker for the parasitophorous vacuole membrane or the parasite plasma membrane. This is a major gap in our information. Further complications arise because profound changes occur in the lipid composition of the red cell membrane. We know that the red cell membrane is modified as well as the parasitophorous vacuolar membrane. There is an enrichment in octadecenoic acid in the parasite membranes, and maybe also in the red cell membrane; also, the ratio of phospholipid to cholesterol in the infected red cell is higher than that of the normal red cell. These changes may affect the biology of the parasitic situation. The differentiation and separation of parasite and host membrane is another major gap, as I see it. We have to develop relevant probes for each. Subcellular fractionation remains unsatisfactory as a tool because of the ambiguity in membrane characterization.

Another point is that the parasitophorous vacuole membrane (PVM) grows as the parasite enlarges within the red cell. The parasite is surrounded by the PVM during its entire intraerythrocytic existence. In fact, it may be necessary that the parasite have the PVM for it to undergo schizogony. I don't think significant compositional differences exist between the PVM and the parasite's plasma membrane. And, these membranes may not be separable by conventional biochemical methods. Indeed, with time the vacuolar membrane becomes modified to such a degree that it takes on the composition of the parasite's plasma membrane.

Bannister: In freeze-fractured preparations the two membranes are very different, so that is one possible marker (McLaren et al 1979); they have different sizes of intramembranous particle, and different particle distributions.

Howard: The surface area of the outer cell membrane appears to increase also. Does this imply a reduced density for the host membrane proteins, which we presume are not added to the membranes of infected cells? And is the spectrin network altered in some way? It interacts with transmembrane proteins which are spread over a larger membrane surface area and is also presumably tightly linked structurally to erythrocyte shape changes.

Cabantchik: I don't think the density change you are suggesting is as dramatic as that. However, changes in the interaction between the cytoskeleton and some of the membrane proteins could lead to changes in membrane functions and, as was recently shown, also to changes in the transmembrane lipid distribution. However, dilution of membrane proteins *per se* will probably have minor functional consequences.

Bannister: We did some crude measurements of the area of the infected schizont stage compared with other stages in *P. knowlesi* (McLaren et al 1979). The volume of the erythrocyte increases as the parasite grows, but the surface area of the erythrocyte plasmalemma remains approximately the same, the cell merely becoming more rounded.

Sherman: Another interesting aspect of the changes shown in these investigations on *P. knowlesi*-infected cells, studied by treatment with purified phospholipase A_2, is that they mimic what is seen in older red cells. This suggests that a precocious ageing of the red cell is induced by the parasite.

Luzzatto: One piece of evidence for a change in some feature of the parasitized cell is the observation that in multiple infections, whether *in vivo* or *in vitro*, the parasites inside a red cell are of the same age or stage. That suggests that once a parasite is infected by one ring, it cannot be infected again. Is this true, in other people's experience? Or do you see a ring and a schizont in the same cell?

Facer: Yes; in non-synchronized *P. falciparum* cultures, we have seen rings and late trophozoites/early schizonts within the same red cell.

Luzzatto: There is also definite evidence of adaptive changes in the parasite. One intriguing example is the change in repetitive DNA, reported by Frontali's group in Rome (Birago et al 1982). They found that the time courses of loss of repetitive DNA and loss of the capacity to make gametocytes go hand in hand when *P. berghei* is passaged serially by syringe in mice. The mechanism is still obscure. This finding may be relevant to the question of what determines the differentiation of the parasite, which must decide, at the trophozoite stage, between gametogenesis and schizogony.

Anders: Is that a process analogous to the *Tetrahymena* system?

Luzzatto: I'm not familiar with that, but the main result is that if Birago et al take parasites from a fresh infection directly from the mosquito there is about 18% repetitive DNA. When they take a strain that has been in mice for 30 years, there is only about 4% repetitive DNA. With a fresh strain, passaged continually, there is a gradual decrease in repetitive DNA, in parallel with a decline in *infective* gametocytes.

Anders: In his summary, Dr Howard talked about dramatic changes in antigenic phenotype. However, this will depend on the method that is being used and consequently the subset of antigens being visualized. If you use schizont-infected cell agglutination you see dramatic changes. The results of several groups including our own have demonstrated great similarities between different *P. falciparum* isolates (Tait 1981, G.V. Brown et al 1981). This is a different situation from that in African trypanosomes or *Babesia bovis*.

McGregor: The role of the knob in binding to endothelial cells during sequestration has been considered. The developing gametocyte of *P. falciparum* remains sequestered for about the first 10 days of its life. Is the surface of this gametocyte covered with knobs?

Aikawa: The gametocyte of *P. falciparum* does not form knobs on the erythrocyte membrane.

McGregor: Yet we talk of the knob as an important sequestration mechanism for the asexual parasite and we think sequestration may be an important means of evading the host's immune defences. Much research in malaria has focused attention on the importance of neutralizing merozoite antibodies which act at the time of schizont rupture—that is, after sequestration. Sequestration may complicate the action of antibodies with merozoite specificity, but it should not negate it completely. I am doubtful that the prime purpose of these knobs is for sequestration and parasite survival.

Pasvol: Does anyone know exactly where in the body reinvasion occurs in *P. falciparum* infections? This would be relevant in terms of anti-merozoite antibody. The only evidence I know is in mice (*P. berghei*). Leon Weiss has scanning electron micrographs of denucleated erythroid cells coming out of the bone marrow, and schizonts sitting waiting to pounce on these young cells. This is interesting, because the known preference for young cells, in that system, can be explained by the young cells being the only ones there. But I can't understand this in the context of *P. falciparum* infections in humans. Where does invasion of red cells by merozites take place?

McGregor: There is no answer to that, any more than to the question of where the parasite is killed. As a hypothesis of how parasites are killed and where all this happens, the most efficient way might be that anti-merozoite antibody functions by stopping invasion of the red cell by the parasite. The merozoite-antibody complex is then carried round to a site where effector mechanisms, either antibody-mediated or not, are concentrated which kill the parasite. That site may be the spleen or the liver. But we haven't specific evidence on this.

Friedman: We need to consider whether the surface modifications studied have any significance, and whether we are looking at qualitative or quantitative modifications to the membrane. That is, are we looking at accelerated degradation, or added factors? Is this being studied? And could these modifications be increased, to make the cell more recognizable as being infected?

Howard: The first problem is to identify the modifications. Then the levels of these new antigens can be measured by quantitative immunoprecipitation or, better, by using monoclonals in a radioimmunoassay measuring antibody binding to the surface of infected cells.

Cabantchik: I think one could amplify the modified properties of the infected cell. The most effective and practical means of increasing the antigenicity of several blood groups on the red blood cell surface is by increasing the ratio of cholesterol to phospholipid. Perhaps by biochemical manipulation *in vitro* of infected red cells one could increase their cholesterol content, and thereby increase their antigenicity, and they would be recognized as foreign cells.

Sherman: In fact, *in vivo* the opposite normally happens; that is, the cholesterol:phospholipid ratio is decreased. Perhaps, as a consequence, the antigenicity of the infected cell is reduced, and the parasite thereby evades immune recognition!

Cabantchik: If so, one should take these cells, load them *in vitro* with cholesterol, and test whether their antigenicity has been amplified. This could perhaps have therapeutic applications.

Weatherall: How would you propose doing that?

Cabantchik: It has been done before, with solid tumours. For the present case, red cells taken from an individual can be concentrated, washed and incubated with cholesterol derivatives, either in serum or in polyvinyl pyrrolidone suspensions. One can increase the cholesterol to phospholipid ratio quite substantially and then reinject the red cells into the same individual.

Weatherall: Red cell cholesterol is in rapid free equilibrium with unesterified plasma cholesterol.

Cabantchik: That is true, but previous studies by Dr M. Shinitzky have indicated that the antigenicity of cells was markedly increased after these treatments.

Wallach: The exchange is extremely rapid in the cancer cell, certainly.

Brown: The parasite, in fact, has no difficulty in making the red cell antigenic. The host, and therefore the parasites, would die if the host didn't make an immune response, so for a viable host–parasite relationship the host has to make an immune response to control the parasitaemia. Malaria parasites are very good at making host cells antigenic. The problem for the parasite is in creating and regulating antigenicity sufficiently to prevent elimination of the infection and, for the host, to produce a response which cuts across variation of parasite antigens. The central issue of parasite immunology is whether there are exposed parasite antigens common to all variants; if there are such antigens, do they stimulate antibody, or T lymphocytes? This is the important question.

Cohen: There are answers here, obtained using monoclonal antibodies. The protective antigen that we are studying on *P. knowlesi* is recognizable in all the variants and in all the strains we have tested. The answer is that there are common antigens that have functional immunological importance.

Anders: The answers are not only coming from monoclonal antibodies. Purified antibody preparations from sera obtained in Papua New Guinea were more inhibitory for *P. falciparum* isolates from Papua New Guinea than for two non-Papua New Guinean isolates, one from Thailand and one from Africa (G.V. Brown et al, unpublished work).

Using inhibitory and non-inhibitory antibodies in immunoprecipitation analyses, we have identified an antigen that is preferentially recognized by inhibitory antibodies (G.V. Brown et al 1982). This particular antigen, M_r 96 000, is in all the *P. falciparum* isolates examined.

Cohen: There has always been evidence that malaria is unlike African trypanosomiasis in the way it evokes clinical immunity. The monoclonals serve to pinpoint the antigens which are common among variants of the malaria parasite.

Holder: Using monoclonal and polyvalent antibodies raised against parasite proteins which are protective when used to immunize against *P. yoelii* YM, we have looked by immunofluorescence for cross-reaction with other species of murine malaria. Within this restricted range of malarial parasites we find a considerable degree of cross-reaction.

Brown: That is contrary to the whole biology of the parasite! Immunity is species-specific and often strain-specific.

Holder: I am not claiming that immunization with either the 230 000 M_r or 235 000 M_r proteins of *P. yoelii* YM will induce a protective immune response *in vivo* against other murine malarias. There are determinants common to different species which can be detected by immunofluorescence, but this does not imply that the immunity which we observe *in vivo* is more than species-specific.

Brown: When you immunize with this protein *in vivo* you get a slightly delayed parasitaemia. I would expect that if you immunize with an antigen in Freund's complete adjuvant and give 1000 or 10 000 parasites, you will not get an infection or, if you do, it will not be a delayed parasitaemia and then a sudden rise to a high level parasitaemia. That doesn't fit any immunological dynamics. You are not taking into account that by destroying parasites initially and delaying the parasitaemia, probably by a variant-specific antigen, you are altering the immune status of the host and sensitizing the host *in vivo*. Therefore you cannot assume that you are immunizing with a protective cross-reacting antigen.

Holder: *P. yoelii* YM is a virulent parasite. If we inject 10 000 parasitized erythrocytes into BALB/c mice, by Day 8 all mice develop a more than 80% parasitaemia and die. If the mice have been immunized with 12 μg of 230 000 M_r *P. yoelii* antigen and its fragments in Freund's complete adjuvant on two occasions followed by an intravenous boost with 20 μg, the challenge infection is suppressed (mean parasitaemia of less than 10%) and then cleared. These results have been discussed more fully elsewhere (Holder & Freeman 1981). If larger amounts of protein (for example, 50 μg) are used for the immunization, no parasites can be detected in blood smears after challenge infection.

Immunization of mice with a 235 000 M_r merozoite antigen of *P. yoelii* appears to restrict a challenge infection to the reticulocyte compartment. The percentage parasitaemia is then a reflection of the number of reticulocytes in the system, until an effective immune response operates. The implication is that immunization with the 235 000 M_r antigen inhibits the invasion of mature red cells but does not affect the course of the reticulocyte-confined infection.

McGregor: We have discussed the specificity of immune responses to malaria infection, but we haven't said much about non-specific mechanisms involved in destruction of parasites, and how the two link up. This area will require future investigation. We have heard briefly about the possible importance of acute-phase proteins and inducers of such proteins. We have also heard about the effects of acid glycoproteins on parasites *in vitro*, from Dr Friedman. This area will be important, once it starts to open up.

REFERENCES

Aikawa M, Miller LH, Rabbege J 1975 Caveola–vesicle complexes in the plasmalemma of erythrocytes infected by *Plasmodium vivax* and *P. cynomolgi*. Am J Pathol 79:285-294

Barnwell JW, Howard RJ, Miller LH 1982 Altered expression of *Plasmodium knowlesi* variant antigen on the erythrocyte membrane of splenectomized rhesus monkeys. J Immunol 128:224-226

Birago C, Bucci A, Dore E, Frontali C, Zenobi P 1982 Gametogenesis is directly related to the amount of repetitive DNA in *Plasmodium berghei*. Exp Parasitol, in press

Brown GV, Anders RF, Stace JD, Alpers MP, Mitchell G F 1981 Immunoprecipitation of biosynthetically-labelled proteins from different Papua New Guinea *Plasmodium falciparum* isolates by sera from individuals in the endemic area. Parasite Immunol (Oxf) 3:283-298

Brown GV, Anders RF, Mitchell GF, Heywood PF 1982 Target antigens of purified human immunoglobulins which inhibit growth of *Plasmodium falciparum in vitro*. Nature (Lond) 297:591-593

Gupta CM, Mishra GC 1981 Transbilayer phospholipid asymmetry in *Plasmodium knowlesi*-infected host cell membrane. Science (Wash DC) 212:1047-1049

Howard RJ 1982 Alterations in the surface membrane of red blood cells during malaria. Immunol Rev 61:67-107

Howard RJ, Sawyer WH 1980 Changes in the membrane microviscosity of mouse red blood cells infected with *Plasmodium berghei* detected using *n*-(9-anthroyloxy) fatty acid fluorescent probes. Parasitology 80:331-342

Langreth SG, Reese RT, Motyl MR, Trager W 1979 *Plasmodium falciparum*: loss of knobs on the infected erythrocyte surface after long-term cultivation. Exp Parasitol 48:213-219

Luse SA, Miller LH 1971 *Plasmodium falciparum* malaria: structure of parasitized erythrocytes in cardiac vessels. Am J Trop Med Hyg 20:655-660

McLaren DJ, Bannister LH, Trigg PI, Butcher GA 1979 Freeze-fracture studies on the interaction between the malaria parasite and the host erythrocyte in *Plasmodium knowlesi* infections. Parasitology 79:125-139

Tait A 1981 Analysis of protein variation in *Plasmodium falciparum* by two-dimensional gel electrophoresis. Mol Biochem Parasitol 2:205-218

Tanner MJA, Jenkins RE, Anstee DJ, Clamp JR 1976 Abnormal carbohydrate composition of the major penetrating membrane protein of En(a–) human erythrocytes. Biochem J 155:701-703

Udeinya IJ, Schmidt JA, Aikawa M, Miller LH, Green FI 1981 Falciparum malaria-infected erythrocytes specifically bind to cultured human endothelial cells. Science (Wash DC) 213:555-557

Closing remarks

D. J. WEATHERALL

Nuffield Department of Clinical Medicine, John Radcliffe Hospital, Headington, Oxford, OX3 9DU, UK

The different aspects of parasite–red cell interactions have been summarized admirably by Russell Howard in his introduction to the final discussion. It appears that we may be closer to an understanding of how malarial parasites recognize and interact with the surface of human red cells, and that we are starting to gain some insight about the general features of the invasion mechanism. Although knowledge about parasite metabolism and the metabolic changes which occur in parasitized red cells is still scanty, considerable progress has been made in defining the changes in parasite antigens that occur during different stages of development and the related structural changes on the surface of parasitized red cells. *In vitro* culture studies are throwing up tantalizing clues about the general nature of the protective mechanisms against malarial parasites which the red cell may mediate through genetic alterations of its membrane, haemoglobin or metabolic pathways. However, it is always going to be extremely difficult to extrapolate these *in vitro* findings to what may be happening in human populations.

The speakers have been naturally reluctant to discuss the possible practical implications of much of the work that has been presented at this meeting. The immunological studies summarized here underline some of the difficulties that will be encountered in any attempts to produce a vaccine against the erythrocytic forms of the parasite. However, it is becoming apparent that a detailed analysis of the interaction of the parasitized red cell with vascular endothelium may be of prime importance in our further understanding of the major clinical features of malaria, particularly its cerebral and renal manifestations. This may have important therapeutic implications.

There was a genuine air of excitement about this meeting. Undoubtedly, this was engendered by a feeling that a better understanding of how malarial parasites interact with red cells may provide information which ultimately may help in the eradication of one of the commonest infectious diseases in the world

1983 Malaria and the red cell. Pitman, London (Ciba Foundation symposium 94) p 246-247

population. Furthermore, it may help us to understand how the commonest genetic disorders have been maintained at such extraordinarily high frequencies. What at first sight appeared to be a rather narrow field of biological interest is turning out to have remarkably far-ranging implications!

Index of contributors

Entries in bold type indicate papers; other entries refer to discussion contributions

Indexes compiled by John Rivers

Subject index